D0185290

Prince Charles Hospital
Merthyr Tydfil

THE EVIDENCE BASE OF
CLINICAL DIAGNOSIS

NORTH GLAMORGAN NHS TRUST LIBRARY

Please return to the library
by the date

DISPOSED OF BY STH
LIBRARY SERVICES
2021
...E INFORMATION
...E AVAILABLE

PC00005494

THE EVIDENCE BASE OF CLINICAL DIAGNOSIS

Edited by

J ANDRÉ KNOTTNERUS
Netherlands School of Primary Care Research, University of Maastricht, The Netherlands

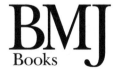

9 **Diagnostic decision support: contributions from medical informatics**   167
JOHAN VAN DER LEI and JAN H VAN BEMMEL

10 **Clinical problem solving and diagnostic decision making: a selective review of the cognitive research literature**   179
ARTHUR S ELSTEIN and ALAN SCHWARTZ

11 **Improving test ordering and diagnostic cost effectiveness in clinical practice – bridging the gap between clinical research and routine health care**   197
RON AG WINKENS and GEERT-JAN DINANT

12 **Epilogue: overview of evaluation strategy and challenges**   209
J ANDRÉ KNOTTNERUS

Index   217

Contributors

Jan H van Bemmel Department of Medical Informatics, Erasmus University Rotterdam, The Netherlands

Patrick M Bossuyt Department of Clinical Epidemiology and Biostatistics, Academic Medical Centre, University of Amsterdam, The Netherlands

Frank Buntinx Department of General Practice, Catholic University Leuven, Belgium

Walter L Devillé Institute for Research in Extramural Medicine, Vrije Universiteit, Amsterdam, The Netherlands

Geert-Jan Dinant Department of General Practice, University of Maastricht, The Netherlands

René Eijkemans Center for Clinical Decision Sciences, Department of Public Health, Erasmus University Rotterdam, The Netherlands

Arthur S Elstein Department of Medical Education, University of Illinois College of Medicine, Chicago, Illinois, USA

Constantine Gatsonis Center for Statistical Sciences, Brown University, Providence, Rhode Island, USA

Paul P Glasziou Department of Social and Preventive Medicine, University of Queensland Medical School, Australia

J Dik F Habbema Center for Clinical Decision Sciences, Department of Public Health, Erasmus Medical Center Rotterdam, The Netherlands

R Brian Haynes Clinical Epidemiology and Biostatistics, McMaster University Medical Centre, Hamilton, Ontario, Canada

Les M Irwig Department of Public Health and Community Medicine, University of Sydney, Australia

J André Knottnerus Netherlands School of Primary Care Research, University of Maastricht, The Netherlands

Pieta Krijnen Center for Clinical Decision Sciences, Department of Public Health, Erasmus Medical Center Rotterdam, The Netherlands

Johan van der Lei Department of Medical Informatics, Erasmus University Rotterdam, The Netherlands

Jeroen G Lijmer Department of Clinical Epidemiology and Biostatistics, Academic Medical Centre, University of Amsterdam, The Netherlands

Jean W Muris Department of General Practice, University of Maastricht, The Netherlands

David L Sackett Trout Research and Education Centre at Irish Lake, Markdale, Ontario, Canada

Onno P van Schayck Institute for Extramural and Transmural Health Care, University of Maastricht, The Netherlands

Alan Schwartz Department of Medical Education, University of Illinois College of Medicine, Chicago, Illinois, USA

Chris van Weel Department of General Practice and Social Medicine, Institute for Evidence-Based Practice, University of Nijmegen, The Netherlands

Ron AG Winkens Transmural and Diagnostic Centre, Academic Hospital Maastricht, The Netherlands

Preface

"I consider much less thinking has gone into the theory underlying diagnosis, or possibly one should say less energy has gone into constructing the correct model of diagnostic procedures, than into therapy or prevention where the concept of 'altering the natural history of the disease' has been generally accepted and a theory has been evolved for testing hypotheses concerning this."[1]

Although seeking an evidence base for medicine is as old as medicine itself, in the past decade the concept of evidence-based medicine (EBM) has strongly stimulated the application of the best available evidence from clinical research into medical practice. At the same time, this process has revealed the need for a more extensive and more valid evidence base as input for EBM. Accordingly, investigators have been encouraged to intensify the production and innovation of clinical knowledge, and clinical research has become more successful in seeing its results implemented in practice more completely in a shorter period.

In developing the evidence base of clinical management it has come forward that, even 3 decades after Archie Cochrane wrote the words cited above, the methodology of diagnostic research lags far behind that of research into the effectiveness of treatment. This is the more challenging because making an adequate diagnostic process is a prime requirement for appropriate clinical decision making, including prognostic assessment and the selection of the most effective treatment options.

In view of this apparent need for further methodological development of the evidence base of clinical diagnosis, this book was initiated. The aim is to provide a comprehensive framework for (future) investigators who want to do diagnostic research, and for clinicians, practitioners and students who are interested to learn more about principles, and about relevant methodological options and pitfalls. Clearly, not all topics relevant for diagnostic research could be covered, nor could the selected subjects be dealt with in all detail. For those who wish to know more, the references in the chapters can be a useful guide. In preparing the work, the contributors were able to profit from the experience and insights collected and reported by many leading clinical researchers in the field.

First, a general outline of diagnostic research is presented. What are the key objectives, the challenges, and the corresponding options for study design? What should the architecture of diagnostic research look like to provide us with an appropriate research strategy, yielding the clinical information we are looking for, with a minimum burden for study patients and an efficient use of resources? Second, important design features for studying the accuracy and clinical impact of diagnostic tests and procedures are dealt with in more detail, addressing the cross-sectional study, the randomised trial, and the before–after study. In addition, it is shown that the impact of diagnostic tests varies with different clinical settings and target populations, and indications are given as how to ensure that estimates of test accuracy will travel and be transferable to other settings. Also, for clinical diagnostic studies, an overview of the most important data-analytic issues is presented, from simple two by two tables to multiple logistic regression analysis.

Nowadays, for both clinical investigators and readers of research articles, it is not enough to understand the methodology of original clinical studies. They must also know more about the techniques to summarise and synthesise results from various clinical studies on a similar topic. Guidelines for diagnostic systematic reviews and meta-analysis are therefore presented.

Learning from accumulated clinical experience and the application of diagnostic knowledge in practice has much in common with retrieving and selecting information from clinical databases. Accordingly, diagnostic decision support using information and communication technology (ICT) is addressed as an increasingly important domain for clinical practice, research, and education. Furthermore, as clinical research results can only be successfully incorporated into diagnostic decision making if the way clinicians tend to solve medical problems is taken into account, an overview of the domain of clinical problem solving is given. Eventually, we have to recognise that improving test use in daily care needs more than clinical research, and presenting guidelines and other supportive materials. Therefore, the strategy of successful implementation – which has become a field of study in itself – is also covered.

This book includes contributions from many authors. In order to allow each chapter to keep a logical structure in itself, a number of topics have been dealt with more than once, albeit to a varying extent. Instead of seeing this as a problem, we think that it may be informative for readers to see important issues considered from different perspectives.

Parallel to the preparation of this book, an initiative to reach international agreement of standards for reporting diagnostic accuracy (STARD) was taken and elaborated. This development can be expected to make a significant contribution to improving the quality of published literature on the value of diagnostic tests. We are happy that members of the group of initiators of STARD have contributed to this book as the authors of chapters 4 and 6, and are looking forward to seeing these standards having an impact.

The field of diagnostic research is developing strongly and an increasing number of talented clinical investigators are working in (the methodology of) diagnostic research. In view of this dynamic field, we welcome comments from readers and suggestions for possible improvements.

The contributors wish to thank Richard Smith from the *BMJ*, who has so positively welcomed the initiative for this book, Trish Groves from the *BMJ* who gave very useful feedback on the proposed outline and stimulated us to work it out, and Mary Banks from BMJ Books, who has provided support and encouragement from the beginning and monitored the progress of the book until the work was done.

André Knottnerus

1 Cochrane AL. Effectiveness and efficiency. Random reflections on health services. The Nuffield Provincial Hospitals Trusts, 1972. Reprinted: London, the Royal Society of Medicine Press Limited, 1999.

laboratory or other technical facilities. Not only a "test" must be considered, but also the specific question the test is supposed to answer. Therefore, the performance of tests must be evaluated in accordance with their intended objectives. Objectives may include:

- *Detecting or excluding disorders, by increasing diagnostic certainty as to their presence or absence.* This can only be achieved if the test has sufficient discrimination. Table 1.1 shows the most common measures of discrimination. Most of these can be simply derived from a 2×2 table comparing the test result with the diagnostic standard, as demonstrated by the example of ankle trauma. A more elaborate and comprehensive explanation of how to calculate these and other measures from collected data is presented in Chapter 7. Examples of tests for which such measures have been assessed are given in Table 1.2. Such a representation allows various tests for the same purpose to be compared. This can show, for example, that less invasive tests (such as ultrasonography) may be as good as or even better diagnostically than more invasive or hazardous ones (for example angiography). Also, it can be shown that history data (for example change in bowel habit) may be at least as valuable as laboratory data. What is important is not just the discrimination per se, but rather what a test may add to what cheaper and less invasive diagnostics already provide to the diagnostic process. This is relevant, for instance, in assessing the added value of liver function tests to history taking and physical examination in ill-defined, non-specific complaints.
- *Contributing to the decision making process with regard to further diagnostic and therapeutic management,* including the indications for therapy (for example by determining the localisation and shape of a lesion) and choosing the preferred therapeutic approach
- *Assessing prognosis* on the basis of the nature and severity of diagnostic findings. This is a starting point for planning the clinical follow up and for informing and – if justified – reassuring the patient
- *Monitoring the clinical course* of a disorder or a state of health such as pregnancy, or the clinical course of an illness during or after treatment
- *Measuring physical fitness* in relation to requirements, for example for sports or employment.

The evaluation of a diagnostic test concentrates on its added value for the intended application, taking into consideration the burden for the patient and any possible complications resulting from the test (such as intestinal perforation in endoscopy). This requires a comparison between the situations with and without the use of the test, or a comparison with the use of other tests.

Prior to evaluation, one must decide whether to focus on maximising the health perspectives of the individual patient (which is usually the

3

Table 1.1 Commonly used measures of the discrimination of a diagnostic test T for disease D, illustrated with physical examination for detecting a fracture in ankle trauma, using x ray film as the reference standard.

T: conclusion of physical examination	D: result of x ray		
	Fracture	No fracture	Total
Fracture	190	80	270
No fracture	10	720	730
Total	200	800	1000

The SENSITIVITY of T is the probability of a positive test result in people with D: $P(T+|D+) = 190/200 = 0.95$.

The SPECIFICITY of T is the probability of a negative test result in people without D: $P(T-|D-) = 720/800 = 0.90$.

Note: sensitivity and specificity together determine the discrimination of a test.

The LIKELIHOOD RATIO (LR) of test result T_X is the probability of test result T_X in people with D, divided by the probability of T_X in people without D.

The general formula for LR_X is: $\dfrac{P(T_X|D+)}{P(T_X|D-)}$

For a positive result, LR+ is: $\dfrac{P(T+|D+)}{P(T+|D-)}$

which is equivalent to: $\dfrac{\text{Sensitivity}}{1-\text{specificity}} = \dfrac{190/200}{1-720/800} = 9.5$

For a negative result, LR− is: $\dfrac{P(T-|D+)}{P(T-|D-)}$

which is equivalent to: $\dfrac{1-\text{sensitivity}}{\text{Specificity}} = \dfrac{1-190/200}{720/800} = 0.06$

Note: LR is an overall measure of the discrimination of test result T_X. The test is useless if LR = 1. The test is better the more LR differs from 1, that is, greater than 1 for LR+ and lower than 1 for LR−.

For tests with multiple outcome categories, LR_X can be calculated for every separate category x as the ratio of the probability of outcome category x among diseased and the probability of outcome category x among non-diseased.

The PREDICTIVE VALUE of a test result T_X is:

for a positive result, the probability of D in persons with a positive test result: $P(D+|T+) = 190/270 = 0.70$.

for a negative result, the probability of absence of D in persons with a negative result: $P(D-|T-) = 720/730 = 0.99$.

Note: the predictive value (posterior or post-test probability) must be compared with the estimated probability of D before T is carried out (the prior or pretest probability). For a good discrimination, the difference between the post-test and the pretest probability should be large.

The ODDS RATIO (OR), or the cross-product ratio, represents the overall discrimination of a dichotomous test T, and is equivalent to the ratio of LR+ and LR−. $OR = (190 \times 270)/(80 \times 10) = 171$

Note: If $OR = 1$, T is useless. T is better the more OR differs from 1.

The RECEIVER OPERATING CHARACTERISTIC (ROC) curve represents the relation between sensitivity and specificity for tests with a variable cut-off point, on an ordinal scale (for example, in case of 5 degrees of suspicion of ankle fracture; or cervical smear) or interval scale (for example, if degree of suspicion of ankle fracture is expressed in a percentage; or ST changes in exercise ECG testing). If the AUC (area under the curve) = 0.5, the test is useless. For a perfect test the AUC = 1.0 (see Chapter 7).

Table 1.2 Discrimination of some diagnostic tests for various target disorders, expressed in sensitivity, specificity, likelihood ratios, and odds ratio (estimates based on several sources).

Test	Target Disorder	Sensitivity (%)	Specificity (%)	Likelihood ratio Positive result	Likelihood ratio Negative result	Odds ratio
Exercise ECG[*9]	Coronary stenosis	65	89	5.9	0.39	15.0
Stress thallium scintigraphy[9]	Coronary stenosis	85	85	5.7	0.18	32.1
Ultrasonography[9]	Pancreatic cancer	70	85	4.7	0.35	13.2
CT scan[9]	Pancreatic cancer	85	90	8.5	0.17	51.0
Angiography[9]	Pancreatic cancer	75	80	3.8	0.31	12.0
ESR $\geq$28 mm/1 h[**10]	Malignancy	78	94	13.0	0.23	56.0
ESR $\geq$28 mm/1 h[**10]	Inflammatory disease	46	95	9.2	0.57	16.2
Intermittent claudication[**11]	Peripheral arterial occlusive disease	31	93	4.4	0.74	5.6
Posterior tibial/dorsalis pedis artery pulse[**11]	Peripheral arterial occlusive disease	73	92	9.1	0.29	30.4
Change in bowel habit[**12]	Colorectal cancer	88	72	3.1	0.17	18.4
Weight loss[**12]	Colorectal cancer	44	85	2.9	0.66	4.6
ESR $\geq$30 mm/1 h[**12]	Colorectal cancer	40	96	10.0	0.42	14.0
White blood cell count >10^9[**12]	Colorectal cancer	75	90	7.5	0.28	26.3
Occult blood test $\geq$1 positive out of 3[**12]	Colorectal cancer	50	82	2.7	0.61	4.6

[*]Cut-off point: ST depression $\geq$1 mm.
[**]In a general practice setting.

physician's aim) or on the best possible cost effectiveness (as economists are likely to do). The latter can be expressed in the amount of money to be invested per number of life years gained, whether or not adjusted for quality of life. Between these two approaches, which do not necessarily yield the same outcome, there is the tension between strictly individual and collective interests. This becomes especially obvious when policy makers have to decide which options would be accepted as the most efficient in a macroeconomic perspective.

Another prior decision is whether one would be satisfied with a qualitative understanding of the diagnostic decision making process, or is also aiming at a detailed quantitative analysis.[13] In the first case one would chart the stages and structure of the decision making process, in relation to the test to be evaluated. This may already provide sufficient insight, for instance if it becomes clear beforehand that the result will not influence the decision to be taken. Examples of useless testing are (1) the value of the routine electrocardiogram in acute chest pain, exploring the likelihood of a suspected myocardial infarction, with the consequent decision whether or not to admit the patient to hospital; and (2) the value of "routine blood tests" in general practice for the decision as to whether or not to refer a patient with acute abdominal pain to a surgeon. In addition to qualitatively mapping the structure of the decision making process, quantitative analysis attempts to assess test discrimination and the ultimate clinical outcome, taking the risks (and the costs) of the test procedure into account. The choice of a qualitative or a quantitative approach depends on the question to be answered and the data available.

If a test has not yet been introduced, the prospects for a good evaluation are better than if it is already in general use. It is then, for example, still possible to define an appropriate control group to whom the test is not applied, so that its influence on the prognosis can be investigated. In addition, at such an early stage the conclusion of the analysis can still be used in the decision regarding introduction. Furthermore, it is possible to plan a procedure for monitoring and evaluation after introduction. All of this emphasises the importance of developing an evaluation programme before a test is introduced.

A common misunderstanding is that only expensive, advanced diagnostic technology cause unacceptable increases in healthcare costs; in fact, cheap but very frequently used (routine) tests account for a major part of direct costs. Moreover, these tests greatly influence other costs, as they often preselect patients for more expensive procedures. Yet the performance of such low-threshold diagnostics has often not been adequately evaluated. Examples include many applications of haematological, clinicochemical, and urine tests.[14-16]

Methodological challenges

In the evaluation of diagnostic procedures a number of methodological challenges have to be considered.

Complex relations

Most diagnostics have more than one indication or are relevant for more than one nosological outcome. In addition, tests are often not applied in isolation but in combinations, for instance in the context of protocols. Ideally, diagnostic research should reflect the healthcare context,[17] but it is generally impossible to investigate all aspects in one study. Therefore, choices must be made as to which issues are the most important. Multivariable statistical techniques are available to allow for the (added) value of various diagnostic data, both separately and in combination, and also in the form of diagnostic prediction rules.[18,19] Such techniques were originally developed for the purpose of analysing aetiologic data, generally focusing on the overall aetiologic impact of a factor adjusted for covariables. Diagnostic analysis aims to specify test performance in clinical subgroups or to identify the set of variables that yield the best individual diagnostic prediction, which is a completely different perspective. Much work remains to be done to improve the methodology of diagnostic data analysis.[20]

Diagnostic data analysis will be discussed further in Chapter 7.

The "gold" standard problem

To evaluate the discriminatory power of a test, its results must be compared with an independently established standard diagnosis. However, a "gold" standard, providing full certainty on the health status, rarely exists. Even x rays, CT scans and pathological preparations may produce false positive and false negative results. The aim must then be to define an adequate reference standard that approximates the "gold" standard as closely as possible.

Sometimes one is faced with the question whether any appropriate reference standard procedure exists at all. For example, in determining the discrimination of liver tests for diagnosing liver pathology, neither imaging techniques nor biopsies can detect all abnormalities. In addition, as a liver biopsy is an invasive procedure it is unsuitable for use as a standard in an evaluation study. A useful independent standard diagnosis may not even exist conceptually, for example when determining the predictive value of symptoms that are themselves part of the disease definition, as in migraine, or when the symptoms and functionality are more important for management decisions than the anatomical status, as in prostatism. Also, in studying the diagnostic value of clinical examination to detect severe pathology in non-acute abdominal complaints, a comprehensive invasive standard diagnostic screening, if at all possible or ethically allowed, would yield many irrelevant findings and not all relevant pathology would be immediately found. An option, then, is diagnostic assessment after a follow up period by an independent panel of experts, representing a "delayed type" cross-sectional study.[21] This may not be perfect, but can be the most acceptable solution.[1]

A further issue is the dominance of prevailing reference standards. For example, as long as classic angiography is considered the standard when validating new vascular imaging techniques, the latter will always seem less valid because perfect agreement is never attainable. However, as soon as the new method comes to be regarded as sufficiently valid to be accepted as the standard, the difference will from then on be explained in favour of this new method. In addition, when comparing advanced ultrasound measurements in blood vessels with angiography, one must accept that the two methods actually measure different concepts: the first measures blood flow, relevant to explain the symptoms clinically, whereas the second reflects the anatomical situation, which is important for the surgeon. Furthermore, the progress of clinicopathological insights is of great importance. For example, although clinical pattern X may first be the standard to evaluate the significance of microbiological findings, it will become of secondary diagnostic importance once the infectious agent causing X has been identified. The agent will then be the diagnostic standard, as illustrated by the history of the diagnosis of tuberculosis.

In Chapters 3 and 6 more will be said about reference standard problems.

Spectrum and selection bias

The evaluation of diagnostics may be flawed by many types of bias.[1,22,23] The most important of these are spectrum bias and selection bias.

Spectrum bias may occur when the discrimination of the diagnostic is assessed in a study population with a different clinical spectrum (for instance in more advanced cases) than will be found among those in whom the test is to be applied in practice. This may, for example, happen with tests calibrated in a hospital setting but applied in general practice. Also, sensitivity may be determined in seriously diseased subjects, whereas specificity is tested in clearly healthy subjects. Both will then be grossly overestimated relative to the practical situation, where testing is really necessary because it is clinically impossible to distinguish in advance who is healthy and who is diseased.

Selection bias is to be expected if there is a relation between the test result and the probability of being included in the study population in which the test is calibrated. For example, subjects with an abnormal exercise electrocardiogram are relatively likely to be preselected for coronary angiography. Consequently, if this exercise test is calibrated among preselected subjects, a higher sensitivity and a lower specificity will be found than if this preselection had not occurred.[24] Similarly, on the basis of referral patterns alone it is to be expected that the sensitivity of many tests is higher in the clinic than in general practice, and the specificity lower.

Although spectrum and selection biases are often related, in the first the clinical picture is the primary point of concern, whereas in the latter the mechanism of selection is the principal issue. These types of bias may affect not only sensitivity and specificity, but also all other measures of discrimination listed in Table 1.1.[25]

Chapters 2 and 6 will further address the issue of dealing with spectrum and selection biases.

"Soft" measures

Subjective factors such as pain, feeling unwell and the need for reassurance are of great importance in diagnostic management. Most decisions for a watchful waiting strategy in the early phase of an episode of illness are based on the valuation of "soft" measures. These often determine the indication for diagnostic examinations, and may themselves be part of the diagnostics (for example a symptom or complaint) to be evaluated. Also, such factors are generally indispensable in the assessment of the overall clinical outcome. Evaluation studies should, on the one hand, aim as much as possible to objectify these subjective factors in a reproducible way. On the other hand, interindividual and even intraindividual differences will always play a part[26] and should be acknowledged in the clinical decision making process.

Observer variability and observer bias

Variability between different observers, as well as for the same observer in reading and interpreting diagnostic data, should not only be acknowledged for "soft" diagnostics such as history taking and physical examination, but also for "harder" ones like x rays, CT scans and pathological slides. Even tests not involving any human factors show inter- and intrainstrument variability. Such variability should be limited if the diagnostic is to produce useful information.

At the same time, evaluation studies should beware of systematic observer bias as a result of prior knowledge about the subjects examined. Clearly, if one wishes to evaluate whether a doctor can accurately diagnose an ankle fracture based on history and clinical examination, it must be certain that he is not aware of an available x ray result; and a pathologist making an independent final diagnosis should not be informed about the most likely clinical diagnosis.[27] In such situations "blinding" is required. A different form of observer bias could occur if the diagnosticians are prejudiced in favour of one of the methods to be compared, as they may unconsciously put greater effort into that technique. A further challenge is that the experience and skill required should be equal for the methods compared, if these are to have a fair chance in the assessment. In this respect, new methods are at risk of being disadvantaged, especially shortly after being introduced.

Discrimination does not mean usefulness

For various reasons, a test with very good discrimination does not necessarily influence management.

To begin with, a test may add too little to what is already known clinically to alter management. Furthermore, the physician may take insufficient account of the information provided by the test. This is a complex problem. For instance, studies of the consequences of routine blood testing have shown that in some cases an unaltered diagnosis still led to changes in the considered policy.[14] In a study on the therapeutic impact of upper gastrointestinal endoscopy, a number of changes (23%) in management were made in the absence of a change in diagnosis, whereas in many patients (30%) in whom the diagnosis was changed management was not altered.[28] Also, a test may detect a disorder for which no effective treatment is available. For example, the MRI scan provides refined diagnostic information with regard to various brain conditions for which no therapy is yet in prospect. Finally, as discussed in the previous section, supplementary test results may not be relevant for treatment decisions.

For this reason we strongly recommend that evaluation studies investigate both the discrimination of a test and its influence on management.

Indication area and prior probability

Whether a test can effectively detect or exclude a particular disorder is influenced by the prior probability of that disorder. A test is generally not useful if the prior probability is either very low or very high: not only will the result rarely influence patient management, but the risk of, respectively, a false positive or a false negative result is relatively high. In other words, there is an "indication area" for the test between these extremes of prior probability.[9,10] Evaluation of diagnostics should therefore address the issue of whether the test could be particularly useful for certain categories of prior probability. For example, tests with a moderate specificity are not useful for screening in an asymptomatic population (with a low prior probability) because of the high risk of false positive results.

Small steps and large numbers

Compared with therapeutic effectiveness studies, evaluation studies of diagnostic procedures have often neglected the question of whether the sample size is adequate to provide the desired information with a sufficient degree of certainty. A problem is that progress in diagnostic decision making often takes the form of a series of small steps so as to gain in certainty, rather than one big breakthrough. Evaluating the importance of a small step, however, requires a relatively large study population.

Changes over time and the mosaic of evidence

Innovations in diagnostic technology may proceed at such a speed that a thorough evaluation may take longer than the development of even more advanced techniques. For example, the results of evaluation studies on the cost effectiveness of the CT scan had not yet crystallised when the MRI and PET scans appeared on the scene. So, the results of evaluation studies may already be lagging behind when they appear. Therefore, there is a need for general models (scenarios) for the evaluation of particular (types of) tests and test procedures, whose overall framework is relatively stable and into which information on new tests can be entered by substituting the relevant piece in the whole mosaic. This allows, for instance, a quick evaluation of the impact of new mammographic or DNA techniques with better discrimination on the cost effectiveness of breast cancer screening, if other pieces of the mosaic (such as treatment efficacy) have not changed. As discrimination itself can often be relatively rapidly assessed by means of a cross-sectional study, this may avoid new prospective studies. The same can be said for the influence of changes in relevant costs, such as fees for medical treatment or the price of drugs.

Research designs

There are various methodological approaches for evaluating diagnostic technologies, including original clinical research on the one hand, and systematically synthesising the findings of already performed empirical studies and clinical expertise on the other.

For empirical clinical studies, a range of design options is available. The appropriate study design depends on the research question to be answered (Table 1.3). In diagnostic accuracy studies the relationship between test result and reference standard has to be assessed cross-sectionally. This can be achieved by a cross-sectional survey, but especially in early validation studies other approaches (case–referent or test result-based sampling) can be most efficient. Design options for studying the impact of diagnostic testing on clinical decision making and patient prognosis are the "diagnostic randomised controlled trial" (RCT), which is methodologically the strongest approach, and the before–after study. Also, cohort and case–control designs have been shown to have a place in this context. In Chapter 2, the most important strategic considerations in choosing the appropriate design in diagnostic research will be specifically addressed.

Current knowledge can be synthesised by systematic reviews, meta-analyses, clinical decision analysis, cost effectiveness studies and consensus methods, with the ultimate aim of integrating and translating research findings for implementation in practice.

In the following, issues of special relevance to diagnostic evaluation studies will be briefly outlined.

Clinical studies

A common type of research is the cross-sectional study, assessing the relationship between diagnostic test results and the presence of particular

Table 1.3 Methodological options in diagnostic research in relation to study objectives.

Study objective	Methodological options
Clinical studies	
Diagnostic accuracy	Cross-sectional study
	survey
	case–referent sampling
	test result-based sampling
Impact of diagnostic testing on prognosis or management	Randomised controlled trial
	Cohort study
	Case–control study
	Before–after study
Synthesising findings and expertise	
Synthesising results of multiple studies	Systematic review
	Meta-analysis
Evaluation of most effective or cost effective diagnostic strategy	Clinical decision analysis
	Cost effectiveness analysis
Translating findings for practice	Integrating results of the above mentioned approaches
	Expert consensus methods
	Developing guidelines
Integrating information in clinical practice	
	ICT support studies
	Studying diagnostic problem solving
	Evaluation of implementation in practice

disorders. This relationship is usually expressed in the measures of discrimination included in Table 1.1. Design options are: (1) a survey in an "indicated population", representing subjects in whom the studied test would be considered in practice; (2) sampling groups with (cases) and without disease (referents) to compare their test distributions; or (3) sampling groups with different test results, between which the occurrence of a disease is compared. It is advisable to include in the evaluation already adopted tests, as this is a direct way to obtain an estimate of the added value of the new test. The cross-sectional study will be dealt with in more detail in Chapter 3.

In an RCT the experimental group undergoes the test to be evaluated, while a control group undergoes a different (for example the usual) or no test. This allows the assessment of not only differences in the percentage of correct diagnoses, but also the influence of the evaluated test on management and prognosis. A variant is to apply the diagnostic test to all patients but to disclose its results to the caregivers for a random half of the patients, if ethically justified. This constitutes an ideal placebo procedure for the patient. Although diagnostic RCTs are not easy to carry out and often not feasible, several have been already carried out some time ago.[29–34] Among the best known are the early trials on the effectiveness of breast cancer screening, which have often linked a standardised management protocol to the screening result.[35,36] The randomised controlled trial in diagnostic research is further discussed in Chapter 4.

If the prognostic value of a test is to be assessed and an RCT is not feasible, its principles can serve as the paradigm in applying other methods, one such being the cohort study. The difference from the RCT is that the diagnostic information is not randomly assigned, but a comparison is made between two previously established groups.[37] It has the methodological problem that one can never be sure, especially regarding unknown or unmeasurable covariables, whether the compared groups have similar disease or prognostic spectra to begin with. A method providing relatively rapid results regarding the clinical impact of a test is the case–control study. This is often carried out retrospectively, that is, after the course and the final status of the patients are known, in subjects who at the time have been eligible for the diagnostic test to be evaluated. It can be studied whether "indicated subjects" showing an adverse outcome (cases) underwent the diagnostic test more or less frequently than indicated subjects without such outcome (controls). A basic requirement is that the diagnostic must have been available to all involved at the time. Well known examples are case–control studies on the relationship between mortality from breast cancer and participation in breast cancer screening programmes.[38,39] This is an efficient approach, although potential bias because of lack of prior comparability of tested and non-tested subjects must once again be borne in mind.

The influence of a diagnostic examination on the physician's management can be also investigated by comparing the intended management policies before and after test results are available. Such before–after comparisons (diagnostic impact studies) have their own applications, limitations and precautionary measures, as reviewed by Guyatt et al.[40] The method has, for example, been applied in determining the added value of the CT scan and in studying the diagnostic impact of haematological tests in general practice.[41,42] The before–after study design will be outlined in Chapter 5.

Although using appropriate inclusion and exclusion criteria for study subjects is as important as in therapeutic research, in diagnostic research defining such criteria is less well developed. However, appropriate criteria are indispensible in order to focus on the clinical question at issue, the relevant spectrum of clinical severity, the disorders to be evaluated and the desired degree of selection of the study population (for example primary care or referred population).[43]

Synthesising research findings and clinical expertise

Often the problem is not so much a lack of research findings but the lack of a good summary and systematic processing of those findings.

13

A diagnostic systematic review, and meta-analysis of the pooled data of a number of diagnostic studies, can synthesise the results of those studies. This provides an overall assessment of the value of diagnostic procedures,[44,45] and can also help to identify differences in test accuracy between clinical subgroups. In this way, an overview of the current state of knowledge is obtained within a relatively short time. At present, this method is very much under development. One is aiming at bridging a methodological backlog, compared to the more established therapeutic systematic review and meta-analysis. The methodology of systematically reviewing studies on the accuracy of diagnostic tests is elaborated in Chapter 8.

Another important approach is clinical decision analysis, systematically comparing various diagnostic strategies as to their clinical outcome or cost effectiveness, supported by probability and decision trees. If good estimates of the discrimination and risks of testing, the occurrence and prognosis of suspected disorders, and the "value" of various clinical outcomes are available, a decision tree can be evaluated quantitatively in order to identify the clinically optimal or most cost effective strategy. An important element in the decision analytic approach is the combined analysis of diagnostic and therapeutic effectivenes. In this context, a qualitative analysis can be very useful. For example, non-invasive techniques nowadays show a high level of discrimination in diagnosing carotid stenoses, even in asymptomatic patients. This allows improved patient selection for the invasive and more hazardous carotid angiography, which is needed to make final decisions regarding surgical intervention. But if surgery has not been proved to influence the prognosis of asymptomatic patients favourably compared to non-surgical management,[46] the decision tree is greatly simplified as it no longer would include either angiography or surgery, and maybe not even non-invasive testing.

Decision analysis does not always provide an answer. The problem may be too complex to be summarised in a tree, essential data may be missing, and there is often a lack of agreement on key assumptions regarding the value of outcomes. Therefore, consensus procedures are often an indispensable step in the translational process from clinical research to guidelines for practice. In these procedures, clinical experts integrate the most recent state of knowledge with their experience to reach agreement on clinical guidelines regarding the preferred diagnostic approach of a particular medical problem, differentiated for relevant subgroups.[47,48]

Integrating information in clinical practice

In order to help clinical investigators harvest essential diagnostic research data from clinical databases and to support clinicians in making and improving diagnostic decisions, medical informatics and ICT (information and communications technology) innovations are indispensible. However, as described in Chapter 9, to use the potentials in this field optimally, specific methodological and practical requirements must be met.

The information processing approaches outlined in the previous section constitute links between research findings and clinical practice, and can be applied in combination to support evidence-based medicine. How such input can have optimal impact on the diagnostic decision making of individual doctors is, however, far from simple or straightforward. Therefore, given the growing cognitive requirements of diagnostic techniques, studies to increase our insight in diagnostic problem solving by clinicians is an increasingly important part of diagnostic research. This topic is discussed in Chapter 10.

Information from good clinical studies, systematic reviews and guideline construction is necessary but in many cases not sufficient for improving routine practice. In view of this, during the last decade, implementation research has been strongly developed to face this challenge and to facilitate the steps from clinical science to patient care. Accordingly, Chapter 11 deals with implementation of (cost-)effective test ordering in clinical practice.

Conclusion

Diagnostic technology assessment would be greatly stimulated if formal standards for the evaluation of diagnostics were to be formulated, as a requirement for market acceptance. Health authorities could take the initiative in assembling panels of experts to promote and monitor the evaluation of both new and traditional diagnostic facilities. Criteria for the acceptance and retention of diagnostics in clinical practice should be developed. Furthermore, professional organisations have a great responsibility to set, implement, maintain, and improve clinical standards. More effective international cooperation would be useful, as it has proved to be in the approval and quality control of drugs. In this way, the availability of resources for industrial, private, and governmental funding for diagnostic technology assessment would also be stimulated.

As regards the feasibility of diagnostic evaluation studies, the required size and duration must be considered in relation to the speed of technological progress. This speed can be very great, for instance in areas where the progress of molecular genetic knowledge and information and communication technology play an important part. Especially in such areas, updating of decision analyses, expert assessments and scenarios by inserting new pieces of the "mosaic" of evidence may be more useful than fully comprehensive, lengthy trials. This may, for example, be very relevant for the evaluation of diagnostic areas where traditional tests will be replaced by

DNA diagnostics in the years to come. Finally, successful integration of "soft" health measures, quality of life aspects, and health economic objectives into clinical evaluations will require much additional research, and methodological and ethical consideration.[49]

References

1 Feinstein AR. *Clinical epidemiology. The architecture of clinical research.* Philadelphia: WB Saunders, 1985.
2 Sackett DL, Haynes RB, Tugwell P. *Clinical epidemiology: a basic science for clinical medicine.* Boston: Little, Brown and Co., 1985.
3 Pocock SJ. *Clinical trials, a practical approach.* New York: John Wiley & Sons, 1983.
4 Kleinbaum DG, Kupper LL, Morgenstern H. *Epidemiologic research, principles and quantitative methods.* Belmont (CA): Wadsworth, 1982.
5 Miettinen OS. *Theoretical epidemiology, principles of occurrence research in medicine.* New York: John Wiley & Sons, 1985.
6 Sheps SB, Schechter MT. The assessment of diagnostic tests. A survey of current medical research. *JAMA* 1984;**252**:2418–22.
7 Reid ML, Lachs MS, Feinstein AR. Use of methodological standards in diagnostic research. Getting better but still not good. *JAMA* 1995;**274**:645–51.
8 Lijmer JG, Mol BW, Heisterkamp S, *et al.* Empirical evidence of design-related bias in studies of diagnostic tests. *JAMA* 1999;**282**:1061–6.
9 Panzer RJ, Black ER, Griner PF, eds. *Diagnostic strategies for common medical problems.* Philadelphia: American College of Physicians, 1991.
10 Dinant GJ, Knottnerus JA, Van Wersch JW. Discriminating ability of the erythrocyte sedimentation rate: a prospective study in general practice. *Br J Gen Pract* 1991; **41**:365–70.
11 Stoffers HEJH, Kester ADM, Kaiser V, Rinkens PELM, Knottnerus JA. Diagnostic value of signs and symptoms associated with peripheral arterial obstructive disease seen in general practice: a multivariable approach. *Med Decision Making* 1997;**17**:61–70.
12 Fijten GHF. *Rectal bleeding, a danger signal?* Amsterdam: Thesis Publishers, 1993.
13 Knottnerus JA, Winkens R. Screening and diagnostic tests. In: Silagy C, Haines A, eds. *Evidence based practice in primary care.* London: BMJ Books, 1998.
14 Dinant GJ. *Diagnostic value of the erythrocyte sedimentation rate in general practice.* PhD thesis, University of Maastricht, 1991.
15 Hobbs FD, Delaney BC, Fitzmaurice DA, *et al.* A review of near patient testing in primary care. *Health Technol Assess* 1997;**1**:i–iv,1–229.
16 Campens D, Buntinx F. Selecting the best renal function tests. A meta-analysis of diagnostic studies. *Int J Technol Assess Health Care* 1997;**13**:343–56.
17 van Weel C, Knottnerus JA. Evidence-based interventions and comprehensive treatment. *Lancet* 1999;**353**:916–18.
18 Spiegelhalter DJ, Crean GP, Holden R, *et al.* Taking a calculated risk: predictive scoring systems in dyspepsia. *Scand J Gastroenterol* 1987;**22**(suppl 128):152–60.
19 Knottnerus JA. Diagnostic prediction rules: principles, requirements, and pitfalls. *Primary Care* 1995;**22**:341–63.
20 Knottnerus JA. Application of logistic regression to the analysis of diagnostic data. *Med Decision Making* 1992;**12**:93–108.
21 Knottnerus JA, Dinant GJ. Medicine based evidence, a prerequisite for evidence based medicine. *BMJ* 1997;**315**:1109–1110.
22 Ransohoff DF, Feinstein AR. Problems of spectrum and bias in evaluating the efficacy of diagnostic tests. *N Engl J Med* 1978;**299**:926–30.
23 Begg CB. Biases in the assessment of diagnostic tests. *Statistics Med* 1987;**6**:411–23.
24 Green MS. The effect of validation group bias on screening tests for coronary artery disease. *Statistics Med* 1985;**4**:53–61.
25 Knottnerus JA, Leffers P. The influence of referral patterns on the characteristics of diagnostic tests. *J Clin Epidemiol* 1992;**45**:1143–54.

26 Zarin OA, Pauker SG. Decision analysis as a basis for medical decision making: the tree of Hippokrates. *J Med Philos* 1984;**9**:181–213.

27 Schwartz WB, Wolfe HJ, Pauker SG. Pathology and probabilities, a new approach to interpreting and reporting biopsies. *N Engl J Med* 1981;**305**:917–23.

28 Liechtenstein JI, Feinstein AR, Suzio KD, DeLuca V, Spiro HM. The effectiveness of pandendoscopy on diagnostic and therapeutic decisions about chronic abdominal pain. *J Clin Gastroenterol* 1980;**2**:31–6.

29 Dronfield MW, Langman MJ, Atkinson M, *et al.* Outcome of endoscopy and barium radiography for acute upper gastrointestinal bleeding: controlled trial in 1037 patients. *BMJ* 1982;**284**:545–8.

30 Brett GZ. The value of lung cancer detection by six-monthly chest radiographs. *Thorax* 1968;**23**:414–20.

31 Brown VA, Sawers RS, Parsons RJ, Duncan SL, Cooke ID. The value of antenatal cardiotocography in the management of high risk pregnancy: a randomised controlled trial. *Br J Obster Gynaecol* 1982;**89**:716–22.

32 Flynn AM, Kelly J, Mansfield H, Needham P, O'Connor M, Viegas O. A randomised controlled trial of non-stress antepartum cardiotocography. *Br J Obster Gynaecol* 1982;**89**:427–33.

33 Durbridge TC, Edwards F, Edwards RG, Atkinson M. An evaluation of multiphasic screening on admission to hospital. *Med J Aust* 1976;**1**:703–5.

34 Hull RD, Hirsch J, Carter CJ, *et al.* Diagnostic efficacy of impedance phletysmography for clinically suspected deep-vein thrombosis. A randomized trial. *Ann Intern Med* 1985; **102**:21–8.

35 Shapiro S, Venet W, Strax Ph, Roeser R. Ten to fourteen year effect of screening on breast cancer mortality. *J Natl Cancer Inst* 1982;**69**:349–55.

36 Tabár L, Fagerberg CJG, Gad A, Badertorp L. Reduction in mortality from breast cancer after mass screening with mammography. *Lancet* 1985;**1**:829–31.

37 Harms LM, Schellevis FG, van Eijk JT, Donker AJ, Bouter LM. Cardiovascular morbidity and mortality among hypertensive patients in general practice: the evaluation of long-term systematic management. *J Clin Epidemiol* 1997;**50**:779–86.

38 Collette HJA, Day NE, Rombach JJ, de Waard F. Evaluation of screening for breast cancer in a non-randomised study (the DOM project) by means of a case control study. *Lancet* 1984;**1**:1224–6.

39 Verbeek ALM, Hendriks JHCL, Holland R, Mravunac M, Sturmans F, Day NE. Reduction of breast cancer mortality through mass-screening with modern mammography. *Lancet* 1984;**1**:1222–4.

40 Guyatt GH, Tugwell P, Feeny DH, Drummond MF, Haynes RB. The role of before–after studies of therapeutic impact in the evaluation of diagnostic technologies. *J Chronic Dis* 1986;**39**:295–304.

41 Fineberg HV, Bauman R. Computerized cranial tomography: effect on diagnostic and therapeutic planns. *JAMA* 1977;**238**:224–7.

42 Dinant GJ, Knottnerus JA, van Wersch JW. Diagnostic impact of the erythrocyte sedimentation rate in general practice: a before–after analysis. *Fam Pract* 1991;**9**:28–31.

43 Knottnerus JA. Medical decision making by general practitioners and specialists. *Fam Pract* 1991;**8**:305–7.

44 Irwig L, Macaskill P, Glasziou P, Fahey M. Meta-analytic methods for diagnostic test accuracy. *J Clin Epidemiol* 1995;**48**:119–130.

45 Buntinx F, Brouwers M. Relation between sampling device and detection of abnormality in cervical smears: a meta-analysis of randomised and quasi-randomised studies. *BMJ* 1996;**313**:1285–90.

46 Benavente O, Moher D, Pham B. Carotid endarterectomy for asymptomatic carotid stenosis: a meta-analysis. *BMJ* 1998;**317**:1477–80.

47 Van Binsbergen JJ, Brouwer A, van Drenth BB, Haverkort AFM, Prins A, van der Weijden T. Dutch College of General Practitioners standard on cholesterol (M20). *Huisarts Wet* 1991;**34**:551–7.

48 Consensus on non-invasive diagnosis of peripheral arterial vascular disease. Utrecht: CBO, 1994.

49 Feinstein AR. *Clinimetrics*. New Haven: Yale University Press, 1987.

2 The architecture of diagnostic research

DAVID L SACKETT, R BRIAN HAYNES

Summary box

- Because diagnostic testing aims to discriminate between clinically "normal" and "abnormal", the definition of "normal" and "the normal range" is a basic issue in diagnostic research. Although the "gaussian" definition is traditionally common, the "therapeutic definition" of normal is the most clinically relevant.
- The diagnostic research question to be answered has to be carefully formulated, and determines the appropriate research approach. The four most relevant types of question are:
- **Phase I questions: Do patients with the target disorder have different test results from normal individuals?** The answer requires a comparison of the distribution of test results among patients known to have the disease and people known not to have the disease.
- **Phase II questions: Are patients with certain test results more likely to have the target disorder than patients with other test results?** This can be studied in the same dataset that generated the Phase I answer, but now test characteristics such as sensitivity and specificity are estimated.
- Only if Phase I and Phase II studies, performed in "ideal circumstances", are sufficiently promising as to possible discrimination between diseased and non-diseased subjects, it is worth evaluating the test under "usual" circumstances. Phase III and IV questions must then be answered.
- **Phase III questions: Among patients in whom it is clinically sensible to suspect the target disorder, does the test result**

distinguish those with and without the target disorder? To get the appropriate answer, a consecutive series of such patients should be studied.

- The validity of Phase III studies is threatened when cases where the reference standard or diagnostic test is lost, not performed, or indeterminate, are frequent or inappropriately dealt with.

- Because of a varying patient mix, test characteristics such as sensitivity, specificity and likelihood ratios may vary between different healthcare settings.

- **Phase IV questions: Do patients who undergo the diagnostic test fare better (in their ultimate health outcomes) than similar patients who do not?** These questions have to be answered by randomising patients to undergo the test of interest or some other (or no) test.

Introduction

When making a diagnosis, clinicians seldom have access to reference or "gold" standard tests for the target disorders they suspect, and often wish to avoid the risks or costs of these reference standards, especially when they are invasive, painful, or dangerous. No wonder, then, that clinical researchers examine relationships between a wide range of more easily measured phenomena and final diagnoses. These phenomena include elements of the patient's history, physical examination, images from all sorts of penetrating waves, and the levels of myriad constituents of body fluids and tissues. Alas, even the most promising phenomena, when nominated as diagnostic tests, almost never exhibit a one-to-one relationship with their respective target disorders, and several different diagnostic tests may compete for primacy in diagnosing the same target disorder. As a result, considerable effort has been expended at the interface between clinical medicine and scientific methods in an effort to maximise the validity and usefulness of diagnostic tests. This book describes the result of those efforts, and this chapter focuses on the specific sorts of questions posed in diagnostic research and the study architectures used to answer them.

At the time that this book was being written, considerable interest was being directed to questions about the usefulness of the plasma concentration of B-type natriuretic peptide in diagnosing left ventricular dysfunction.[1] These questions were justified on two grounds: first, left ventricular dysfunction is difficult to diagnose on clinical examination; and second, randomised trials have shown that treating it (with angiotensin converting enzyme inhibitors) reduces its morbidity and mortality. Because real examples are far better than hypothetical ones in illustrating not just the overall strategies but also the down-to-earth tactics of clinical research, we will employ this one in the following paragraphs. To save space and tongue twisting we will refer to the diagnostic test, B-type natriuretic peptide, as BNP and the target disorder it is intended to diagnose, left ventricular dysfunction, as LVD. The starting point in evaluating this or any other promising diagnostic test is to decide how we will define its normal range.

What do you mean by "normal" and "the normal range"?

This chapter deals with the strategies (a lot) and tactics (a little) of research that attempts to distinguish patients who are "normal" from those who have a specific target disorder. Before we begin, however, we need to acknowledge that several different definitions of normal are used in clinical medicine, and we confuse them at our (and patients') peril. We know six of them[2] and credit Tony Murphy for pointing out five.[3] A common "*gaussian*" definition (fortunately falling into disuse) assumes that the diagnostic test results for BNP (or some arithmetic manipulation of them) for everyone, or for a group of presumably normal people, or for a carefully characterised "reference" population, will fit a specific theoretical distribution known as the *normal* or *gaussian* distribution. Because the mean of a gaussian distribution plus or minus 2 standard deviations encloses 95% of its contents, it became a tempting way to define the normal several years ago, and came into general use. It is unfortunate that it did, for three logical consequences of its use have led to enormous confusion and the creation of a new field of medicine: the diagnosis of non-disease. First, diagnostic test results simply do not fit the gaussian distribution (actually, we should be grateful that they do not; the gaussian distribution extends to infinity in both directions, necessitating occasional patients with impossibly high BNP results and others on the minus side of zero!). Second, if the highest and lowest 2.5% of diagnostic test results are called abnormal, then all the diseases they represent have exactly the same frequency, a conclusion that is also clinically nonsensical.

The third harmful consequence of the use of the gaussian definition of normal is shared by its more recent replacement, the *percentile*. Recognising the failure of diagnostic test results to fit a theoretical distribution such as the gaussian, some laboratorians have suggested that we ignore the shape of the distribution and simply refer (for example) to the lower (or upper) 95% of BNP or other test results as normal. Although this percentile definition does avoid the problems of infinite and negative test values, it still suggests

21

that the underlying prevalence of all diseases is similar – about 5% – which is silly, and still contributes to the "upper-limit syndrome" of non-disease because its use means that the only "normal" patients are the ones who are not yet sufficiently worked up. This inevitable consequence arises as follows: if the normal range for a given diagnostic test is defined as including the lower 95% of its results, then the probability that a given patient will be called "normal" when subjected to this test is 95%, or 0.95. If this same patient undergoes two independent diagnostic tests (independent in the sense that they are probing totally different organs or functions), the likelihood of this patient being called normal is now $(0.95) \times (0.95) = 0.90$. So, the likelihood of any patient being called normal is 0.95 raised to the power of the number of independent diagnostic tests performed on them. Thus, a patient who undergoes 20 tests has only 0.95 to the 20th power, or about one chance in three, of being called normal; a patient undergoing 100 such tests has only about six chances in 1000 of being called normal at the end of the work up.[*]

Other definitions of normal, in avoiding the foregoing pitfalls, present other problems. The *risk factor* definition is based on studies of precursors or statistical predictors of subsequent clinical events; by this definition, the normal range for BNP or serum cholesterol or blood pressure consists of those levels that carry no additional risk of morbidity or mortality. Unfortunately, however, many of these risk factors exhibit steady increases in risk throughout their range of values; indeed, some hold that the "normal" total serum cholesterol (defined by cardiovascular risk) might lie well below 3.9 mmol/L (150 mg%), whereas our local laboratories employ an upper limit of normal of 5.2 mmol/L (200 mg%), and other institutions employ still other definitions.

Another shortcoming of this risk factor definition becomes apparent when we examine the health consequences of acting upon a test result that lies beyond the normal range: will altering BNP or any other risk factor really change risk? For example, although obesity is a risk factor for hypertension, controversy continues over whether weight reduction improves mild hypertension. One of us led a randomised trial in which we peeled 4.1 kg (on average) from obese, mildly hypertensive women with a behaviourally oriented weight reduction programme the (control women lost less than 1 kg).[4] Despite both their and our efforts (the cost of the experimental group's behaviourally oriented weight reduction programme came to US$60 per kilo), there was no accompanying decline in blood pressure.

A related approach defines the normal as that which is *culturally desirable*, providing an opportunity for what HL Mencken called "the corruption of

---

[*]This consequence of such definitions helps explain the results of a randomised trial of hospital admission multitest screening that found no patient benefits, but increased healthcare costs, when such screening was carried out.[20]

medicine by morality" through the "confusion of the theory of the healthy with the theory of the virtuous".[5] Although this definition does not fit our BNP example, one sees such definitions in their mostly benign form at the fringes of the current lifestyle movement (for example, "It is better to be slim than fat,"[†] and "Exercise and fitness are better than sedentary living and lack of fitness"), and in its malignant form in the healthcare system of the Third Reich. Such a definition has the potential for considerable harm, and may also serve to subvert the role of medicine in society.

Two final definitions are highly relevant and useful to the clinician because they focus directly on the clinical acts of diagnosis and therapy. The *diagnostic* definition identifies a range of BNP (or other diagnostic test) results beyond which LVD (or another specific target disorder) is (with known probability) present. It is this definition that we focus on in this book. The "known probability" with which a target disorder is present is known formally as the positive predictive value, and depends on where we set the limits for the normal range of diagnostic test results. This definition has real clinical value and is a distinct improvement over the definitions described above. It does, however, require that clinicians keep track of diagnostic ranges and cut-offs.

The final definition of normal sets its limits at the level of BNP beyond which specific treatments for LVD (such as ACE inhibitors) have been shown conclusively to do more good than harm. This *therapeutic* definition is attractive because of its link with action. The therapeutic definition of the normal range of blood pressure, for example, avoids the hazards of labelling patients as diseased unless they are going to be treated. Thus, in the early 1960s the only levels of blood pressure conclusively shown to benefit from antihypertensive drugs were diastolic pressures in excess of 130 mmHg (phase V). Then, in 1967, the first of a series of randomised trials demonstrated the clear advantages of initiating drugs at 115 mmHg, and the upper limit of normal blood pressure, under the therapeutic definition, fell to that level. In 1970 it was lowered further to 105 mmHg with a second convincing trial, and current guidelines about which patients have abnormal blood pressures that require treatment add an element of the risk factor definition and recommend treatment based on the combination of blood pressure with age, sex, cholesterol level, blood sugar, and smoking habit. These days one can even obtain evidence for blood pressure treatment levels based on the presence of a second disease: for example, in type 2 diabetes the "tight control" of blood pressure reduces the risk of major complications in a cost effective way. Obviously, the use of this therapeutic definition requires that clinicians (and guideline developers) keep abreast of advances in therapeutics, and that is as it should be.

---

†But the tragic consequences of anorexia nervosa teach us that even this definition can do harm.

In summary, then, before you start any diagnostic study you need to define what you mean by normal, and be confident that you have done so in a sensible and clinically useful fashion.

The question is everything

As in other forms of clinical research, there are several different ways in which one could carry out a study into the potential or real diagnostic usefulness of a physical sign or laboratory test, and each of them is appropriate to one sort of question and inappropriate for others. Among the questions one might pose about the relation between a putative diagnostic test (say, BNP) and a target disorder (say, LVD), four are most relevant:

- **Phase I questions**: Do patients with the target disorder have different test results from normal individuals? (Do patients with LVD have higher BNP than normal individuals?)
- **Phase II questions**: Are patients with certain test results more likely to have the target disorder than patients with other test results? (Are patients with higher BNP more likely to have LVD than patients with lower BNP?)
- **Phase III questions**: Among patients in whom it is clinically sensible to suspect the target disorder, does the level of the test result distinguish those with and without the target disorder? (Among patients in whom it is clinically sensible to suspect LVD, does the level of BNP distinguish those with and without LVD?)
- **Phase IV questions**: Do patients who undergo this diagnostic test fare better (in their ultimate health outcomes) than similar patients who do not? (Of greatest interest in evaluating early diagnosis through screening tests, this might be phrased: Do patients screened with BNP (in the hope of achieving the early diagnosis of LVD) have better health outcomes (mortality, function, quality of life) than those who do not undergo screening?).

At first glance the first three questions may appear indistinguishable or even identical. They are not, because the strategies and tactics employed in answering them are crucially different, and so are the conclusions that can be drawn from their answers. The first two differ in the "direction" in which their results are analysed and interpreted, and the third differs from the first two as well in the fashion in which study patients are assembled. The fourth question gets at what we and our patients would most like to know: are they better off for having undergone it? The conclusions that can (and, more importantly, cannot) be drawn from the answers to these questions are crucially different, and there are plenty of examples of the price paid by patients and providers when the answers to Phase I or II questions are interpreted as if they were answering a Phase III (or even a Phase IV) question.

These questions also nicely describe an orderly and efficient progression of research into the potential usefulness of a clinical sign, symptom, or laboratory result, and we will use the BNP story to show this sequence.

Phase I questions: Do patients with the target disorder have different test results from normal individuals?

Question 1 often can be answered with a minimum of effort, time, and expense, and its architecture is displayed in Table 2.1.

For example, a group of investigators at a British university hospital measured BNP precursor in convenience samples of "normal controls" and in patients who had various combinations of hypertension, ventricular hypertrophy, and LVD.[6] They found statistically significant differences in median BNP precursors between patients with and normal individuals without LVD, and no overlap in their range of BNP precursor results. It was not surprising, therefore, that they concluded that BNP was "a useful diagnostic aid for LVD".

Note, however, that the direction of interpretation here is from known diagnosis back to diagnostic test. Answers to Phase I questions cannot be applied directly to patients because they are presented as overall (usually average) test results. They are not analysed in terms of the diagnostic test's sensitivity, specificity, or likelihood ratios. Moreover, Phase I studies are typically conducted among patients known to have the disease and people known not to have the disease (rather than among patients who are suspected of having, but not known to have, the disease). As a result, this phase of diagnostic test evaluation cannot be translated into diagnostic action.

Why, then, ask Phase I questions at all? There are two reasons. First, such studies add to our biologic insights about the mechanisms of disease, and may serve later research into therapy as well as diagnosis. Second, such studies are quick and relatively cheap, and a negative answer to their question removes the need to ask the tougher, more time-consuming, and costlier questions of Phases II–IV. Thus, if a convenience (or "grab")

Table 2.1 Answering a Phase I question: Do patients with LVD have higher BNP than normal individuals?

	Patients known to have the target disorder (LVD)	Normal controls
Average diagnostic test (BNP precursor) result (and its range)	493.5 (range from 248.9 to 909)	129.4 (range from 53.6 to 159.7)

25

sample of patients with LVD already known to the investigators displays the same average levels and distribution of BNP as apparently healthy laboratory technicians or captive medical students, it is time to abandon it as a diagnostic test and devote scarce resources to some other lead.

Phase II questions: Are patients with certain test results more likely to have the target disorder than patients with other test results?

Following a positive answer to a Phase I question, it is logical to ask a Phase II question, this time changing the direction of interpretation so that it runs from diagnostic test result forward to diagnosis. Although the Phase II questions often can be asked in the same dataset that generated the Phase I answer, the architecture of asking and answering them differs. For example, a second group of investigators at a Belgian university hospital measured BNP in "normal subjects" and 3 groups of patients with coronary artery disease and varying degrees of LVD.[7] Among the analyses they performed (including the creation of ROC curves; see Chapter 7) was a simple plot of individual BNP results, generating the results shown in Table 2.2 by picking the cut-off that best distinguished their patients with severe LVD from their normal controls.

As you can see, the results in Table 2.2 are extremely encouraging. Whether it is used to "rule out" LVD on the basis of its high sensitivity (SnNout)[8] or to "rule in" LVD with its high specificity (SpPin),[9] BNP looks useful, so it is no wonder that the authors concluded: "BNP concentrations are good indicators of the severity and prognosis of

Table 2.2 Answering a Phase II question: Are patients with higher BNP more likely to have LVD than patients with lower BNP?

	Patients known to have the target disorder (LVD)	Normal controls
High BNP	39	2
Normal BNP	1	25
Test characteristics and their 95% confidence intervals	Lower	Upper
Sensitivity = 98%	87%	100%
Specificity = 92%	77%	98%
Positive predictive value = 95%	84%	99%
Negative predictive value = 96%	81%	100%
Likelihood ratio for an abnormal test result = 13	3.5	50
Likelihood ratio for a normal test result = 0.03	0.0003	0.19

congestive heart failure". But is Table 2.2 overly encouraging? It compares test results between groups of patients who already have established diagnoses (rather than those who are merely suspected of the target disorder), and contrasts extreme groups of normals and those with severe disease. Thus, it tells us whether the test shows diagnostic promise under ideal conditions. A useful way to think about this difference between Phase II

Table 2.3 Explanatory and pragmatic studies of diagnostic tests and treatments.

	Promising diagnostic test		Promising treatment	
Feature	Explanatory (Phase II study)	Pragmatic (Phase III study)	Explanatory	Pragmatic
Question	Can this test discriminate under ideal circumstances?	Does this test discriminate in routine practice?	Efficacy: Can this treatment work under ideal circumstances?	Effectiveness: Does this treatment work in routine practice?
Selection of patients	Preselected groups of normal individuals and of those who clearly have the target disorder	Consecutive patients in whom it is clinically sensible to suspect the target disorder	Highly compliant, high-risk, high-response patients	All comers, regardless of compliance, risk or responsiveness
Application of manoeuvre	Carried out by expert clinician or operator on best equipment	Carried out by usual clinician or operator on usual equipment	Administered by experts with great attention to compliance	Administered by usual clinicians under usual circumstances
Definition of outcomes	Same reference standard for those with and without the target disorder	Often different standards for patients with and without the target disorder; may invoke good treatment-free prognosis as proof of absence of target disorder	May focus on pathophysiology, surrogate outcomes, or cause-specific mortality	"Hard" clinical events or death (often all-cause mortality)
Exclusion of patients or events	Often exclude patients with lost results and indeterminate diagnoses	Include all patients, regardless of lost results or indeterminate diagnoses	May exclude events before or after treatment is applied	Includes all events after randomisation
Results confirmed in a second, independent ("test") sample of patients	Usually not	Ideally yes		
Incorporation into systematic review	Usually not	Ideally yes	Sometimes	Ideal

and Phase III studies is by analogy with randomised clinical trials, which range from addressing explanatory (efficacy) issues of therapy (can the new treatment work under ideal circumstances?) to management (pragmatic, effectiveness) issues (does the new treatment work under usual circumstances?). We have summarised this analogy in Table 2.3.

As shown in Table 2.3, the Phase II study summarised in Table 2.2 is explanatory in nature: preselected groups of normal individuals (ducks) and those who clearly have the target disorder (yaks) undergo testing under the most rigorous circumstances possible, with the presence or absence of the target disorder being determined by the same reference standard. No attempt is made to validate these initial ("training set") results (especially the cut-off used to set the upper limit of normal BNP) in a second, independent "test" set of ducks and yaks. On the other hand, and as with the Phase I study, this relatively easy Phase II investigation tells us whether the promising diagnostic test is worth further, costlier evaluation; as we have said elsewhere,[10] if the test cannot tell the difference between a duck and a yak it is worthless in diagnosing either one. As long as the writers and readers of a Phase II explanatory study report make no pragmatic claims about its usefulness in routine clinical practice, no harm is done. Furthermore, criticisms of Phase II explanatory studies for their failure to satisfy the methodological standards employed in Phase III pragmatic studies do not make sense.

Phase III questions: Among patients in whom it is clinically sensible to suspect the target disorder, does the level of the test result distinguish those with and without the target disorder?

Given its promise in Phase I and II studies, it is understandable that BNP would be tested in the much costlier and more time-consuming Phase III study, in order to determine whether it was really useful among patients in whom it is clinically sensible to suspect LVD. As we were writing this chapter, an Oxfordshire group of clinical investigators reported that they did just that by inviting area general practitioners "to refer patients with suspected heart failure to our clinic".[11] Once there, these 126 patients underwent independent, blind BNP measurements and echocardiography. Their results are summarised in Table 2.4.

About one third of the patients referred by their general practitioners had LVD on echocardiography. These investigators documented that BNP measurements did not look nearly as promising when tested in a Phase III study in the pragmatic real-world setting of routine clinical practice, and concluded that "introducing routine measurement [of BNP] would be unlikely to improve the diagnosis of symptomatic [LVD] in the

Table 2.4 Answering a Phase III question: Among patients in whom it is clinically sensible to suspect LVD, does the level of BNP distinguish patients with and without LVD?

	Patients with LVD on echocardiography	Patients with normal echoes
High BNP (>17.9 pg/ml)	35	57
Normal BNP (<18 pg/ml)	5	29
Prevalence or pretest probability of LVD	40/126 = 32%	
Test characteristics and their 95% confidence intervals	Lower	Upper
Sensitivity = 88%	74%	94%
Specificity = 34%	25%	44%
Positive predictive value = 38%	29%	48%
Negative predictive value = 85%	70%	94%
Likelihood ratio for an abnormal test result = 1.3	1.1	1.6
Likelihood ratio for a normal test result = 0.4	0.2	0.9

Table 2.5 Answering a Phase III question with likelihood ratios.

	Patients with LVD on echocardiography	Patients with normal echoes	Likelihood ratio and 95% CI
High BNP (>76 pg/ml)	26 (0.650)	11 (0.128)	5.1 (2.8–9.2)
Mid BNP (10–75 pg/ml)	11 (0.275)	60 (0.698)	0.4 (0.2–0.7)
Low BNP (<10 pg/ml)	3 (0.075)	15 (0.174)	0.4 (0.1–1)
Total	40 (1.000)	86 (1.000)	

community". However, their report of the study also documented the effect of two other cut-points for BNP. This led both to a counterclaim on the usefulness of BNP in the subsequent email letters to the editor, and to an opportunity for us to describe an alternative way of presenting information about the accuracy of a diagnostic test: the multilevel likelihood ratio (LR). The original report makes it possible for us to construct Table 2.5.

By using multilevel likelihood ratios to take advantage of the full range of BNP results, we can be slightly more optimistic about the diagnostic usefulness of higher levels: the LR for BNP results >76 pg/ml was 5.1. These levels were found in 29% of the patients in this study, and their presence raised the pretest probability of LVD in the average patient from 32% to a post-test probability of 70%. This can be determined directly from Table 2.5 for this "average" patient with a pretest probability of 32% and a high BNP: reading horizontally across the top row, the result is 26/(26+11) = 70%.

However, if the patient has a different pretest likelihood, say 50%, then either the table must be reconstructed for this higher figure, or the pretest probability needs to be converted to a pretest odds (50% is a pretest odds of $(1-0.5)/0.5 = 1$), and then multiplied by the likelihood ratio for the test result (5.1 in this case), giving a post-test odds of 5.1, which then can be converted back into a post-test probability of $5.1/(1+5.1) = 84\%$. These calculations are rendered unnecessary by using a nomogram, as in Figure 2.1.

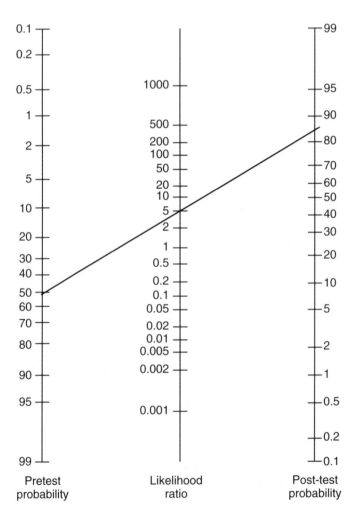

Pretest probability   Likelihood ratio   Post-test probability

Figure 2.1 Nomogram for converting pretest likelihoods (left column) to post-test likelihoods (right column) by drawing a straight line from the pretest likelihood through the likelihood ratio for the test result.

Given the quite wide confidence intervals around these LRs, further type III studies may be fruitful (and readers can check to see whether this was done after this chapter was published).

Threats to the validity of Phase III studies

There are several threats to the validity of Phase III studies that distort their estimates of the accuracy of the diagnostic test, and the first batch are violations of the old critical appraisal guide: "Has there been an independent, blind comparison with a gold standard of diagnosis?"[12] By *independence* we mean that *all* study patients have undergone *both* the diagnostic test *and* the reference ("gold") standard evaluation and, more specifically, that the reference standard is applied *regardless of the diagnostic test result*. By *blind* we mean that the reference standard is applied and interpreted in total ignorance of the diagnostic test result, and vice versa. By anticipating these threats at the initial question forming phase of a study, they can be avoided or minimised.

Although we prefer to conceptualise diagnostic test evaluations in terms of 2×2 tables such as the upper panel of Table 2.6 (and this is the way that most Phase II studies are performed), in reality Phase III studies generate the 3×3 tables shown in the lower panel of Table 2.6. Reports get lost, their results are sometimes incapable of interpretation, and sometimes we are unwilling to apply the reference standard to all the study patients.

The magnitude of the cells *v–z* and the method of handling patients who fall into these cells will affect the validity of the study. In the perfect study these cells are kept empty, or so small that they cannot exert any important

Table 2.6 The ideal Phase III study meets the real world.

The ideal study	Reference standard	
	Target disorder present	Target disorder absent
Diagnostic test result		
Positive	*a*	*b*
Negative	*c*	*d*

The real study	Reference standard		
	Target disorder present	Lost, not performed, or indeterminate	Target disorder absent
Diagnostic test result			
Positive	*a*	*v*	*b*
Lost, not performed, or indeterminate	*w*	*x*	*y*
Negative	*c*	*z*	*d*

effect on the study conclusions. However, there are 6 situations in which they become large enough to bias the measures of test accuracy. First, when the reference standard is expensive, painful, or risky, investigators will not wish to apply it to patients with negative diagnostic test results. As a consequence, such patients risk winding up in cell z. Furthermore, there is an understandable temptation to shift them to cell d in the analysis. Because no diagnostic test is perfect, some of them surely belong in cell c. Shifting all of them to cell d falsely inflates both sensitivity and specificity. If this potential problem is recognised before the study begins, investigators can design their reference standard to prevent such patients from falling into cell z. This is accomplished by moving to a more pragmatic study and adding another, prognostic dimension to the reference standard, namely the clinical course of patients with negative test results who receive no intervention for the target disorder. If patients who otherwise would end up in cell z develop the target disorder during this treatment-free follow up, they belong in cell c. If they remain free of disease, they join cell d. The result is an unbiased and pragmatic estimate of sensitivity and specificity.

Second, the reference standard may be lost; and third, it may generate an uninterpretable or indeterminate result. As before, arbitrarily analysing such patients as if they really did or did not have the target disorder will distort measures of diagnostic test accuracy. Once again, if these potential biases are identified in the planning stages they can be minimised, a pragmatic solution such as that proposed above for cell z considered, and clinically sensible rules established for shifting them to the definitive columns in a manner that confers the greatest benefit (in terms of treatment) and the least harm (in terms of labelling) to later patients.

Fourth, fifth, and sixth, the diagnostic test result may be lost, never performed, or indeterminate, so that the patient winds up in cells w, x, or y. Here the only unforgivable action is to exclude such patients from the analysis of accuracy. As before, anticipation of these problems before the study begins should minimise tests that are lost or never performed to the point where they would not affect the study conclusion regardless of how they were classified. If indeterminate results are likely to be frequent, a decision can be made before the study begins as to whether they will be classified as positive or negative. Alternatively, if multilevel likelihood ratios are to be used, these patients can form their own stratum.

In addition to the 6 threats to validity related to cells v–z, there are two more. The seventh threat to validity noted in the above critical appraisal guide arises when a patient's reference standard is applied or interpreted by someone who already knows that patient's diagnostic test result (and vice versa). This is a risk whenever there is any degree of interpretation (even in reading off a scale) involved in generating the result of the diagnostic test or reference standard. We know that these situations lead to biased inflations of sensitivity and specificity.

The eighth and final threat to the validity of accuracy estimates generated in Phase III studies arises whenever the selection of the "upper limit of normal" or cut-point for the diagnostic test is under the control of the investigator. When they can place the cut-point wherever they want, it is natural for them to select the point where it maximises sensitivity (for use as a SnNout), specificity (for use as a SpPin), or the total number of patients correctly classified in that particular "training" set. If the study were repeated in a second, independent "test" set of patients, employing that same cut-point, the diagnostic test would be found to function a little or a lot worse. Thus, the true accuracy of a promising diagnostic test is not known until it has been evaluated in one or more independent studies.

The foregoing threats apply whether the diagnostic test comprises a single measurement of a single phenomenon or a multivariate combination of several phenomena. For example, Philip Wells and his colleagues determined the diagnostic accuracy of the combination of several items from the medical history, physical examination, and non-invasive testing in the diagnosis of deep vein thrombosis.[13] Although their study generated similar results in three different centres (two in Canada and one in Italy), even they recommended further prospective testing before widespread use.

Limits to the applicability of Phase III studies

Introductory courses in epidemiology introduce the concept that predictive values change as we move back and forth between screening or primary care settings (with their low prevalence or pretest probability of the target disorder) to secondary and tertiary care (with their higher probability of the target disorder). This point is usually made by assuming that sensitivity and specificity remain constant across all settings. However, the mix (or spectrum) of patients also varies between these locations; for example, screening is applied to asymptomatic individuals with early disease, whereas tertiary care settings deal with patients with advanced or florid disease. No wonder, then, that sensitivity and specificity often vary between these settings. Moreover, because primary care patients with positive diagnostic test results (which comprise false positive as well as true positive results) are referred forward to secondary and tertiary care, we might expect specificity to fall as we move along the referral pathway. There is very little empirical evidence addressing this issue, and we acknowledge our debt to Dr James Wagner of the University of Texas at Dallas for tracking down and systematically reviewing diagnostic data from over 2000 patients with clinically suspected appendicitis seen in primary care and on inpatient surgical wards (personal communication, 2000). The diagnostic tests comprised the clinical signs that are sought when clinicians suspect appendicitis, and the reference standard is a combination of pathology

33

Table 2.7 The accuracy of right lower quadrant tenderness in the diagnosis of appendicitis.

	Primary care settings Appendicitis		Tertiary care settings Appendicitis	
	Yes (%)	No (%)	Yes (%)	No (%)
Right lower quadrant tenderness				
Present	84	11	81	84
Absent	16	89	19	16
Total	100	100	100	100
Frequency of appendicitis	14%		63%	
Frequency of positive sign	21%		82%	
Sensitivity	84%		81%	
Specificity	89%		16%	
LR+	7.6		1	
LR−	0.2		1	

reports on appendices when operations were performed, and a benign clinical course when they were not. The results for the diagnostic test of right lower quadrant tenderness are shown in Table 2.7.

A comparison of the results in primary and tertiary care shows, as we might expect, an increase in the proportions of patients with appendicitis (from 14% to 63%). But, of course, this increase in prevalence occurred partly because patients with right lower quadrant tenderness (regardless of whether this was a true positive or false positive finding) tended to be referred to the next level of care, whereas patients without this sign tended not to be referred onward; this is confirmed by the rise in the frequency of this sign from 21% of patients in primary care to 82% of patients in tertiary care. Although this sort of increase in a positive diagnostic test result is widely recognised, its effect on the accuracy of the test is not. The forward referral of patients with false positive test results leads to a fall in specificity, in this case a dramatic one from 89% down to 16%. As a result, a diagnostic sign of real value in primary care (LR+ of 8, LR− of 0.2) is useless in tertiary care (LR+ and LR− both 1); in other words, its diagnostic value has been "used up" along the way.[‡]

This phenomenon can place major limitations on the applicability of Phase III studies carried out in one sort of setting to another setting where

---

[‡]Although not germane to this book on research methods, there are two major clinical ramifications of this phenomenon. First, because clinical signs and other diagnostic tests often lose their value along the referral pathway, tertiary care clinicians might be forgiven for proceeding immediately to applying invasive reference standards. Second, tertiary care teachers should be careful what they teach primary care trainees about the uselessness of clinical signs.

Table 2.8 The accuracy of abdominal rigidity in the diagnosis of appendicitis.

	Primary care settings Appendicitis		Tertiary care settings Appendicitis	
	Yes (%)	No (%)	Yes (%)	No (%)
Rigid abdomen				
Present	40	26	23	6
Absent	60	74	77	94
Total	100	100	100	100
Frequency of appendicitis	14%		47%	
Frequency of positive sign	28%		14%	
Sensitivity	40%		24%	
Specificity	74%		94%	
LR+	1.5		5	
LR−	0.8		0.8	

the mix of test results may differ. Overcoming this limitation is another bonus that attends the replication of a promising Phase III study in a second "test" setting attended by patients of the sort that the test is claimed to benefit.

Does specificity always fall between primary care and tertiary care settings? Might this be employed to generate a "standardised correction factor" for extrapolating test accuracy between settings? Have a look at the clinical sign of abdominal rigidity in Table 2.8.

In this case, a clinical sign that is useless in primary care (LR+ barely above 1 and LR− close to 1) is highly useful in tertiary care (LR+ of 5), and in this case specificity has risen (from 74% to 95%), not fallen, along the referral pathway. The solution to this paradox is revealed in the frequency of the sign in these two settings; it has fallen (from 28% to 14%), not risen, along the pathway from primary to tertiary care. We think that the explanation is that primary care clinicians, who do not want to miss any patient's appendicitis, are "over-reading" abdominal rigidity compared to their colleagues in tertiary care. At this stage in our knowledge of this phenomenon we do not think the "standard correction factors" noted in the previous paragraph are advisable, and this paradox once again points to the need to replicate promising Phase III study results in "test" settings attended by patients (and clinicians!) of the sort that the test is claimed to benefit. In this regard we welcome the creation of the CARE consortium of over 800 clinicians from over 70 countries[14] for their performance of web-based, large, simple, fast studies of the clinical examination.[15] It is hoped that this group, which can be contacted at www.carestudy.com, can make a large contribution to determining the wide applicability of the

35

diagnostic test information obtained from the medical history and physical examination.

For clinicians who wish to apply the bayesian properties of diagnostic tests, accurate estimates of the pretest probability of target disorders in their locale and setting are required. These can come from five sources: personal experience, population prevalence statistics, practice databases, the publication that described the test, or one of a growing number of primary studies of pretest probability in different settings.[16]

Phase IV questions: Do patients who undergo this diagnostic test fare better (in their ultimate health outcomes) than similar patients who do not?

The ultimate value of a diagnostic test is measured in the health outcomes produced by the further diagnostic and therapeutic interventions it precipitates. Sometimes this benefit is self-evident, as in the correct diagnosis of patients with life threatening target disorders who thereby receive life saving treatments. At other times these outcomes can be hinted at in Phase III studies if the reference standard for the absence of the target disorder is a benign clinical course despite the withholding of treatment. More often, however, Phase IV questions are posed about diagnostic tests that achieve the early detection of asymptomatic disease, and can only be answered by the follow up of patients randomised to undergo the diagnostic test of interest or some other (or no) test.

Methods for conducting randomised trials are discussed elsewhere,[17] and we will confine this discussion to an example of the most powerful sort, a systematic review of several randomised trials of faecal occult blood testing.[18] In these trials, over 400 000 patients were randomised to undergo annual or biennial screening or no screening, and then carefully followed for up to 13 years in order to determine their mortality from colorectal cancer. The results are summarised in Table 2.9.

Table 2.9 A systematic review of randomised trials of screening for colorectal cancer.

Outcome	Unscreened group	Screened group	Relative risk reduction	Absolute risk reduction	Number needed to screen to prevent one more colorectal cancer death
Colorectal cancer mortality	0.58%	0.50%	16%	0.08%	1237

In this example, patients were randomised to undergo or not undergo the diagnostic test. Because most of them remained cancer free, the sample size requirement was huge and the study architecture is relatively inefficient. It would have been far more efficient (but unacceptable) to randomise the disclosure of positive test results, and this latter strategy was employed in a randomised trial of a developmental screening test in childhood.[19] In this study, the experimental children whose positive test results were revealed and who subsequently received the best available counselling and interventions fared no better in their subsequent academic, cognitive or developmental performance than control children whose positive test results were concealed. However, parents of the "labelled" experimental children were more likely to worry about their school performance, and their teachers tended to report more behavioural problems among them. This warning that diagnostic tests can harm as well as help those who undergo them is a suitable stopping point for this chapter.

References

1 Hobbs R. Can heart failure be diagnosed in primary care? *BMJ* 2000;**321**:188–9.

2 Sackett DL, Haynes RB, Guyatt GH, Tugwell P. *Clinical Epidemiology: a Basic Science for Clinical Medicine*, 2nd edn. Boston: Little, Brown and Company, 1991; pp. 58–61.

3 Murphy EA. The normal, and perils of the sylleptic argument. *Perspect Biol Med* 1972;**15**:566.

4 Haynes RB, Harper AC, Costley SR, *et al*. Failure of weight reduction to reduce mildly elevated blood pressure: a randomized trial. *J Hypertension* 1984;**2**:535.

5 Mencken HL. *A Mencken chrestomathy*. Westminster: Knopf, 1949;12.

6 Talwar S, Siebenhofer A, Williams B, Ng L. Influence of hypertension, left ventricular hypertrophy, and left ventricular systolic dysfunction on plasma N terminal pre-BNP. *Heart* 2000;**83**:278–82.

7 Selvais PL, Donickier JE, Robert A, *et al*. Cardiac natriuretic peptides for diagnosis and risk stratification in heart failure. *Eur J Clin Invest* 1998;**28**:636–42.

8 Sackett DL, Haynes RB, Guyatt GH, Tugwell P. op cit; p. 83.

9 Sackett DL, Haynes RB, Guyatt GH, Tugwell P. op cit; p. 77.

10 Sackett DL, Haynes RB, Guyatt GH, Tugwell P. op cit; p. 57.

11 Landray MJ, Lehman R, Arnold I. Measuring brain natriuretic peptide in suspected left ventricular systolic dysfunction in general practice: cross-sectional study. *BMJ* 2000; **320**:985–6.

12 Sackett DL, Haynes RB, Guyatt GH, Tugwell P. op cit; p. 52.

13 Wells PS, Hirsh J, Anderson DR, *et al*. A simple clinical model for the diagnosis of deep-vein thrombosis combined with impedance plethysmography: potential for an improvement in the diagnostic process. *J Intern Med* 1998;**243**:15–23.

14 McAlister FA, Straus SE, Sackett DL, on behalf of the CARE-COAD group. Why we need large, simple studies of the clinical examination: the problem and a proposed solution. *Lancet* 1999;**354**:1721–4.

15 Straus SE, McAlister FA, Sackett DL, Deeks JJ. The accuracy of patient history, wheezing, and laryngeal measurements in diagnosing obstructive airway disease. *JAMA* 2000; **283**:1853–7.

16 Sackett DL, Straus SE, Richardson WS, Rosenberg W, Haynes RB. *Evidence-Based Medicine: how to Practise and Teach EBM*, 2nd edn. Edinburgh: Churchill Livingstone, 2000;82–4.

17 Shapiro SH, Louis TA. *Clinical Trials: Issues and Approaches*, 2nd edn. New York: Marcel Dekker, 2000; (in press).

18 Towler BP, Irwig L, Glasziou P, Weller D, Kewenter J. *Screening for colorectal cancer using the faecal occult blood test, Hemoccult.* Cochrane Review, latest version 16 Jan 1998. In: The Cochrane Library, Oxford: Update Software.
19 Cadman D, Chambers LW, Walter SD, Ferguson R, Johnston N, McNamee J. Evaluation of public health preschool child development screening: The process and outcomes of a community program. *Am J Public Health* 1987;77:45–51.
20 Dunbridge TC, Edwards F, Edwards RG, Atkinson M. *An evaluation of multiphasic screening on admission to hospital.* Précis of a report to the National Health and Medical Research Council. *Med J Aust* 1976;1:703–5.

3 Assessment of the accuracy of diagnostic tests: the cross-sectional study

J ANDRÉ KNOTTNERUS, JEAN W MURIS

Summary box

- In determining the accuracy of diagnostic testing, the first step is to appropriately define the contrast to be evaluated. Options are: to evaluate one single test contrast; to compare two or more single tests; to evaluate further testing in addition to previous diagnostics; and to compare alternative diagnostic strategies. In addition, the clinical diagnostic problem under study must be specified. Finally, distinction should be made between evaluating testing in "extreme contrast" or "clinical practice" settings.
- For accuracy studies, general design types are (1) a survey of the total study population, (2) a case–referent approach, or (3) a test-based enrolment. The direction of the data collection should generally be prospective, but ambispective and retrospective approaches are sometimes appropriate.
- One should specify the determinants of primary interest (the test(s) under study) and other potentially important determinants (possible modifiers of test accuracy and confounding variables).
- The reference standard procedure to measure the target disorder should be applied on all included subjects, independently of the result of the test under study. Applying a reference standard procedure can be difficult because of classification errors, lack of a

well defined pathophysiological concept, incorporation bias, or too invasive or too complex patient investigations. Possible solutions are: an independent expert panel, and the delayed-type cross-sectional study (clinical follow up). Also, a prognostic criterion can be chosen to define clinical outcome.

- Inclusion criteria must be based on "the intention to diagnose" or "intention to screen" with respect to the studied clinical problem. The recruitment procedure is preferably a consecutive series of presenting patients or a target population screening, respectively.
- In the design phase, sample size estimation should be routine. Both Bivariate and multivariate techniques can be used in the analysis, based on the evaluated contrast. Estimating test accuracy and prediction of outcome require different approaches.
- External (clinical) validation should preferably be based on repeated studies in other, similar populations. Also, systematic reviews and meta-analysis have a role.

Introduction

Although the ultimate objective of the diagnostic phase is to optimise the patient's prognosis by enabling the clinician to choose an adequate therapeutic strategy, an accurate diagnostic assessment is a first and indispensable step in the process of clinical management.

Making a useful clinical diagnosis implies classifying the presented health problem of a patient in the context of accepted nosological knowledge. This diagnostic classification may result in confirmation or exclusion of the presence of a certain disease, in the selection of one disease from a set of possibly present diseases, or in the conclusion that a number of diseases are present simultaneously.[1] Also, it can be concluded that, given present knowledge, a further diagnostic classification than the observed symptomatology cannot be achieved. Sometimes such a classification is not worthwhile, considering the balance between expected gain in certainty, the burden of making a definitive diagnosis, and relevant therapeutic consequences.

Apart from making a diagnostic classification, the diagnostic process may be aimed at assessing the clinical severity or monitoring the clinical course of a diagnosed condition. Another very important clinical application is documenting the precise localisation or shape of a diagnosed lesion to support further, for example surgical, decision making.

A potential new diagnostic test must first go through a phase of pathophysiological and technical development, before its clinical effectiveness in terms of diagnostic accuracy or prognostic impact can be evaluated. The methodology discussed in this book, focused on clinical effectiveness, is applicable to the further evaluation of tests that have succesfully passed this early development.

A basic question to be anwered, then, is: what is the probability that this particular patient with this particular symptomatology or test result has a certain disorder or a combination of disorders? Obtaining an evidence-based answer, using clinical epidemiological research data, requires an analysis of the association between the presented symptomatology or test result and the appropriate diagnostic classification, that is, the presence or absence of certain diagnoses.

This chapter deals with principles, design and pitfalls of cross-sectional diagnostic research. In this context, cross-sectional research includes studies in which the measured test results and the health status to be diagnosed essentially represent one point in time for each study subject.[2]

Diagnostic research on test accuracy: the basic steps to take

All measures of diagnostic association[3] (Chapters 1 and 7) can be derived from research data on the relation between test results and a reference standard diagnosis. A valid data collection on this relation is the main point of concern,[4] and the various measures can be calculated by applying straightforward analytical methods. Research data for the purpose of diagnostic discrimination are generally collected in cross-sectional research, irrespective of the diagnostic parameters to be used.

As usual in research, a first requirement is to specify the research question. Second, the most appropriate study design to answer this question has to be outlined. A third step is to operationalise the determinants (test(s) to be evaluated, relevant modifiers of diagnostic accuracy, and possible confounding variables) and outcome (generally the presence or absence of the disorder to be diagnosed). Further, the study population, the corresponding inclusion and exclusion criteria, and the most appropriate recruitment procedure have to be further specified. Finally, an adequate data analysis must be planned and achieved.

The research question: contrast to be evaluated

In short, the diagnostic research question should define:

- The test or test set to be evaluated
- The clinical problem for which the use of these test(s) is considered possibly relevant

41

- Whether the planned study should evaluate (1) the potential of the test procedure to discriminate between subjects with and without a target disorder in an ideal situation of extreme contrast, or (2) to what extent it could be useful in a daily practice clinical setting (where discrimination is, by definition, more difficult).

Box 3.1   The research question

(a) *Contrast to be evaluated*
  - single test
  - comparing single tests
  - additional testing
  - comparing diagnostic strategies
(b) *Define the clinical problem*
(c) *Extreme contrast or practice setting*

A key issue is the specific contrast to be evaluated (a). The question can be, for example, What is the discriminative power of one specific test or test procedure to be applied for a certain clinical diagnostic problem (single test)? However, the focus may also be on the discriminative power of a new test compared to the best test(s) already available for a similar clinical diagnostic problem (comparing single tests). For clinical practice, it is important to determine the added value of further (for example more invasive) testing, given the tests already performed (additional testing),[5] or to evaluate the most accurate or efficient diagnostic test set or test sequence (diagnostic strategy) for a certain diagnostic problem. In general, we recommend that in studying a new, more invasive or more expensive test, already available less invasive or less expensive tests with fewer adverse effects should be also included. This makes it possible to critically evaluate the new test's net contribution, if any. Also, it is informative to include the clinician's diagnostic assessment (without knowing the test result) as a separate test. The performance of the new approach can then be evaluated as to its added value compared to the doctor's usual diagnostic performance or "black box".

Regarding the clinical problem studied (b), it is of key importance not only to define the target disorder(s) to be diagnosed, but also the clinical setting and clinical spectrum (for example, early or later in the development of the disorder, and degree of severity) at which one is primarily aiming. It is crucial whether the investigator wants to evaluate the validity of a test for diagnosing a possible disease in its early phase in a primary care setting, or to diagnose more advanced disease in an outpatient clinic or hospital setting, with patients selected by referral based on suspect symptoms or previous tests.[6,7] This is dealt with in more detail in Chapters 2 and 6.

As to (c), critical appraisal of the state of current knowledge is important for defining an optimally efficient research strategy. For instance, if nothing at all is known yet about the discriminative power of a test, it is more efficient – in terms of reducing the burden for study patients, the sample size, the resources, and the time needed for the study – first to evaluate whether the test discriminates between clearly diseased and clearly non-diseased subjects. If the test does not discriminate in such a Phase I study (Feinstein[2], Sackett and Haynes, Chapter 2 of this book) any further, usually larger and longer, studies evaluating a more difficult contrast between clinically similar study subjects will be useless: the index test cannot be expected to add anything valuable to clinical practice anyhow.

The specification of these three aspects of the research question is decisive for designing the optimal study methodology. Aspect (c) was extensively addressed in Chapter 2.

Outline of the study design

Because study questions on diagnostic accuracy generally evaluate the association between (combinations of) test results and health status (mostly the presence or absence of a target disorder), a cross-sectional design is a natural basic design option. However, this basic design has various modifications, each with specific pros and cons in terms of scientific requirements, burden for the study subjects, and efficient use of resources.

Box 3.2   Study design

General approach
- survey of total study population
- case–referent approach
- test based enrolment

Direction of data collection
- prospective
- ambispective
- retrospective

General approach

The most straightforward approach of the cross-sectional design is a survey of the study population to determine the test distribution and the presence of the target disorder simultaneously. Examples are a survey on the relationship between intermittent claudication and peripheral arterial occlusive disease in an elderly population,[8] and a study in a consecutive series of sciatica patients to determine the accuracy of history and clinical examination.[9]

Another option is the case–referent approach, starting from an already known disease status (for example present or absent) as the criterion for enrolment, the test result being determined afterwards in the study patients. This design type may be more efficient or more acceptable when the disease under study is infrequent or when the reference standard procedure is highly invasive to the patient, for example in pancreatic cancer, or very expensive.

A further approach is test based enrolment, where the available test result (such as positive or negative) is the criterion for recruitment, with the disease status being determined afterwards. This modification may be preferable when test results are easily available from routine health care. An example regarding the latter is a study on the diagnostic value of "fatigue" for detecting anaemia in primary care, comparing patients presenting with fatigue and a control group as to haematological parameters.[10]

In the context of the cross-sectional design, efficient sampling of the studied distributions may be artificially facilitated at the determinant (test) or the outcome (target disorder) side. For example, in order to achieve a balanced data collection over the relevant categories, a stratified sample can be drawn from the various test result levels or from various parts of the whole disease spectrum, from clearly no disease to most severe disease. Also, the contrast between the categories of the diseased and non-diseased subjects can be enhanced by limiting the sampling to those who have been proved to be clearly diseased and those proved to be completely healthy. The latter approach is applied in planning a Phase I study (Chapter 2), which is essentially a case–referent study. Because of a sharp contrast in disease spectrum between diseased and non-diseased, sensitivity and specificity will be optimal, and as by sampling of cases and referents the "prevalence" in the study population can also be artificially optimised (with, for example, a disease prevalence of 50%), Phase I studies generally need a relatively small number of subjects to be included. Moreover, for a Phase I study the subjects in the "case group" (the diseased) and those in the reference group (the healthy or non-diseased subjects) can be specifically selected from populations consisting of subjects who have already undergone a "reference standard" procedure with maximum certainty.

Direction of data collection

Whereas Phase I and Phase II studies (according to Sackett and Haynes, Chapter 2) may be based on either retrospective or prospective identification of subjects with a certain diagnosis or test status, Phase III studies must usually be prospectively planned. The latter start from a study population of subjects comparable with those who will be tested in clinical practice. In such studies it is not known in advance who is diseased and who is not, and the clinical characteristics of the two are therefore very similar (which in fact is the reason that testing is clinically necessary at all). Because the clinical contrast is much less pronounced, and as the prevalence of diseased subjects is usually much lower than 50%, substantially larger sample sizes are generally needed than in Phase I studies.

Also, when the subject selection is prospective the data collection can be partly retrospective (ambispective approach). For instance, if patient history is an important element of the diagnostic test to be evaluated (such as when studying the diagnostic value of rectal bleeding, palpitations, or psychiatric symptoms in the preceding 6 months), information about the past is included in the test result. Essential, however, is that the test result status, albeit based on historical information, is evaluated and interpreted as to its diagnostic accuracy at the very moment that the patient "history" is taken.

The "direction" of the sampling and the data collection must be decided upon in advance. In addition, and secondary to scientific considerations, practical issues may play a role, such as the availability of data and the efficiency of its collection. Prospectively planned data collections often take more time but are generally more valid, as the procedure and the quality of the data collection can be optimised beforehand. But this is not necessarily always the case. Valid data may be already available in a well documented database of an appropriate study population with an adequately described epidemiological (morbidity) numerator and (population) denominator, and with all relevant covariables present. Especially when the clinical indication to perform the test is appropriately defined (for example coronary angiography in instable angina pectoris) and recorded, and when all eligible patients can be assumed to be included, this is an option. Moreover, a prospective data collection may sometimes imply a higher risk of bias than a retrospective approach. For example, if participating clinicians know that they are being observed in a study of the accuracy of their usual diagnostic assessment compared to an independent standard or panel, their behaviour will be easily be influenced in the context of a prospective design (Hawthorne effect). However, in a retrospective design the availability of complete and well standardised data and the controlling of the subject selection process are often problematic.

Operationalising determinants and outcome

Determinants

As in any (clinical) epidemiological study, research questions on diagnostic accuracy can be operationalised in a central "occurrence relation"[11] between independent and dependent variables.

45

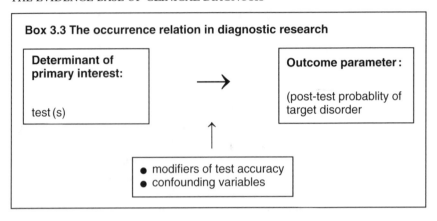

The independent variable or determinant of primary interest is the test result to be evaluated, and the primary dependent or outcome variable is (presence or absence of) the target disorder. When evaluating a single test, the test results in all study subjects are related to the reference standard. In fact, we are then comparing testing (yielding the post-test probabilities of the disorder D, for example for positive and negative test results) with not testing (expressed in the pretest probability of D). When two or more tests are compared, we have a number of separate determinants that are contrasted as to their discriminatory power. In studying the value of an additional (for example more invasive) test, given the tests already performed, the discrimination of applying all other tests is compared with that of applying all other tests plus the additional one. And to evaluate the most accurate or efficient diagnostic test set or strategy for a certain clinical problem, the performances of all the considered test combinations and sequences must be compared. To be able to make these comparisons, all separate tests have to be performed in all study subjects.

The accuracy of diagnostic tests may vary in relation to subject characteristics, such as gender, age, and comorbidity. For example, in studying the diagnostic accuracy of mammography in the detection of breast cancer, it is important to consider that this accuracy depends on age, gender, and the possible presence of fibroadenomatosis of the breasts. To evaluate the influence of such modifiers of test accuracy, these have to be measured and included in the analysis. In fact, we are dealing here with various subgroups where the diagnostic accuracy may be different. Effect modifying variables can be accounted for later in the analysis, for example by stratified analysis (subgroup analysis) of the measures of diagnostic association, or by introducing interaction terms in the logistic regression analysis (Chapter 7).[12,13] Because diagnostic assessment can be seen as optimal discrimination between subgroups with a different probability of disease, effect modifying variables can also be considered as additional diagnostic tests themselves.

Confounding variables are independent extraneous determinants of the outcome that may obscure or inflate an association between the test and the disorder. They are essentially related to both the test result and the outcome. For example, in studying whether the symptom fatigue is predictive for a low blood haemoglobin level, it is important to know which study subjects have previously taken oral iron, as this can improve the fatigue symptoms and enhance the haemoglobin level as well. A confounder can only be controlled for if it is considered beforehand and measured, which requires insight into relevant external influences. In diagnostic research the term "confounding variable" is used in a different, more pragmatic sense than in aetiologic research, as consistent diagnostic correlations do not need to be fully causally understood to be useful.

Generally, according to Bayes' theorem, the pretest probability of the target disorder is seen as a basic determinant of the post-test probability, independent of the accuracy of the applied tests. However, the clinical spectrum of the disorder may be essentially different in high and low prevalence situations. Because the clinical spectrum can influence test accuracy (Chapters 1, 2, and 6), it is then crucial to measure separately spectrum characteristics, such as disease severity, and frequency of occurrence as such. Spectrum characteristics can then be analysed as modifiers of test accuracy.

Good test reproducibility is a requirement for good accuracy in practice. Therefore, when the test under study is sensitive to inter- or intraobserver variability, documentation and, if possible, reduction of this variability is important. Documentation can be achieved in a pilot study or in the context of the main study. For example, in a study of the accuracy and reproducibility of erythrocyte sedimentation rate (ESR) measurements in general practice centres, for measuring an identical specimen a clinically relevant range between practices from 4 to 40 mm/1 h was observed. The average coefficient of variation (CV: standard deviation as a percentage of the mean) was 37% between practices and 28% within practices.[9] Observer variability can be reduced by training. In the same ESR study, the average inter- and intrapractice CVs were reduced by training to 17% and 7%, respectively. The accuracy of a test can be evaluated in relation to the achieved reproducibility. This reproducibility must then, for practical purposes, be judged as to its clinical acceptability and feasibility.

Outcome: the reference standard

Principles

Establishing a final and "gold standard" diagnosis of the target disorder is generally more invasive and expensive than applying the studied diagnostic test. It is exactly for this reason that good test accuracy (for example a very high sensitivity and specificity) would be very useful in clinical practice to make a satisfactory diagnostic assessment without having to perform the reference standard. However, in performing diagnostic research the central outcome variable – the presence or absence of the target disorder – must be measured, as it is the reference standard for estimating the test accuracy. A real gold – that is, perfect – standard test, with 100% sensitivity and specificity, is exceptional. Even histological classification and MRI imaging are not infallible, and may yield false positive, false negative and uninterpretable conclusions. Therefore, the term "reference standard" is nowadays considered better than "gold standard".

Box 3.4   The reference standard

Principles
- to be applied on all included subjects
- independent assessment of test and standard
- standardised protocol

Possible problems with the reference standard
- imperfect: classification errors
- pathophysiological concept not well defined (independent from clinical presentation)
- incorporation bias
- too invasive
- too complex

Possible solutions
- pragmatic criteria
- independent expert panel
- clinical follow up: delayed-type cross-sectional study
- tailormade standard protocol
- prognostic criterion

The reference standard to establish the final diagnosis (outcome) should be applied for all included subjects. Applying different standard procedures for different patients may yield an inconsistent reference for the evaluated test, as each of the "standards" will have its own idiosyncratic error rate.

The results of the test for each patient should be interpreted without knowledge of the reference standard results. Similarly, the reference standard result should be established without knowing the outcome of the test under study. Where such blinding is not maintained, "test review bias" and "diagnosis review bias" may occur: non-independent assessment of test and reference standard, mostly resulting in overestimation of test accuracy.

The reference standard must be properly performed and interpreted using standardised criteria. This is especially important when the standard diagnosis depends on subjective interpretations, for example by a psychiatrist, a pathologist, or a radiologist. In such cases inter- and even intraobserver variability in establishing the standard can occur. For example, in evaluating the intraobserver variability of MRI assessment as the standard for nerve root compression in sciatica patients, the same radiologist repeatedly scored the presence of root compression as such consistently (κ: 1.0) but the site of root compression only moderately (κ: 0.60).[14] In these situations, training sessions and permanent documentation of performance are important.

Problems and solutions

Apart from the limitations in reaching a 100% perfect standard diagnosis, meeting the requirements for a reference standard can be problematic in various ways.

For many conditions a reference standard cannot be measured on the basis of a well defined pathophysiological concept, independent of the clinical presentation. Examples are sinusitis, migraine, depression, irritable bowel syndrome, and benign prostatic hyperplasia. When, in such cases, information related to the test result (for example symptom status) is incorporated into the diagnostic criteria, "incorporation bias" may result in overestimation of test accuracy. Furthermore, a defined reference standard procedure may sometimes be too invasive for research purposes. For instance, when validating urinary flow measurement it would be unacceptable to apply invasive urodynamic studies to those with normal flow results.[15] And in studying the diagnostic value of non-acute abdominal pain in primary care for diagnosing intra-abdominal cancer, one cannot imagine that all patients presenting with non-acute abdominal pain would be routinely offered laparotomy.[16] In addition, one may doubt whether such laparotomy, if it were to be performed, could always provide an accurate final diagnosis in the very early stage of a malignancy. Another problem can be that a complex reference standard might include a large number of laboratory tests, so that many false positive test results could occur by chance.

For these problems, practical solutions have been sought.

Pragmatic criteria

The absence of a well defined pathophysiological concept can sometimes be overcome by defining consensus based pragmatic criteria. However, if applying such reference standard criteria (such as a cut-off value on a

49

depression questionnaire) is no more difficult than applying the test under study, evaluating and introducing the test will not be very useful.

Independent expert panel

Another method is the composition of an independent expert panel that, given general criteria and decision rules for clinical agreement, can assign a final diagnosis to each patient, based on the available clinical information. To achieve a reasonably consistent classification it is important that the panel is well prepared for its task, and a training session or pilot study using patients with an already established diagnosis is recommended. The agreement of the primary assessments of the individual panel members, prior to reaching to consensus, can be documented.

Clinical follow up: delayed-type cross-sectional study

When applying a definitive reference standard is too invasive or otherwise inapplicable at the very moment that the test should be predictive for the presence of the target disorder, a good alternative can be follow up of the clinical course during a suitable predefined period. Most diseases that are not self-limiting, such as cancers and chronic degenerative diseases, will usually become clinically manifest a period of months or a year or so after the first diagnostic suspicion (generally the moment of enrolment in the study) was raised. The follow up period should not be too short, in order to give early phase disorders the chance to become manifest and therefore to have a minimum number of "false negative" final diagnoses. Nor should it be too long, so as to avoid the final diagnosis after follow up being related to a new disease episode started after the baseline "cross-section" (false positives).[16,17] In addition, it would be ideal to collect the follow up data that are decisive for making the final diagnosis independently from and blinded to the health status and test results at time zero, and also to blind the final outcome assessment for these test results.

One should take into account that "confounding by indication" can occur: management decisions during follow up are possibly related to the health status at baseline, and might therefore influence the clinical course and the probability of detecting the target disorder. This is especially a point of concern in studying target disorders with a rather variable clinical course, becoming clinically manifest dependent on management decisions.

In contrast to what is commonly thought, it has to be acknowledged that the described method of clinical follow up should not be considered as a "follow up" or "cohort" study, as the focus is not on relating the time zero data to a subsequently developing (incident) disorder. In fact, the follow up procedure is aimed at retrospectively assessing the (prevalent) health status at time zero, as a substitute for establishing the reference standard diagnosis of the target disorder immediately at time zero itself. Therefore, this design modification can be designated a "delayed-type cross-sectional study", instead of a follow up study.[18]

The expert panel and the clinical follow up can be combined in a composite reference standard procedure, in which the outcome after follow up is evaluated and established by the panel.[15]

Tailormade standard protocol

In some situations, for example in diagnostic research on psychiatric illnesses, it might be difficult to separate test data at time zero (for example the presence of anxiety) from the information needed to make a final assessment (anxiety disorder). As mentioned earlier, in such situations incorporation bias may be the result. If test data are indeed an essential part of the diagnostic criteria, one cannot avoid balancing a certain risk of incorporation bias against not being able to perform diagnostic research at all, or making a final diagnosis while ignoring an important element of the criteria. Often, one can find a practical compromise in considering that for clinical purposes it is sufficient to know to what extent the available diagnostic tests at time zero are able to predict the target disorder's becoming clinically manifest during a reasonably chosen follow up period.[17] There is also the option to ask the expert panel to establish the final diagnosis first without the baseline test data, and then to repeat it with these data incorporated. This can be done while adding an extra blinding step, such as randomly rearranging the order of anonymised patient records. If there then appear to be important differences in the research conclusions, this should be transparently reported and discussed as to the clinical implications.

When it is impossible to meet the principle that the reference standard should be similarly applied to all study subjects irrespective of their health or test result status, "next best" solutions can be considered. For example, to determine the accuracy of the exercise electrocardiogram (ECG) in primary care settings, it might be considered medically and ethically unjustified to submit those with a negative test result to coronary angiography. For these test negatives a well standardised clinical follow up protocol (delayed-type cross-sectional study) might be acceptable. This option is particularly important when the focus is on exercise ECG in patients who have a relatively low prior probability of coronary heart disease. For this spectrum of patients, results of a study limited to those who would be clinically selected for coronary angiography would be clearly not applicable.[19–21] If one would still prefer an identical standard procedure for primary care patients, irrespective of previous test results, one could also consider submitting all patients to the clinical follow up standard procedure. In order to have some validation of this procedure, for the subgroup who had an angiography one can compare the standard diagnoses based on the follow up with the angiography results.

In summary, although a completely identical and "hard" reference standard for all included study subjects is the general methodological paradigm, this is not always achievable. In such situations, given the described limitations and the suggested alternative approaches, establishing a well documented and reproducible reference standard protocol – indicating the optimal procedure for each type of patient – may be not only the best one can get but also sufficient for clinical purposes.

Prognostic criterion

Diagnostic testing should ultimately be in favour of the patient's health, rather than just an assessment of the probability of the presence of disease. In view of this, the reference standard procedure can sometimes incorporate prognosis or consequences for clinical management.[22,23] It is then a starting point for further decision making (for example, whether treatment is useful or not) rather than a diagnostic endpoint. This is especially relevant in situations where an exhaustive nosological classification is less important, and when management is based primarily on the clinical assessment (for example in deciding about physiotherapy in low back pain, or referral to a neurosurgeon in sciatica[14]). Sometimes making a final diagnosis is less important than a prognosis, in view of the clinical consequences (incidental fever) or the lack of a solid diagnostic consensus (the pyriformis syndrome). In establishing a "prognostic reference criterion", a pitfall is that prognosis can be influenced by interfering treatments. In this context, methods for unbiased assessment of the impact of testing on patient prognosis are important (Chapter 4). It is to be expected that with the progress of DNA testing for disease, prognostic relevance will increasingly be the reference standard.

Standard shift as a result of new insights

At certain moments during the progress of pathophysiological knowledge on diagnosis, new diagnostic tests may be developed that are better than the currently prevailing reference standard. However, if this possibility is systematically ignored by reducing diagnostic accuracy research to just comparing new tests with traditional standards, possible new reference standards would never be recognised, as they would always seem less accurate than the traditional ones. Therefore, pathophysiological expertise should be involved in the evaluation of diagnostic accuracy. Examples of a shift in reference standard are the replacement of the clinical definition of tuberculosis by the identification of *Mycobacterium tuberculosis*, and of old imaging techniques by new ones (see also Chapter 1).

Specifying the study population

As in all clinical research, the study population for diagnostic research should be appropriately chosen, defined, and recruited. The selection of patients is crucial for the study outcome and its external (clinical) validity. For example, as has already been emphasised, it is widely recognised that diagnostic accuracy is very much dependent on the spectrum of included patients and the results of relevant tests performed earlier, and may differ for primary care patients and patients referred to a hospital.[6,7,21]

Given that the test has successfully passed Phase I and Phase II studies (Chapter 2), the starting point is the clinical problem for which the test under study should be evaluated as to its diagnostic accuracy, taking the relevant healthcare setting into account. For example, the study can address the diagnostic accuracy of clinical tests for sciatica in general practice, the accuracy of ECG recording in outpatients with palpitations without a compelling clinical reason for immediate referral, or the diagnostic accuracy of the MRI scan in diagnosing intracerebral pathology in an academic neurological centre. The study population should be representative for the "indicated", "candidate", or "intended" patient population, also called the target population, thereby being clinically similar to the group of patients in whom the validated test is to be applied in practice.[24,25] The "intention to diagnose" should be the key criterion for the study of presented clinical problems. For the evaluation of population screening of asymptomatic subjects, such as in the context of breast cancer screening or hypertension case finding, a study population similar to the target population "intended to be screened" is required.

Box 3.5 Study population

- In accordance with studied clinical problem
- "Intention to diagnose" or "intention to screen"
- Inclusion criteria corresponding with "indicated" population
- Consecutive series ("iatrotropic") or target population survey

---

The next step is generally straightforward: the specification of the relevant process of selection of patients for the study (preferably corresponding with the clinical problem and the healthcare setting requirements), and the relevant inclusion citeria (in accordance with the indicated population and the relevant patient spectrum). Exclusion criteria may also be defined, for example identifying those patients for whom the reference standard procedure is too risky or too burdensome. The importance of explicitly formulated entry criteria is demonstrated by a study on the diagnostic value of reported collapse for the diagnosis of clinically relevant arrhythmias in general practice: if the inclusion was based on presented symptoms the odds ratio (OR) was 1.9, whereas for an inclusion based on coincidentally finding a pulse < 60 or > 100 bpm or an irregular pulse, the OR was 10.1.[26] Investigators should include "indicated" patients as long as there is no compelling reason not to do so, in order that after the study a non-evidence-based testing practice will not be introduced or maintained for relevant parts of the "real life" patient spectrum. In this context it is emphasised that, for example in the elderly, comorbidity in addition to the possible presence of the target disorder is often an important aspect of clinical reality.[27] For the clinical applicability of the study measuring comorbidity and studying it as a modifier of diagnostic accuracy is the preferred approach, instead of excluding it.

In the section on study design we discussed the choice between population survey and disorder- or test-oriented subject selection, covering the principal starting point of patient recruitment. In addition, the pros and cons of the various options for practical patient recruitment should be considered. When problems presented to clinicians are studied, recruiting (a random sample of) a series of consecutively presenting patients who meet the criteria of the indicated population is most sensible for clinical validity purposes. This should preferably be supported by a description of the patient flow in health care prior to presentation. Sometimes, however, it may take too long to await the enrolment of a sufficiently large consecutive series – for example when the clinical problem or target disorder is very rare, or when a useful contribution to rapidly progressing diagnostic knowledge can only be made within a limited period. In such situations, active surveys of the target population or sampling from a patient register can be alternatives. However, it should be borne in mind that such methods may yield a population of study subjects with a different clinical spectrum. Also, for such subjects the indication to test is less clear than for patients who experienced an "iatrotropic" stimulus[2] to visit a doctor at the very moment that they want their health problem to be solved.

Of course, for validating test procedures to be used in population screening, an active survey of a study population similar to the target population is the best approach.

In order to enhance external validity, it is essential to add key demographic and clinical characteristics of the identified study population, and to evaluate non-response in relation to these characteristics. Furthermore, all important steps in the study protocol, with data on specific subgroups, including subgroup non-response, should be documented. This can be supported by a flow diagram.

54

Adverse effects of test and reference standard

Apart from its accuracy, the performance of a test has to be evaluated as to its (dis)comfort to both patient and doctor. In particular, a test should be minimally invasive and have a minimal risk of adverse effects and serious complications. Measuring these aspects in the context of a diagnostic accuracy study can add to the comparison with other tests as to their clinical pros and cons.

For the research community, it is also important to learn about the invasiveness and risks of the reference standard used. For example, if in the evaluation of the positive test results of Haemoccult screening colonoscopy, sigmoidoscopy or double contrast barium enema were to be used, one might expect complications (perforation or haemorrhage) once in 300–900 subjects investigated.[28] Researchers can use the experience reported by colleagues studying similar problems, in order to make an optimal choice of reference standard procedure, taking possible adverse events into consideration.

Statistical aspects

Box 3.6   Statistical aspects

- Sample size
- Bivariate and multivariable analysis
- Test accuracy or prediction of outcome
- Single test; comparing tests or strategies; additional testing
- Difference between diagnostic and aetiologic data analysis

In the planning phase of the study the required sample size should be considered. To evaluate the relationship between a dichotomous test and the presence of a disorder, one can use the usual programs for sample size estimation. For example, for a case–referent study with equal group sizes, accepting certain values for type I and type II errors (for example 0.05 and 0.20, respectively) and using two-sided testing, one can calculate the number of subjects needed per group to detect a minimum sensitivity (proportion of test positives among the diseased, for example at least 0.60) assuming a certain maximum proportion of test positives among non-diseased (for example 0.20, implying a specificity of at least 0.80). For the example above the calculation using the program EPI-Info[29] would yield a required number of 27 cases and 27 referents. Of course, when performing a cross-sectional study prospectively in a consecutive series with a low expected prevalence of the target disorder (unequal group sizes), the required sample will be much higher. Also, if a number of determinants is simultaneously included in the analysis, the required sample size is higher: as a rule of thumb, for each determinant at least 10 subjects with the target disorder are needed.[30]

Data analysis in diagnostic research follows the general lines of that in clinical epidemiological research. For single tests the first step is a Bivariate analysis focused on one predictive variable only, for example in a 2×2 table in the case of a dichotomous test. It is possible to stratify for modifiers of accuracy, thereby distinguishing relevant clinical subgroups, and to adjust for potential confounding variables. Point estimates and confidence intervals for the measures of diagnostic accuracy can be determined. Subsequently, there are various options for multivariable analysis, taking the influence of multiple independent variables into account simultaneously. Multiple logistic regression is especially useful for analysing accuracy data.[12,13] These data analytical challenges in diagnostic research are discussed in detail in Chapter 7.

It is important to distinguish the analytical approach focusing on the accuracy of individual tests from the analysis where an optimal prediction of the presence of the studied disorder in patients is at stake. In the first, the dependent variable may even be test accuracy itself, as a function of various determinants. In the latter, a diagnostic prediction model can be derived with disease probability as the dependent variable, and with various tests, demographic, and clinical covariables as independent variables.[18,31]

When a number of tests are applied there are various analytical options. First, the accuracy of all tests can be determined and compared. Furthermore, using multivariate analysis such as multiple logistic regression, the combined predictive power of sets of test variables can be determined. Moreover, starting from the least invasive and most easily available test (such as history taking), it can be evaluated whether adding more invasive or more expensive tests contributes to the diagnosis. For example, the subsequent contributions of history, physical examination, laboratory testing, and more elaborate additional investigations can be analysed, supported by displaying the ROC curves (with areas under the curve) of the respectively extended test sets (see Chapter 7).[8,26]

It must be acknowledged that data analysis in diagnostic research is essentially different from aetiologic data analysis. The principal difference is that aetiologic analysis usually focuses on the effect of a hypothesised aetiologic factor adjusted for the influence of possible confounders, thereby aiming at a causal interpretation. In diagnostic research the focus is on identifying the best correlates of the target disorder irrespective of any causal interpretations. It is sufficient if these correlates (tests) can be systematically and reproducibly used for diagnostic prediction. Whereas in aetiologic analysis there is a natural hierarchical relation between the possible aetiologic factor of interest and the covariables to be adjusted for, such a hierarchy is absent for the possible predictors in diagnostic research. This implies that diagnostic data analysis can be more pragmatic, seeking for the best correlates.

External validation

Analyses of diagnostic accuracy in the collected data set, especially the results of multivariable analyses, may produce too optimistic results that may not be reproducible in clinical practice or similar study populations.[32] Therefore, it is advisable to perform one or more separate external validation studies in independent but clinically similar populations.

Box 3.7   External (clinical) validation

- Results based on study data may be too optimistic
- "Split-half" analysis is no external validation
- Repeated studies in other, similar populations are preferred
- First exploration: compare first included half with second half
- Role of systematic reviews and meta-analysis

Sometimes authors derive a diagnostic model in a random half of the research data set and test its performance in the other half (split-half analysis). This approach is not addressing the issue of external validation: in fact, it only evaluates the degree of random error at the cost of possibly increasing such error by reducing the available sample size by 50%.[18] Also, other methods using one and the same database do not provide a real external validation. An exploratory approximation, however, could be to compare the performance of the diagnostic model in the chronologically first enrolled half of the patients, with that in the second half. The justification is that the second half is not a random sample of the total, but rather a subsequent clinically similar study population. However, totally independent studies in other, clinically similar settings will be more convincing. In fact, over time, various studies can be done in comparable settings, enabling diagnostic systematic reviews and meta-analyses to be performed. This may yield a constantly increasing insight into the performance of the studied diagnostic test, both in general and in relevant clinical subgroups (Chapter 8).

References

1 van den Akker M, Buntinx F, Metsemakers JF, Roos S, Knottnerus JA. Multimorbidity in general practice: prevalence, incidence, and determinants of co-occurring chronic and recurrent diseases. *J Clin Epidemiol* 1998;**51**:367–75.

2 Feinstein AR. *Clinical Epidemiology. The architecture of clinical research.* Philadelphia: WB Saunders, 1985.

3 Sackett DL, Haynes RB, Guyatt GH, Tugwell P. *Clinical epidemiology. A basic science for clinical medicine.* Boston: Little, Brown and Company, 1991.

4 Lijmer JG, Mol BW, Heisterkamp S *et al.* Empirical evidence of design-related bias in studies of diagnostic tests. *JAMA* 1999;**282**:1061–6.

5 Moons KGM, van Es GA, Deckers JW, Habbema JDF, Grobbee DE. Limitations of sensitivity, specificity, likelihood ratio, and Bayes's theorem in assessing diagnostic probabilities: a clinical example. *Epidemiology* 1997;**8**:12–17.

6 Ransohoff DF, Feinstein AR. Problems of spectrum and bias in evaluating the efficacy of diagnostic tests. *N Engl J Med* 1978;**299**:926–30.

7 Knottnerus JA, Leffers P. The influence of referral patterns on the characteristics of diagnostic tests. *J Clin Epidemiol* 1992;**45**:1143–54.

8 Stoffers HEJH. *Peripheral arterial occlusive disease. Prevalence and diagnostic management in general practice.* Thesis. Maastricht: Datawyse, 1995.

9 Dinant GJ, Knottnerus JA, van Aubel PGJ, van Wersch JWJ. Reliability of the erythrocyte sedimentation rate in general practice. *Scand J Prim Health Care* 1989;**7**:231–5.

10 Knottnerus JA, Knipschild PG, van Wersch JWJ, Sijstermanns AHJ. Unexplained fatigue and hemoglobin, a primary care study. *Can Fam Phys* 1986;**32**:1601–4.

11 Miettinen OS. *Theoretical Epidemiology. Principles of occurrence research in medicine.* New York: John Wiley & Sons, 1985.

12 Spiegelhalter DJ, Knill-Jones RD. Statistical and knowledge-based approaches to clinical decision support systems, with an application to gastroenterology. *J Roy Stat Soc* Ser A 1984;**147**:35–76.

13 Knottnerus JA. Application of logistic regression to the analysis of diagnostic data: exact modeling of a probability tree of multiple binary variables. *Med Decision Making* 1992;**12**:93–108.

14 Vroomen PCAJ. *The diagnosis and conservative treatment of sciatica.* Maastricht: Datawyse, 1998.

15 Wolfs GGMC. *Obstructive micturition problems in elderly males, prevalence and diagnosis in general practice.* Maastricht: Datawyse, 1997.

16 Muris JW, Starmans R. *Non acute abdominal complaints. Diagnostic studies in general practice and outpatient clinic.* Thesis. Maastricht, 1993.

17 Warndorff DK, Knottnerus JA, Huijnen LG, Starmans R. How well do general practitioners manage dyspepsia? *J Roy Coll Gen Pract* 1989;**39**:499–502.

18 Knottnerus JA. Diagnostic prediction rules: principles, requirements and pitfalls. *Primary Care* 1995;**22**:341–63.

19 Green MS. The effect of validation group bias on screening tests for coronary artery disease. *Stat Med* 1985;**4**:53–61.

20 Knottnerus JA. The effects of disease verification and referral on the relationship between symptoms and diseases. *Med Decision Making* 1987;**7**:139–48.

21 Begg CB, Greenes RA. Assessment of diagnostic tests when disease verification is subject to selection bias. *Biometrics* 1983;**39**:207–16.

22 Hunink MG. Outcome research and cost-effectiveness analysis in radiology. *Eur Radiol* 1996;**6**:615–20.

23 Moons KGM. *Diagnostic research: theory and application.* Thesis. Rotterdam 1996.

24 Dinant GJ. *Diagnostic value of the erythrocyte sedimentation rate in general practice.* Thesis. Maastricht, 1991.

25 van der Schouw YT, Verbeek AL, Ruijs SH. Guidelines for the assessment of new diagnostic tests. *Invest Radiol* 1995;**30**:334–40.

26 Zwietering P. *Arrhythmias in general practice, prevalence and clinical diagnosis.* Maastricht: Datawyse, 2000.

27 Schellevis FG, van der Velden J, van de Lisdonk E, van Eijk JT, van Weel C. Comorbidity of chronic diseases in general practice. *J Clin Epidemiol* 1993;**46**:469–73.

28 Towler BP, Irwig L, Glasziou P, Weller D, Kewenter J. *Screening for colorectal cancer using the faecal occult blood test, hemoccult.* Cochrane Database Syst Rev 2000;(2):CD001216.

29 Dean AG. *The Epi Info Manual.* Brixton Books, 1996.

30 Harrell FE Jr, Lee KL, Mark DB. Multivariable prognostic models: issues in developing models, evaluating assumptions and adequacy, and measuring and reducing errors. *Stat Med* 1996;**15**:361–87.

31 Laupacis A, Sekar N, Stiell IG. Clinical prediction rules. A review and suggested modifications of methodological standards. *JAMA* 1997;**277**:488–94.

32 Starmans R, Muris JW, Fijten GH, Schouten HJ, Pop P, Knottnerus JA. The diagnostic value of scoring models for organic and non-organic gastrointestinal disease, including the irritable-bowel syndrome. *Med Decision Making* 1994;**14**:208–16.

4 Diagnostic testing and prognosis: the randomised controlled trial in diagnostic research

JEROEN G LIJMER, PATRICK M BOSSUYT

Summary box

- From the patient's perspective the contribution of diagnostic tests to a better health outcome is of primary importance, rather than their correspondence with the "truth".
- Diagnostic test evaluations should therefore focus on the likelihood that tests detect clinical events of interest and the effect that tests can have on those events by way in which the results affect subsequent management decisions.
- Randomised controlled trials of diagnostic tests are feasible, and several designs are possible.
- Each trial design option has its own advantages and disadvantages. Depending on the clinical problem under study, the type of information needed, and the costs of tests or follow up, one design can be preferred over another.
- Whereas in most randomised controlled trials of diagnostic tests so far the point of randomisation coincided with the clinical decision as to whether or not to perform the test, the trial design can be made more efficient by randomising only patients with the test result of interest.
- The randomised trial design can be elaborated both for evaluating the (additional) prognostic value of a single test, and for comparing different test strategies.

- A randomised controlled trial of diagnostic tests should incorporate a prespecified link between test and treatment options to ascertain validity and generalisability.
- Methods to preserve allocation concealment and blinding deserve special attention.
- Sample size calculations need special attention, and must include an estimation of the discordance rate.

Why bother about the prognostic impact of a diagnostic test?

For scientific purposes it is worth knowing whether or not a result from a medical test corresponds to the truth. Can this value be trusted? Is this truly a sign of disease? These are the first questions that come to the mind in the evaluation of medical tests.

From a patient perspective, mere knowledge about the present, true state of things is in most cases not enough. In relieving health problems, information in itself will not suffice. Patients will only benefit from diagnostic tests if the information generated by those tests is correctly used in subsequent decisions on action to restore or maintain the patient's health.

There are several ways in which medical tests can affect a patient's health. First, undergoing the test itself can have an impact. The adverse effects range from slight discomfort and temporary unpleasantness to lasting side effects or death. On the other hand, undergoing an elaborate procedure can also have a non-specific positive effect on patient complaints, regardless of the information that results from it. This can be called the "placebo" effect of testing, and we know very little about its magnitude and modifying factors.

In addition to the effects of the diagnostic procedure itself, the information generated by the test also influences patients. Information on the likely cause of one's health problems or other aspects of health status can have both a positive and a negative effect, albeit limited. As patients, we want to be informed about the origin of our complaints, even in the absence of a cure. Such information may enable us to find better ways of handling them, by developing strategies to limit their disabling impact on our daily activities.

In these cases it is not just the present state of health that is of interest, but also the future course of disease. It follows, then, that the value of information from diagnostic tests lies not only in the past (where did this come from?) or the present (how is it?), but also in the future. Hence, the relevance of diagnostic information is closely related to prognosis: the implications for the future course of the patient's condition.

The first section of this chapter discusses the evaluation of a single test, starting from an evaluation of its prognostic value and then moving on to the consequences for treatment. It closes with a presentation of randomised designs for evaluating test–treatment combinations. The second section contains an elaboration of the methods for comparing and evaluating multiple test strategies, also including randomised clinical trials. The chapter ends with a discussion on practical issues.

How to measure the prognostic impact of a test

A recent example of the assessment of the prognostic value of a test can be found in the literature on the management of carotid disease. Several studies have examined the need to perform duplex ultrasonography in patients with a cervical bruit without further symptoms of cerebrovascular disease. To answer this question, an assessment has to be made of the value of duplex ultrasonography. Such an evaluation will often look at the amount of agreement between the index test (duplex ultrasonography) and the reference test (the best available method to reveal the true condition of the carotid arteries). In this case, the reference test will mostly likely be conventional angiography. If properly conducted, a 2×2 table can be constructed after the study is done and all indicators of diagnostic accuracy can be calculated. Unfortunately, many of the evaluation studies in diagnostic techniques for carotid stenosis performed so far did not meet the design requirements for an unbiased and useful evaluation.[1]

From a patient perspective, one could successfully argue that it is not so much the correspondence with the "truth" that should be of concern, especially not in asymptomatic patients. For these patients, the true value of the information should come from the strength of the association between data on the presence and severity of carotid stenosis and the likelihood of vascular events in the near future. The appropriate reference standard for such an evaluation will not be a diagnostic procedure. Instead, one should look for clinical information collected through a meticulous follow up of all patients subjected to the index test.

Figure 4.1 illustrates the general design of such a study. All patients with cervical bruits without previous cerebrovascular disease are eligible for the

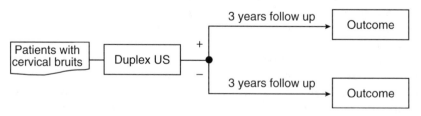

Figure 4.1 Prognostic study.

Table 4.1 Prognostic value of duplex ultrasonography.

	Poor outcome	Favourable outcome	
Stenosis ≥ 80%	63 (47%)	72 (53%)	135
Stenosis < 80%	113 (20%)	451 (80%)	564
Total	176	523	699

study. A duplex ultrasonogram of the right and left common and internal carotid arteries is performed in all patients and the percentage of stenosis measured. Ideally, none of the patients receives treatment. Subsequently patients are followed by regular outpatient visits and telephone interviews. The following clinical indicators of poor outcome are recorded: TIA (transient ischaemic attack), stroke, myocardial infarction, unstable angina, vascular deaths, and other deaths.

With data recorded in such a study standard diagnostic accuracy measures can be calculated to express the prognostic value of a test. Table 4.1, based on data published by Lewis et al.,[2] shows positive and negative predictive values of 47% and 80%, respectively, in predicting a poor outcome for a stenosis ≥ 80%, as detected on duplex ultrasound. The data also showed that the relative risk of a stenosis ≥ 50% for a TIA or stroke was 2.3. However, insufficient data were presented to reconstruct the 2 × 2 table for this cut-off point.

The study in Figure 4.1 can provide an answer to the question whether or not a test is able to discriminate between different risk categories for a specific event. Such prognostic information, although of value to patients and healthcare professionals, does not answer the question as to whether there is an intervention that can improve the prognosis of these patients. To respond to this it is necessary to compare the prognosis for different treatment strategies.

Randomised designs for a single test

A slight modification of the design in Figure 4.1 allows us to measure the prognostic value of a test within the context of subsequent clinical decision making. Instead of treating all patients identically one can randomly allocate them to one of the two treatment strategies, establishing the prognostic value of the test in each arm in a way that is similar to the previous example.

A straightforward comparison of patient outcome in the two treatment arms provides an answer as to which treatment is the most effective for all patients included in the trial. Moreover, an analysis stratified by test result offers the possibility of comparing the effectiveness of the treatment options for groups with identical test results.

This type of design and analysis can be illustrated with another example from the field of cerebrovascular disease. In the management of acute stroke the role of intravenous anticoagulation and duplex ultrasonography of the carotid arteries is unclear. A large trial has been performed with as its primary objective the documentation of the efficacy of unfractionated heparin in the treatment of acute stroke. A secondary objective was an evaluation of the role of duplex ultrasonography in selecting patients for anticoagulation.[3,4] A simplified version of the design of this trial is outlined in Figure 4.2. Patients with evidence of an ischaemic stroke, with symptoms present for more than 1 hour but less than 24 hours, were eligible for the study. A duplex ultrasonogram of the right and left common and internal carotid arteries was performed in all included patients. Subsequently, patients were randomised to treatment with unfractionated heparin or placebo, and followed for 3 months. A favourable outcome after stroke was defined as a score of I or II on the Glasgow Coma Scale and a score of 12–20 on the modified Barthel Index.

Tables 4.2(a) and (b) shows the prognostic value of Duplex ultra-sonography in each trial arm. An odds ratio can be calculated for each table. These odds ratios can be interpreted as measures of the *natural prognostic value* (Table 4.2(b)) and the *prognostic value with intervention* (Table 4.2(a)), respectively. Another presentation of the same data gives us Tables 4.2(c) and (d), which provide us with information on the treatment effect in both test result categories. We will call the odds ratios of the latter two tables *treatment effect in test normals* (Table 4.2(d)) and *treatment effect in test abnormals* (Table 4.2(c)). When the test discriminates well between patients that benefit from treatment and those that do not, the treatment effect in test abnormals will differ from that in test normals. The ratio of the odds ratios of Tables 4.2(c) and 4.2(d) can therefore be used as a measure of the prognostic impact of the test.

The study in Figure 4.2 provides information on the treatment effect in all test result categories. In practice, it will not always be necessary or ethical to randomise all patients, as uncertainty may exist only for patients with a specific – say, abnormal – test result. This will be the case when there is information available that the prognosis for normal test results is good and

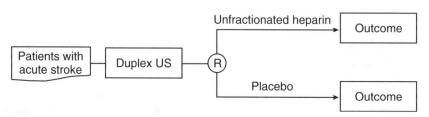

Figure 4.2 Basic RCT of a single diagnostic test.

Table 4.2 Analysis of an RCT of a single diagnostic test.

(a) Unfractionated heparin

	Poor outcome	Favourable outcome	
Stenosis ≥50%	38 (32%)	82 (68%)	120
Stenosis <50%	121 (23%)	400 (77%)	521
Total	159	482	641

(b) Placebo

	Poor outcome	Favourable outcome	
Stenosis ≥50%	51 (47%)	58 (53%)	109
Stenosis <50%	116 (22%)	409 (78%)	525
Total	167	467	634

(c) Stenosis larger than 50% or occlusion

	Poor outcome	Favourable outcome	
Unfract. heparin	38 (32%)	82 (68%)	120
Placebo	51 (47%)	58 (53%)	109
Total	89	140	229

(d) Stenosis smaller than 50%

	Poor outcome	Favourable outcome	
Unfract. heparin	121 (23%)	400 (77%)	521
Placebo	116 (22%)	409 (78%)	525
Total	237	809	1046

(e) Comparison of strategies

	Poor outcome	Favourable outcome	
Duplex US	154 (24%)	491 (76%)	645
No duplex US	167 (26%)	467 (74%)	634
Total	321	958	1279

Duplex US in (e): Decision whether or not to give UFH is based on duplex ultrasonography. The odds ratios and their 95% CI of (a) to (e) are: 1.5 (0.99–2.4), 3.1 (2.0–4.8), 0.53 (0.31–0.90), 1.1 (0.80–1.4), and 0.88 (0.68–1.1). The relative odds ratio of (a)/(b) or (c)/(d) is 0.48.

that patients with such results need no intervention. A logical translation of such a question into a study design would be to randomise only patients with abnormal test results between the different treatment options.

Consider the first example of duplex ultrasonography in patients with cervical bruits. Such a trial could provide evidence that the natural history of patients with a stenosis of less than 50% has a good prognosis. The trial outlined in Figure 4.3 can subsequently answer the question as to whether therapy can improve the prognosis of patients with a stenosis of 50% or more. As in the first example, all patients with cervical bruits without previous cerebrovascular disease are eligible for the study. A duplex ultrasonography of the right and left common and internal carotid arteries is performed in all patients to measure the percentage of stenosis. Subsequently, if the stenosis is 50% or more patients are randomly assigned to receive either aspirin 325 mg a day or placebo. The clinical endpoints – TIA, stroke, myocardial infarction, unstable angina, vascular deaths, and other deaths – are recorded during follow up.

Cote and colleagues performed such a trial in 1995.[5] They randomised 372 neurologically asymptomatic patients with a carotid stenosis of 50% or more between aspirin and placebo. By comparing the outcomes in both treatment arms the effectiveness of treating patients with a stenosis of 50% or more with aspirin was evaluated (treatment effect in test abnormals). In 50 of the 188 patients receiving aspirin and 54 of the 184 receiving placebo a clinical event was measured during follow up, yielding an adjusted hazard ratio (aspirin versus placebo) of 0.99 (95% CI, 0.67–1.46). The authors concluded that aspirin did not have a significant long term protective effect in asymptomatic patients with high grade stenosis (more than 50%).

The trial in Figure 4.3 can also provide information on the accuracy of duplex US in predicting the outcomes of interest (natural prognostic value). This can be done by comparing the outcome in patients in the placebo arm, who all had an abnormal test result, with the outcome in those with a normal test result. A prerequisite for this comparison is that patient management in both of these arms is similar. Table 4.3(a) and (b) shows the crude results and possible comparisons. Note that to calculate the diagnostic accuracy of duplex US it is necessary to correct for the sampling rate of patients with high grade stenosis.[6]

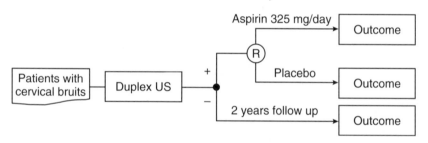

Figure 4.3 Randomising abnormal test results.

Table 4.3 Analysis of an RCT, randomising only abnormal test results

(a) Natural prognostic value	Poor outcome	Favourable outcome		(b) Treatment effect in case of ≥ 50% stenosis	Poor outcome	Favourable outcome	
Stenosis ≥50%*	130 (71%)	54 (29%)	184	Aspirin	138 (73%)	50 (27%)	188
Stenosis <50%	255 (78%)	72 (22%)	327	Placebo	130 (71%)	54 (29%)	184
Total	385	126	511	Total	268	104	372

*Random sample of patients with a stenosis ≥50%.

Alternative randomised designs

An alternative to the design in Figure 4.3 would be to move the point of randomisation back in time to the point where the test results are not yet known. This comes down to the randomisation of all patients to either disclosure or non-disclosure of the test results.

The latter design was used to evaluate Doppler ultrasonography of the umbilical artery in the management of women with intrauterine growth retardation (IUGR).[7] A total of 150 pregnant women with IUGR underwent Doppler ultrasonography and were subsequently randomised to disclosure or non-disclosure of the test results (Figure 4.4(a)). In the group in which the results of the test were revealed, women were hospitalised in case of abnormal flow and discharged with outpatient management in case of normal flow. In the non-disclosure group all patients received the conventional strategy for women with IUGR, of hospitalisation regardless of their test results. The trial compared perinatal outcome, neurological development and postnatal growth between the two strategies. The trial design, depicted in Figure 4.4(a), allows us to determine the natural prognostic value and the treatment effect in test abnormals. Unfortunately the authors did not report sufficient data to reconstruct the necessary 2×2 tables.

One could move the point of randomisation further back in time, to the decision whether or not to perform the test. A translation of this

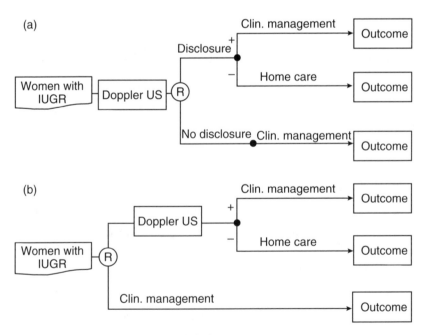

Figure 4.4 Alternative randomised designs.

comparison for the Doppler US in IUGR is the RCT in Figure 4.4(b). Women in whom IUGR has been diagnosed are randomly allocated to two strategies. The first consists of applying the test of interest, Doppler ultrasonography, in all women with IUGR. In case of abnormal flow a patient is hospitalised. In case of normal flow they are discharged with outpatient management. In the second strategy all women with IUGR are hospitalised. Subsequently, neonatal outcome is observed in each trial arm. A comparison of the outcomes in the two arms offers a measure of the effectiveness of using Doppler ultrasonography in making decisions on hospitalisation. Such a design evaluates both the test and the treatment effect; it is, however, not possible to distinguish the treatment effect from the prognostic value of the test.

Similar outcomes in both arms will be observed if there is no difference in outcome with either home care or clinical management in all patients satisfying the inclusion criteria for this trial. Differences in outcome are not necessarily attributed to the test. In case of a wrong choice of treatment, the outcome of the Doppler ultrasonography arm can turn out to be inferior to the conventional strategy, no matter how good or reliable the test actually is. This same line of reasoning can also be applied in case of a superior outcome in the Doppler arm. If there is a (sub)group of patients that is better off with home care, then the expected outcome in the Doppler ultrasonography group will always be superior, regardless of the intrinsic quality or accuracy of the test.

These examples demonstrate that it is not possible to make conclusions on the prognostic impact of the test itself using the design in figure 4(b), as long as it remains unclear to what degree results of such a trial depend on the new treatment, on accurate selection through the test, or both.

How to compare test strategies

In many clinical situations there are multiple tests available to examine the presence of the target condition. When one wishes to compare two competing tests the first three designs introduced earlier for the evaluation of a single test have to be adapted slightly.

To compare the prognostic value of two tests, a straightforward translation of Figure 4.1 is to perform both tests in all patients and to monitor the outcome of interest during a follow up period. Such a design is outlined in Figure 4.5(a). The data from such a study can be used to calculate and compare the prognostic value of each test, using conventional measures of diagnostic accuracy. One can also analyse the data by stratifying the results according to the possible test combinations. With two dichotomous tests this will result in a 4×2 table (Table 4.4). Note that each possible combination of results on test A and test B is treated as a separate test result category, analogously to a single test with four possible result categories. Subsequently, the predictive value or the likelihood ratio of each result category can be calculated as a measure of prognostic value.[8]

To examine both tests in the context of subsequent clinical decision making, it is possible to randomise all patients between two treatment

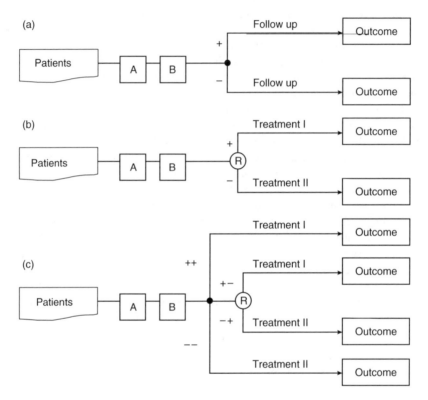

Figure 4.5 Designs to compare diagnostic strategies.

Table 4.4 A 4 × 2 table of the results of two dichotomous tests.

		Outcome	
A	B	+	−
+	+		
+	−		
−	+		
−	−		
Total			

strategies, similar to the design in Figure 4.2, regardless of their test results. Figure 4.5(b) shows an example of such a design: both tests are performed and all patients are randomly allocated to one of the two treatment options. This allows one to explore the prognostic value of both tests in each treatment arm. In addition, the data from such a trial can be used to find the most effective treatment for all patients included in the trial. If statistical power allows it, subgroup analysis of the treatment effect in the four possible test result categories offers the possibility of identifying the most effective treatment option for patients in the respective categories.

Although the previous design allows for many different explorations, only some are relevant from a clinical perspective. When two tests are compared, one of them is often already used in clinical practice and decisions on subsequent management are made based on this test. Let us assume that, in clinical practice, test positive patients are treated and test negative patients are not. If future decisions are to be made under the guidance of the new test, patients who are positive on the new test will be treated and those who are negative will not. This means that the only patients that will be managed differently are the ones who are test positive on the existing test but negative on the new one, and those who are test negative on the existing test but positive on the new one.

As patients with concordant test results ($++$ or $--$) will receive the same management, it is unnecessary and in some circumstances even unethical to examine the treatment effect in these two subgroups. If a new test (B) is then examined with the goal of substituting the old, possibly more invasive, and/or costly test (A), the design in Figure 4.5(c), randomising only the discordant test results, is more efficient. Subsequently, the treatment effect and the predictive values of the discordant result categories (A+B− and A−B+) can be examined (see Table 4.5(a–d)).

By transposing these tables it is possible to examine the effect of a clinical pathway based on test A or test B for patients with discordant test results (Tables 4.5(e) to 4.5(f)). The difference in poor outcome rate between these two tables, after correcting for the frequency of discordant results, is equal to the absolute risk difference of a clinical pathway based on test A compared to a pathway based on test B. To calculate the relative risk or the total risk of each strategy separately it is necessary to have information on the clinical event rate in each concordant group.

An alternative design, using the random disclosure principle, is outlined in Figure 4.6(a). Both test A and test B are performed in all patients. Subsequently, patients are randomised between a clinical pathway based on test A without disclosing the results of test B, and a pathway based on test B with non-disclosure of the results of test A. The same measures and tables can be obtained from such a design as discussed for the design in Figure 4.5.

In some situations one might wish to let the point of randomisation coincide with that of the clinical decision to choose either test A or test B and

Table 4.5 Analysis of an RCT of two tests randomising only discordant results.

(a) Treatment effect A+B−					(b) Treatment effect A−B+			
A+	B−	Poor outcome	Favourable outcome		A−	B+	Poor outcome	Favourable outcome
Treatment I					Treatment I			
Treatment II					Treatment II			
Total					Total			

(c) Treatment					(d) No treatment			
A	B	Poor outcome	Favourable outcome		A	B	Poor outcome	Favourable outcome
+	−				+	−		
−	+				−	+		
Total								

(e) Strategy based on A					(f) Strategy based on B			
A	B	Poor outcome	Favourable outcome		A	B	Poor outcome	Favourable outcome
+	−				+	−		
−	+				−	+		
Total								

act on the respective results. A recent trial used this design to study two different diagnostic approaches for the management of outpatients with dysphagia.[9] Patients with dysphagia are at risk for aspiration pneumonia. A modified barium swallow test (MBS) and flexible endoscopic evaluation of swallowing with sensory testing (FEESST) are supposed to distinguish patients who can benefit from behavioural and dietary management from those who will need a percutaneous endoscopic gastrostomy (PEG) tube. For the discussion we consider a simplified design as outlined in Figure 4.6(b). Outpatients presenting with dysphagia were randomly allocated to either a strategy using MBS or a strategy using FEESST to guide subsequent management. During 1 year of follow up the occurrence of pneumonia was recorded in both trial arms. There were six cases of pneumonia in the 50 (12%) patients allocated to the FEESST strategy and 14 in the 76 (18%) patients allocated to the MBS strategy. The absolute risk difference was not significantly different from zero (risk difference 6%; 95% CI −6% to 19%). As no patient received both tests it is not possible to distinguish the

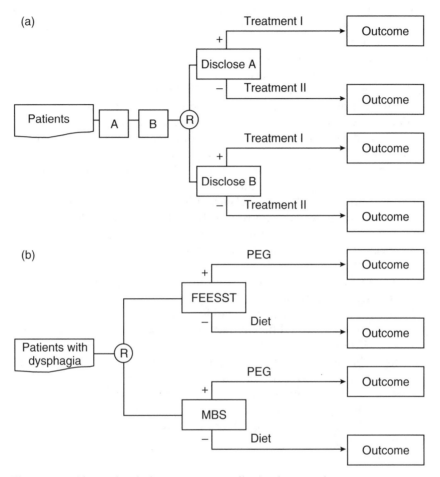

Figure 4.6 Alternative designs to compare diagnostic strategies.

treatment effect from the prognostic value of the tests, nor is it possible to compare the outcome in the subgroups with discordant test results.

Often a new test is introduced to complement rather than to replace existing tests. One example is where the new test is to be added to the diagnostic pathway before an older test as a triage instrument. Patients with a particular test result (say, negative) on the new test will not be subjected to the existing test. Alternatively, the new test is added after the existing test, making further refinement in diagnosis or treatment decisions possible. We refer to these two options as pre- and postaddition.

If a test is added at the end of a diagnostic work up to further classify disease (postaddition) all the designs presented in Figures 4.2 to 4.4 for the single test evaluation can be used to evaluate this new classification. For example, to evaluate the prognostic impact of a genetic test for the classification of women with breast cancer in two different subgroups, one could use a design similar to the one in Figure 4.3. Women suspected of breast cancer are evaluated with the conventional diagnostic work up. Subsequently, only women with breast cancer are eligible for the trial. In all these women genetic tests are performed. Depending on the results, they are subsequently randomised between two types of treatment.

When the goal of a new test is to limit the number of people undergoing the classic diagnostic work up (triage or preaddition), the designs in Figures 4.5(b)–(c) and 4.6(a) can be used to evaluate the prognostic impact of such a strategy. Using the principle that only patients with test results that will actually account for the difference are randomised, one could also adapt the design of Figure 4.5(b), randomising only patients with the pair of discordant test results that will be treated differently if the new strategy is adopted. Another option is shown in Figure 4.7(a). As the difference between the two strategies comes from the group of patients who are not selected for the classic diagnostic work up, one can randomise only these patients to either the classic work up and treatment, or management based on the results of the new test.

Many studies to evaluate the preaddition of a test have randomised all patients between the two different diagnostic work ups.[10,11] One such study evaluated *Helicobacter pylori* serology as a way to reduce the number of patients subjected to endoscopy. Lassen et al.[10] performed the trial outlined in Figure 4.7(b). Patients presenting in primary care with dyspepsia were randomly assigned to either *H. pylori* and eradication therapy or prompt endoscopy. In case of a negative *H. pylori* test patients were still subjected to endoscopy. During a 1 year follow up the symptoms were recorded on a Likert scale.

Choice of design

Each of the designs discussed in Figures 4.1 to 4.7 has its own advantages and disadvantages. Depending on the clinical problem one wishes to answer, the type of information needed, and the costs of tests or follow up, one design can be preferred over another.

The outlines in Figures 4.2 to 4.4 can be used to evaluate a strategy with a new test compared to a classic strategy without such a test. In case of postaddition the classic strategy will consist of the classic diagnostic work up and treatment. In case of a substitution problem, any of the trial designs outlined in Figures 4.5(b) to 4.6(b) can provide an answer. The designs outlined in Figures 4.5(b), 4.6(a), 4.7(a), and 4.7(b) can provide an answer in case of a preaddition problem.

Table 4.6 gives an overview of the information that can be deduced from the different designs. The designs in Figures 4.2 and 4.5(b), testing all

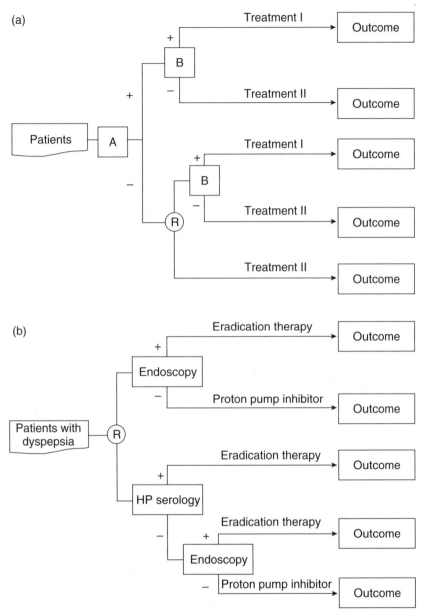

Figure 4.7 Designs to evaluate preaddition.

patients and randomising all between two treatment strategies, provide the most information. In addition to data on the effects of the two evaluated strategies, they provide information on the treatment effect and prognostic value of all possible test result categories. Yet these designs are not always

Table 4.6 Possible analyses of each randomised design.

Figure	1, 5(a)	2	3, 4(a)	5(b)	5(c) 6(a)	4(b) 6(b) 7(a) 7(b)
Natural prognostic value	×	×	×	×		
Prognostic value under intervention		×		×		
Treatment effect test abnormals		×	×	×		
Treatment effect test normals		×		×		
Treatment effect discordant tests				×	×	
Strategy effect		×	×	×	×	×

ethical, as there is often evidence that one treatment is better for some of the test result categories. In that case a better alternative are the designs outlined in Figures 4.3, 4.5(c) and 4.7(a), in which only the patients for whom there is uncertainty in the subsequent management are randomised.

The designs in Figures 4.4(b), 4.6(b) and 4.7(b) have frequently been used in the medical literature, probably because of their pragmatic attractiveness. In these designs the point of randomisation coincides with the decision to perform either test A or test B. From a cost perspective these designs can be more be economical than the other designs, in case of an expensive test, as on average fewer patients are tested than with the other designs. If follow up is expensive, designs randomising only patients with the test category of interest (Figures 4.3, 4.5(c) and 4.7) are more efficient, as fewer patients will be needed to achieve the same amount of statistical precision.[12] However, the latter designs are not feasible when tests that influence each other's performance are being compared. For example, it is not possible to compare two surgical diagnostic procedures, mediastinoscopy and anterior mediastinotomy, for the detection of mediastinal lymphomas by performing them both in all patients as suspected lymph nodes are removed.[13]

Practical issues

We have discussed the pros and cons of different designs to evaluate the prognostic impact of a single test or to compare different test strategies. In the design of a trial there are several other issues that should be considered in advance. In all of the examples we have presented here there was a prespecified link between test results and management decisions. Test positive patients were to receive one treatment, test negative another. If such a link is absent, and clinicians are free to select therapy for each test result, it will remain unclear to what extent poor trial results reflect deficiencies of the test itself, ineffective treatment options or, alternatively, incorrect management decisions. Detailed information on the treatment protocol is also necessary for others to implement the possible findings of the study.

A clear specification of the treatment options and their relation with the different test results is an absolute necessity for any diagnostic study.[12]

As for each randomised controlled trial, methods to preserve allocation concealment and blinding deserve special attention. It has been shown empirically that inadequate concealment of allocation, as well as inadequate blinding, can lead to exaggerated estimates of a strategy's effectiveness.[14] One way to guard adequate allocation concealment is a central randomisation procedure. In some situations the use of sealed opaque envelopes, with monitoring of the concealment process, may be more feasible.[15] Blinding of the outcome measurement for the randomisation outcome is of greater importance for some outcomes than for others, but can be implemented with the same methods as developed for therapeutic trials. Blinding of the clinician or patient to the allocation is more difficult. When two different strategies are randomised (Figure 4.6(b)) one can imagine that the knowledge of the type of test influences subsequent management decisions, despite a prespecified link. For example, an obstetrician might be more reassured with the results of magnetic resonance pelvimetry in a breech presentation at term, than with manual pelvimetry, which will influence subsequent decisions to perform an emergency section.[16] One could choose a design that randomises test results to overcome this problem. Alternatively, one could try to mask the clinician by only presenting standardised test results, without any reference to the type of test.

The *a priori* calculation of the necessary sample size for a randomised diagnostic study is not straightforward. When discussing Figure 4.5(c) we showed that the expected difference in outcome between the two test strategies resulted from the expected difference in the category with discordant test results only. In trials in which patients are randomised to one of two test strategies (Figure 4.6(b)) a large group of participants will also not contribute to the final difference. Let us explain this with another randomised diagnostic trial from the literature, in which ultrasonography was compared with clinical assessment for the diagnosis of appendicitis.[17] The authors report a power of 80% to detect a reduction in the non-therapeutic operation rate from 11% to 2%, by randomising 302 patients. What are the nominator and denominator of these estimated rates?

Figure 4.8 shows the two trial arms. A large group of patients with abnormal results in the ultrasound group, indicating operation, would also have been detected at clinical examination. The same argument stands for a subgroup of patients with a normal ultrasound. The sum of these two groups forms the total with concordant test results. As patients with concordant test results will receive the same management, their event rates will be identical except for chance differences. The rate of 11% results from $(x+n+o)/151$. The rate of 2% results from $(y+n+o)/151$. The rate difference, 9%, results solely from the events in the discordant group. By

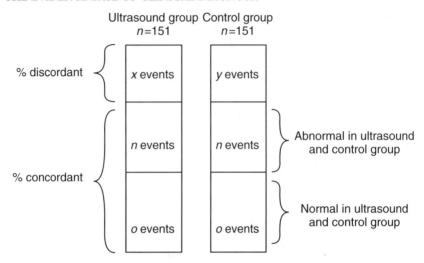

Figure 4.8 Sample size calculation.

assuming a concordance rate of ultrasonography with clinical assessment of 80%, one can calculate the postulated rate difference in this discordant group: 9%/20% is 45%. This could result from a rate of non-therapeutic operations of 55% in patients with a positive clinical assessment and otherwise negative ultrasound, and a rate of 10% in patients with a positive ultrasound and otherwise negative clinical examination. (This implies that the event rate is 0% in the concordant group, which is not very likely, as the authors discuss in their introduction that 15–30% of all operations are non-therapeutic.) With some extra calculations we can show that the difference assumed by the authors implies a discordance rate of at least 80%. It would be very strange to expect such a high discordance rate in advance. This example shows that it is important to incorporate the discordance rate in sample size calculations of randomised trials of diagnostic tests.

Conclusions

In this chapter we discuss the evaluation of the prognostic impact of tests. From a patient perspective one could argue that it is not so much the correspondence with the "truth" that should be the focus of a diagnostic test evaluation, but the likelihood that such a test detects events of clinical interest, and the possibilities that exist to let test results guide subsequent clinical decision making to reduce the likelihood of such events occurring. The latter can be evaluated by evaluating a test–treatment combination in a clinical trial, for which several possible designs are discussed.

The examples of published randomised diagnostic trials in this chapter show that it is feasible to perform such a thorough evaluation of a diagnostic test. Several additional examples can be found in the literature, such as trials of mediastinoscopy, cardiotocography and MRI,[11,18,19] and of a number of screening tests.[20–22] These date back as far as 1975.[23]

In most of these trials the point of randomisation coincided with the clinical decision as to whether or not to perform the tests. This makes it impossible to differentiate between the treatment effect and the prognostic value of the test. Power analyses of any diagnostic trial should incorporate an estimation of the discordance rate, as differences in outcome can only be expected for patients who have discordant test results. In this chapter we have shown that a design incorporating randomisation of discordant test results is more efficient, provides more information, and is less prone to bias. Most importantly, all of these designs require a prespecified test–treatment link. This is to allow for the application of the study results in other settings, and to guard the internal validity of the study.

References

1 Rothwell PM, Pendlebury ST, Wardlaw J, Warlow CP. Critical appraisal of the design and reporting of studies of imaging and measurement of carotid stenosis. *Stroke* 2000;**31**:1444–50.
2 Lewis RF, Abrahamowicz M, Cote R, Battista RN. Predictive power of duplex ultrasonography in asymptomatic carotid disease. *Ann Intern Med* 1997;**127**:13–20.
3 Adams HP Jr, Bendixen BH, Leira E, *et al*. Antithrombotic treatment of ischemic stroke among patients with occlusion or severe stenosis of the internal carotid artery: a report of the Trial of Org 10172 in Acute Stroke Treatment (TOAST). *Neurology* 1999;**53**:122–5.
4 Anonymous. Low molecular weight heparinoid, ORG 10172 (danaparoid), and outcome after acute ischemic stroke: a randomized controlled trial. The Publications Committee for the Trial of ORG 10172 in Acute Stroke Treatment (TOAST) Investigators [see comments]. *JAMA* 1998;**279**:1265–72.
5 Cote R, Battista RN, Abrahamowicz M, Langlois Y, Bourque F, Mackey A. Lack of effect of aspirin in asymptomatic patients with carotid bruits and substantial carotid narrowing. The Asymptomatic Cervical Bruit Study Group. *Ann Intern Med* 1995;**123**:649–55.
6 Kraemer HC. *Evaluating medical tests: objective and quantitative guidelines*. Newbury Park: SAGE Publications, 1992:295.
7 Nienhuis SJ, Vles JS, Gerver WJ, Hoogland HJ. Doppler ultrasonography in suspected intrauterine growth retardation: a randomized clinical trial. *Ultrasound Obstet Gynecol* 1997;**9**:6–13.
8 Simel DL, Samsa GP, Matchar DB. Likelihood ratios with confidence: sample size estimation for diagnostic test studies. *J Clin Epidemiol* 1991;**44**:763–70.
9 Aviv JE. Prospective, randomized outcome study of endoscopy versus modified barium swallow in patients with dysphagia. *Laryngoscope* 2000;**110**:563–74.
10 Lassen AT, Pedersen FM, Bytzer P, de Muckadell OBS. *Helicobacter pylori* test-and-eradicate versus prompt endoscopy for management of dyspeptic patients: a randomised trial. *Lancet* 2000;**356**:455–60.
11 Anonymous. Investigation for mediastinal disease in patients with apparently operable lung cancer. Canadian Lung Oncology Group. *Ann Thorac Surg* 1995;**60**:1382–9.
12 Bossuyt P, Lijmer J, Mol B. Randomised comparisons of medical tests: sometimes invalid, not always efficient. *Lancet* 2000;**356**:1844–7.
13 Elia S, Cecere C, Giampaglia F, Ferrante G. Mediastinoscopy vs. anterior mediastinotomy in the diagnosis of mediastinal lymphoma: a randomized trial. *Eur J Cardiothorac Surg* 1992;**6**:361–5.

14 Schulz KF, Chalmers I, Hayes RJ, Altman DG. Empirical evidence of bias. Dimensions of methodological quality associated with estimates of treatment effects in controlled trials. *JAMA* 1995;**273**:408–12.

15 Swingler GH, Zwarenstein M. An effectiveness trial of a diagnostic test in a busy outpatients department in a developing country: issues around allocation concealment and envelope randomization. *J Clin Epidemiol* 2000;**53**:702–6.

16 van der Post JA, Maathuis JB. Magnetic-resonance pelvimetry in breech presentation [letter; comment]. *Lancet* 1998;**351**:913.

17 Douglas C, Macpherson N, Davidson P, Gani J. Randomised controlled trial of ultrasonography in diagnosis of acute appendicitis, incorporating the Alvarado score. *BMJ* 2000;**321**:1–7.

18 Strachan BK, van Wijngaarden WJ, Sahota D, Chang A, James DK. Cardiotocography only versus cardiotocography plus PR-interval analysis in intrapartum surveillance: a randomised, multicentre trial. FECG Study Group. *Lancet* 2000;**355**:456–9.

19 Dixon AK, Wheeler TK, Lomas DJ, Mackenzie R. Computed tomography or magnetic resonance imaging for axillary symptoms following treatment of breast carcinoma? A randomized trial. *Clin Radiol* 1993;**48**:371–6.

20 Kronborg O, Fenger C, Olsen J, Jorgensen OD, Sondergaard O. Randomised study of screening for colorectal cancer with faecal-occult-blood test. *Lancet* 1996;**348**:1467–71.

21 Anonymous. Controlled trial of universal neonatal screening for early identification of permanent childhood hearing impairment. Wessex Universal Neonatal Hearing Screening Trial Group. *Lancet* 1998;**352**:1957–64.

22 Miller AB, To T, Baines CJ, Wall C. Canadian National Breast Screening Study-2: 13-Year Results of a Randomized Trial in Women Aged 50–59 Years. *J Natl Cancer Inst* 2000;**92**:1490–9.

23 Morris DW, Levine GM, Soloway RD, Miller WT, Marin GA. Prospective, randomized study of diagnosis and outcome in acute upper-gastrointestinal bleeding: endoscopy versus conventional radiography. *Am J Dig Dis* 1975;**20**:1103–9.

5 The diagnostic before–after study to assess clinical impact

J ANDRÉ KNOTTNERUS, GEERT-JAN DINANT, ONNO P van SCHAYCK

Summary box

- The before–after design is more appropriate for evaluating the clinical impact of additional testing than to compare the impact of different diagnostic options.
- Demonstrating an effect of diagnostic testing on the patient's health outcome is more difficult than showing a change in the doctor's assessment and management plan.
- Whether and what specific blinding procedures have to be applied depends on the study objective.
- To optimise the assessment of the independent effect of the test information, performance of the test or disclosure of the test result can be randomised. This would change the before–after design in a randomised trial.
- The therapeutic consequences of the various test results can be standardised in the research protocol, provided that such therapy options are clinically rational and have a well documented evidence base. The study will then evaluate the impact of the test result connected with a defined therapeutic consequence, rather than the test result per se.
- If evaluating the doctor's assessment is the primary study objective, the assessment should preferably take place immediately after

disclosure of the test result, with a minimal risk of interfering factors influencing the doctor's judgement.

- Because a rather long follow up is mostly needed to estimate the impact of testing on the clinical course, the risk of interfering influences is substantial.
- Given that before–after studies can be carried out relatively fast, largely embedded in daily care, while RCTs are more complex or expensive, a well designed before–after study may sometimes be used to explore whether and how a diagnostic RCT should be performed. If an RCT is impossible or infeasible, or ethically unacceptable, a well designed before–after study can be the most suitable alternative.

Introduction

Apart from facilitating an accurate diagnosis, a test is aimed at causing change: starting from a baseline situation, applying the test and interpreting its outcome should result in a new situation. In fact, the most important justification for diagnostic testing is that it is expected to make a difference, by influencing clinical management and ultimately benefiting the patient's wellbeing. Accordingly, performing a test can be seen as an intervention that should be effective in bringing about a clinically relevant change.

In studying the clinical effect of a test result, the randomised controlled trial (RCT) is the strongest methodological design option,[1] and is dealt with in Chapter 4. However, although it is the paradigm for effectiveness research, an RCT cannot always be achieved. This is, for example, the case if randomly withholding a test or test result from patients or doctors is considered medically or ethically unacceptable. Difficulties may also arise if the diagnostic test is integrated in the general skills of the clinician, so that performing it cannot be randomly switched on and off in his or her head, nor simply assigned to a different doctor. This is especially problematic if at the same time patients cannot be randomly assigned to a doctor. This situation may, for instance, occur in studying the impact of diagnostic reasoning skills in general practice. Also, when an RCT is complex and expensive, or will last too long to still be relevant when the results become available, one may wish to consider a more feasible alternative.

One alternative that may be considered is the diagnostic before–after study.[2] This approach seems attractive, as it fits naturally within the clinical process and is easier to perform than the randomised trial. Therefore, this chapter will discuss the potentials, limitations, and pitfalls of this design option.

82

The research question

Example

In a study to assess the diagnostic impact of erythrocyte sedimentation rate (ESR) in general practice, 305 consecutive patients with aspecific symptoms for whom general practitioners (GPs) considered ESR testing necessary were included.[3] Before testing, the GPs were asked to specify the most likely diagnosis in each patient, and to assess whether or not this diagnosis was severe in the sense of malignant or inflammatory disease for which further management would be urgently needed. Subsequently, the ESR was independently performed and the result was made available to the GPs, who then again specified their (revised) diagnostic assessment. After 3 months, based on all the available medical information, a clinical assessment was carried out for each patient by an independent clinician not knowing about the pre- and post-test assessments for each patient, in order to establish a final diagnosis (reference standard).[4]

In Figure 5.1 the percentage of patients most likely having severe pathology according to the GP is presented before and after disclosure of the ESR result. There seems to be no relevant pre–post-test change. However, looking at Table 5.1, it is clear that there was a change in 32 patients: 17 from severe pathology to "other", and 15 from "other" to severe pathology.

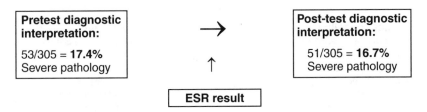

Figure 5.1 Pre- and post-test diagnostic assessment in studying the impact of ESR.

Table 5.1 Relation between pre- and post-test diagnostic assessments in studying the impact of ESR.

	Post-test interpretation		
Pretest interpretation	Severe pathology	Other	Total
Severe pathology	36	17	53
Other	15	237	252
Total	51	254	305

Whether these changes had indeed resulted in a more accurate diagnostic assessment could be determined after correlating the GPs' pre- and post-test findings with the reference standard procedure. It appeared that the pretest accuracy of the GPs' assessment was 69% (that is, 69% of cases were correctly classified), whereas the post-test accuracy was 76%, implying an increase of 7%.

Furthermore, of the 32 patients with a diagnostic classification changed by the GP, nine with a positive (severe) post-test diagnosis proved to be "false positives", and two with a negative (other) post-test diagnosis were "false negatives".

The test characteristics of the ESR (cut-off value $\geq 27\,mm/1h$) could be also determined in relation to the reference diagnosis, yielding a sensitivity of 53%, a specificity of 94%, a positive predictive value of 46%, and a negative predictive value of 91%.

The general model

The basic question in the diagnostic before–after study is whether applying a certain diagnostic test favourably influences the doctor's (a) diagnostic or (b) prognostic assessment of a presented clinical problem; (c) the further management; and, ultimately, (d) the patient's health. It essentially comprises the baseline (pretest) situation, a determinant (the test), and the outcome (post-test situation) (Figure 5.2).

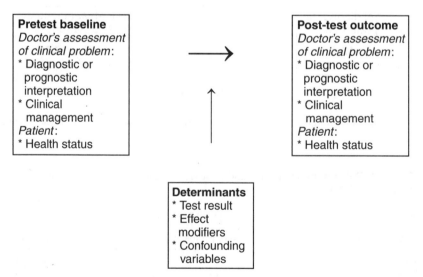

Figure 5.2 General representation of the research question in a diagnostic before–after study.

The point of departure can be characterised by a clinical problem, with the doctor's assessment regarding the possible diagnosis, prognosis, or the preferred management option, and the patient's health status at baseline, without knowing the information from the test to be evaluated. The patient's health status at baseline is important, not only as a starting point for possible outcome assessment but also as a reference for generalising the study results to comparable patient groups.

The determinant of primary interest is performing the diagnostic test and disclosure of its result, which is in fact the intended intervention. Furthermore, because diagnostic classification is essentially involved with distinguishing clinically relevant subgroups, it is often useful to consider the influence of effect modifying variables, such as the doctor's skills and experience, the patient's age and gender, and pre-existing comorbidity. In addition, the effect of possible confounding variables should be taken into account. For example, extraneous factors such as reading publications or attending professional meetings may affect the clinician's assessment. But also the time needed to do the test and obtain its result may be important, as it may be used to think and study on the clinical problem, and this will independently influence the assessment. Moreover, the patient's health status may have changed as a result of the clinical course of the illness, by interfering comorbidity and related interventions, by environmental factors, or by visiting other therapists. The patient's symptom perception may have been influenced by information from family, friends, or the media, or by consulting the internet. Also, the patient may claim to have benefited from a diagnostic intervention because he does not wish to disappoint the doctor.

The key challenge for the investigator is now to evaluate the extent to which applying the diagnostic test has independently changed the doctor's diagnostic or prognostic assessment of the presented clinical problem, the preferred management option, or the patient's health status. The latter will generally be influenced indirectly, via clinical management, but can sometimes also be directly affected, for example because the patient feels himself being taken more seriously by the testing per se. Moreover, patient self testing, which is nowadays becoming more common, can influence patient self management.

At this point, two important limitations of the before–after design must be emphasised. First, the design is more appropriate to evaluate the impact of "add on" technologies[2] (that is, the effect of additional testing) than to compare the impact of different diagnostic technologies or strategies. For the latter purpose one could, in principle, apply both studied technologies, for example colonoscopy and double contrast barium enema, in randomised order, to all included patients, and then compare the impact of disclosing the test results, again in random order, on the clinicians' assessment. Another example would be to subject patients to both CT and

NMR head scanning to study their influence on clinicians' management plans in those with suspected intracranial pathology. However, such comparisons are unrealistic, as the two tests would never be applied simultaneously in practice. Moreover, such studies are very burdensome for patients, not to say ethically unacceptable, and would make it virtually impossible to study the complication rate of each procedure separately.[5] When the various options are mutually exclusive, for example when comparing diagnostic laparotomy with endoscopy in assessing intra-abdominal pathology as to their adverse effects, a before–after design is clearly inappropriate. In such situations, a randomised controlled trial is by far the preferred option. Only when the compared tests can be easily carried out together without any problem for the patient, can they be applied simultaneously. This can be done, for instance, when comparing the impact of different blood tests using the same blood sample. However, when the disclosure of the results of the compared tests to the clinicians is then randomised, which would be a good idea, we are in fact in the RCT option.

Second, demonstrating an effect of diagnostic testing on the patient's health outcome is much more difficult than showing a change in the doctor's assessment and management plan. In fact, this is often impossible, as it usually takes quite some time to observe a health effect that might be ascribed to performance of the test. Controlling for the influence of the many possible confounders over time generally requires a concurrent control group of similar patients not receiving the test. However, a diagnostic before–after study could be convincing in case of: (1) studying a clinical problem with a highly predictable outcome in the absence of testing (such as unavoidable death in the case of imminent rupture of an aneurysm of the aorta), (2) while adding specific diagnostic information (an appropriate imaging technique) leading to a specific therapeutic decision (whether and how to operate) (3), which is aimed at a clearly defined short term effect (prevention of a rupture and survival), possibly followed by less specific long term effects (rehabilitation). However, such opportunities are extraordinary. Besides, although on the one hand some clinicians would consider such clinical situations to be self evident and not needing evaluation by research, others may still see room for dispute as to what extent clinical events are predictable or unavoidable.

Working out the study

Pretest baseline

The study protocol follows the elements of the research question.

At baseline, the clinical problem and the study question are defined. The clinical problem could be aspecific symptoms as presented in primary care, with the question being whether the ESR would contribute to the doctor's diagnostic assessment,[3,4] or sciatica, in order to study whether radiography would affect therapeutic decision making.

The health status of each patient to be included is systematically documented, using standardised measurement instruments for the presented symptoms, patient history, physical examination, and further relevant clinical data.

Overseeing all available patient data, the doctor makes a first clinical assessment of the probability of certain diagnoses or diagnostic categories. In primary care, for example, the probability of a severe organic malignant or inflammatory, disorder can be assessed. This can be done for one specified diagnostic category, for a list of specified diagnoses, or in an open approach, just asking the differential diagnosis the doctor has in mind, with the estimated probability of each specific diagnostic hypothesis being considered.

Furthermore, the doctor is asked to describe the preferred diagnostic or therapeutic management plan, which can be done, again, according to a prepared list of items or as an open question.

At baseline, possibly relevant effect modifying variables should be considered. Often the general clinical experience of the clinicians and their specific expertise regarding the test under study are important. Furthermore, variables characterising important clinical subgroups can be assessed, and potential confounding factors have to be measured in order to be able to take these into account in the data analysis. Recording of covariables is sometimes difficult, for example for extraneous variables such as media exposure. Moreover, it cannot be excluded that important or even decisive factors are not identified or even foreseen.

Diagnostic testing

In performing the diagnostic test or procedure under study and revealing its outcome after the baseline assessment, different options can be considered depending on the specific study objective.

- If one wishes to assess the specific effect of the test information on the outcome, in addition to the pretest clinical information, the test result should be determined independently from the pretest information. This is especially relevant for test procedures with a subjective element in the interpretation of the result, such as patient interviews, auscultation, imaging, x ray films, and pathological specimens. Accordingly, those who interpret the test should not be aware of the pretest information. However, when patient history itself is the test to be evaluated, this will generally not be feasible.
- When it is important to limit possible confounding effects of a preoccupation of participating doctors with the expected relevance of a

certain test, the investigator may wish to obscure the performing of the evaluated test itself. This can theoretically be achieved by not telling the doctor in advance about what specifically is being evaluated, and by disclosing the test result while also providing information on a number of other items irrelevant for the studied comparison. However, such masking is difficult and often not feasible, or may be so much in conflict with clinical reality that the findings will not be relevant for practice. Finally, intentional obscuring of the specific research question will need the explicit approval of the medical ethics review board.

- If the investigator wishes to assess the diagnostic process as it is usually embedded in clinical practice, the interpretation of the test result can be carried out as usual without specific blinding procedures. However, particularly for tests with subjective elements in reading or interpretation of the results, this will imply that the independent contribution of the test cannot be reliably determined.

- To optimise the assessment of the independent effect of the test information, performance of the test or, even more precisely, disclosure of the test result, can be randomised so that half of the participants would and half would not get the result. In fact, this would change the before–after design into a randomised trial, which is discussed in Chapter 4.

Because a test is almost never perfect, applying it may produce mis-classification. Even when most patients are more accurately classified if the clinician uses the test information, some patients with a correct pretest diagnosis may be incorrectly classified after testing, for example because of a false positive or false negative result. As this may have important negative consequences for those patients – for example when a false positive mammography would lead to unnecessary surgery – it is recommended to include evaluation of the actual disease status in the context of the before–after study. This also enables the investigator to determine test accuracy by relating the test result cross-sectionally to the disease status, established according to an acceptable reference standard.[5]

Post-test outcome

The measurement of the final post-test outcome after disclosure of the test result (diagnostic assessment, preferred management plan, and/or patient health status) should follow the same procedure as the baseline measurement. In doing so, both the doctor and the patient will generally remember the baseline status, implying that the post-test assessment of the doctor's differential diagnosis and management options cannot be blinded for the pretest assessment. This has probably been the case in the example of the diagnostic impact of the ESR measurement.

When one is evaluating the impact of adding the test information to already known clinical information at baseline in order to make a comprehensive assessment, lack of blinding is not always a principal problem. In fact, it is clinically natural and supported by Bayes's theorem to study the impact of the test result in the light of the prior probability. However, when clinicians are more or less "anchored" to their initial diagnostic assessment, they are biased in that they do not sufficiently respond to the test information in revising their diagnostic assessment. But even this can sometimes be acceptable for an investigator who deliberately aims to assess the impact of the test in clinical reality, where such anchoring is a common phenomenon,[6,7] and to study the influence of the test result in terms of confirming or refuting this anchoring. As doctors will vary in "anchoring", such evaluations need to include sufficient participating clinicians.

When the post-test outcome is patient status, objective assessment independent of both pretest status and the doctor's interpretations is a basic requirement.

If one evaluates a test which is already firmly accepted among the medical profession, the response of clinicians is in fact "programmed" by medical education, continuing medical education, or clinical guidelines. In such cases the investigator is studying the adherence to agreed guidelines rather than the independent clinical impact of the test result. On the other hand, the clinical impact of testing will not be easily detected if there is no clear relationship between revision of the diagnostic classification based on the test information, and the revision of the management plan.[2] This relation can indeed be unclear when doctors ignore the test information, or when the same test result may lead to a variety of management decisions, including doing nothing. The latter can, for example, be the case when laboratory tests are carried out in asymptomatic patients. As a remedy, the therapeutic consequences of the various test results can be standardised in the research protocol, provided that such therapy options are clinically rational and have a well documented evidence base. Accordingly, the study will then evaluate the impact of the test result connected with a defined therapeutic consequence, rather than the test result per se. On the other hand, when there is a lack of clarity beforehand as to the potential management consequences of performing a test, we should ask ourselves whether such testing should be evaluated or used at all.

The time factor

The interval between the pre- and post-test assessments should be carefully chosen. Generally, the interassessment period should be short if evaluating the doctor's assessment is the primary study objective: the assessment should preferably take place immediately after disclosure of the test result, with a minimal risk of interfering factors influencing the doctor's

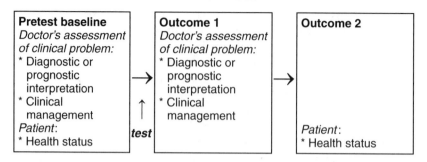

Figure 5.3 Separate post-test measurements of doctor's assessment (immediately) and patient health outcome (later).

judgement. Sometimes, however, this may take some days (bacterial culture) or longer (cervical smear). A rather long period until the final post-test assessment is mostly needed if estimating the impact of testing on the clinical course is the objective, although this longer period will be associated with an increased risk of interfering interventions and influences during follow up. A combined approach can be chosen, with a pretest measurement, a post-test measurement of the clinician's assessment, and a longer follow up period for measuring patient health outcome, respectively (Figure 5.3). In the analysis, then, the relation between the test's impact on the clinician's assessment and patient outcome could be studied if extraneous factors and changes in the clinical condition can be sufficiently controlled for. However, as outlined in the section on the research question, this is mostly impossible in the context of the before–after design. For the purpose of studying the test's impact on patient health, the randomised controlled trial is a more valid option.

Selection of the study subjects

Regarding the selection of the study subjects, similar methodological criteria to those discussed in Chapter 3 should be met: the study patient population should be representative for the "indicated", "candidate" or "intended" patient population, or target population, with a well defined clinical problem, clinically similar to the group of patients in whom the test would be applied in practice. Accordingly, the healthcare setting from where the patients come, the inclusion criteria, and the procedure for patient recruitment must be specified. Regarding the selection of participating doctors, the study objective is decisive. If the aim is to evaluate what the test adds to current practice, the pre- and post-test assessments should be made by clinicians representing usual clinical standards. However, if one wishes to ensure that the test's contribution is analysed using a maximum of available expertise, top experts in the specific clinical field must be recruited.

Generally, in clinical studies a prospectively included consecutive series of patients with a clearly defined clinical presentation will be the most appropriate option with the lowest selection bias. If one were to retrospectively select patients who had already had the test in the past, one would generally not be able to be certain whether those patients really had a similar clinical problem, and whether all candidate patients in the source population would have non-selectively entered the study population. Apart from this, a valid before–after comparison of the doctors' assessments (with the doctors first not knowing and subsequently knowing the test result) is not possible afterwards, as a change in diagnostic assessment and the planning of management cannot be reliably reconstructed post hoc.

Sample size and analysis

Sample size requirements for the before–after study design need to be met according to general conventions. Point of departure can be the size of the before–after difference in estimated disease probability or other effectiveness parameters, for example, the decrease in the rate of (diagnostic) referrals, which would be sufficiently relevant to be detected. If the basic phenomenon to be studied is the clinical assessment of doctors, the latter are the units of analysis. When the consequences for the patients are considered the main outcome, their number is of specific interest.

The data analysis of the basic before–after comparison can follow the principles of the analysis of paired data. In view of the relevance of evaluating differences of test impact in various subgroups of patients, and given the observational nature of the before–after study, studying the effect of effect modifying variables and adjusting for confounding factors using multivariable analytical methods, may add to the value of the study. When the clinician and patient "levels" are to be considered simultaneously, multilevel analysis can be used.

As it is often difficult to reach sufficient statistical power in studies with doctors as the units of analysis, and because of the expected heterogeneity in observational clinical studies, before–after studies are more appropriate to confirm or exclude a substantial clinical impact than to find subtle differences.

Modified approaches

Given the potential sources of uncontrollable bias in all phases of the study, investigators may choose to use "paper" or videotaped patients or clinical vignettes, interactive computer simulated cases, or "standardised patients" especially trained to simulate a specific role consistently over time.

Standardised (simulated) patients can consult the doctor even without being recognised as "non-real".[8] Furthermore, the pre- and post-test assessments can also be done by an independent expert panel in order to ensure that the evaluation of the clinical impact is based on best available clinical knowledge. The limitations of such approaches are that they do not always sufficiently reflect clinical reality, are less suitable (vignettes) for an interactive diagnostic work up, cannot be used to evaluate more invasive diagnostics (standardised patients), and are not appropriate for additionally assessing diagnostic accuracy.

A before–after comparison in a group of doctors applying the test to an indicated patient population can be extended with a concurrent observational control group of doctors assessing indicated patients, without receiving the test information (quasi experimental comparison). However, given the substantial risk of clinical and prognostic incomparability of the participating doctors and patients in the parallel groups compared, and of possibly incorrectable extraneous influences, this will often not strengthen the design substantially. If a controlled design is considered, a randomised trial is to be preferred (Chapter 4).

Concluding remarks

As Guyatt et al.[2] have brilliantly pointed out, in considering a before–after design to study the clinical impact of diagnostic testing, two types of methodological problem must be acknowledged. First, we have to deal with problems for which, in principle, reasonable solutions can be found in order to optimise the study design. In this chapter, some of these "challenges" have been discussed. Examples are appropriate specifications of the clinical problem to be studied and the candidate patient population, and the concomitant documentation of test accuracy. Second, the before–after design has inherent limitations that cannot be avoided nor solved. If these are not acceptable, another design should be chosen. The most important of these limitations are: (1) the before–after design is especially appropriate for evaluating additional testing, rather than comparing two essentially different (mutually exclusive) diagnostic strategies; (2) the reported pretest management options may be different from the real strategy the clinicians would have followed if the test had not been available, or if they would not have known that there is a second (post-test) chance for assessment; (3) the pre- and post-test assessments by the same clinicians for the same patients are generally not independent; and (4) an unbiased evaluation of the impact of testing on the patients' health status can mostly not be achieved.

Acknowledging the large number of difficulties and pitfalls of the before–after design, as outlined in previous sections, we conclude that the design can have a place especially if the pre–post-test assessment interval can be relatively short (evaluation of the test's impact on the doctor's assessment), and if the relation between the diagnostic assessment, the subsequent therapeutic decision making, and therapeutic effectiveness is well understood. If impact on patient outcome is studied, it is important that the clinical course of the studied problem in the absence of testing is well known and highly predictable.

Given the various limitations for studying the clinical impact of diagnostic tests, the randomised controlled trial design, if feasible, will in most cases be superior. However, given that before–after studies can be carried out relatively fast, largely embedded in daily care, whereas RCTs are more complex or expensive, a well designed before–after study may be useful to explore whether a diagnostic RCT could be worthwhile, or how it should be performed. In addition, if an RCT is impossible or infeasible, or ethically unacceptable, a before–after study may be the most suitable alternative. Other options, which could provide a more uniform clinical presentation and a better control of interfering variables, are before–after studies using written patient vignettes, interactive computer simulations, or standardised patients. The specific potentials and limitations (for example representing less clinical reality) of these alternative approaches will then have to be taken into account.

References

1 Alperovitch A. Controlled assessment of diagnostic techniques: methodological problems. *Effective Health Care* 1983;**1**:187–90.
2 Guyatt GH, Tugwell PX, Feeney DH, Drummond MF, Haynes RB. The role of before–after studies in the evaluation of therapeutic impact of diagnostic technology. *J Chronic Dis* 1986;**39**:295–304.
3 Dinant GJ, Knottnerus JA, van Wersch JWJ. Diagnostic impact of the erythrocyte sedimentation rate in general practice: a before–after analysis. *Fam Pract* 1992;**9**:28–31.
4 Dinant GJ. *Diagnostic value of the erythrocyte sedimentation rate in general practice*. Thesis. Maastricht: University of Maastricht, 1991.
5 Guyatt G, Drummond M. Guideline for the clinical and economic assessment of health technologies: the case of magnetic resonance. *Intl J Health Tech Assess Health Care* 1985;**1**: 551–66.
6 Tversky A, Kahneman D. Judgment under uncertainty: heuristics and biases. *Science* 1974; **185**:1124–31.
7 Elstein AS, Shulman LS, Sprafka SA. *Medical problem solving: an analysis of clinical reasoning*. Cambridge, MA: Harvard University Press, 1978.
8 Rethans JJ, Sturmans F, Drop R, van der Vleuten C. Assessment of the performance of general practitioners by the use of standardized (simulated) patients. *Br J Gen Pract* 1991; **41**:97–9.

6 Designing studies to ensure that estimates of test accuracy will travel

LES M IRWIG, PATRICK M BOSSUYT,
PAUL P GLASZIOU, CONSTANTINE GATSONIS,
JEROEN G LIJMER

Summary box

- There may be genuine differences between test accuracies in different settings, such as primary care or hospital, in different types of hospital, or between countries.
- Deciding whether estimates of test accuracy are transferable to other settings depends on an understanding of the possible reasons for variability in test discrimination and calibration across settings.
- The transferability of measures of test performance from one setting to another depends on which indicator of test performance is to be used.
- Real variation in the performance of diagnostic tests (such as different test types, or a different spectrum of disease) needs to be distinguished from artefactual variation resulting from study design features. These features include the target condition and reference standard used, the population and the clinical question studied, the evaluated comparison, and the way the index test was performed, calibrated, and interpreted.
- In preparing studies on diagnostic accuracy, a key question is how to design studies that carry more information about the transferability of results.

- In order to ensure that estimates of diagnostic accuracy will travel, before starting to design a study the following questions must be answered:
  - How are the target condition and reference standard defined?
  - Is the objective to estimate global test performance or to estimate probability of disease in individuals?
  - What is the population and clinical problem?
  - Is the test being considered as a replacement or incremental test?
  - To what extent do you want to study the reasons for variability of the results within your population?
  - To what extent do you want to study the transferability of the results to other settings?
- Designing studies with heterogeneous study populations allows exploration of the transferability of diagnostic performance in different settings. This will require larger studies than have generally been carried out in the past for diagnostic tests.

Introduction

Measures of test accuracy are often thought of as fixed characteristics that can be determined by research and then applied in practice. Yet even when tests are evaluated in a study with adequate quality – including features such as consecutive patients, a good reference standard, and independent, blinded assessments of tests and the reference standard[1] – diagnostic test performance in one setting may vary from the results reported elsewhere. This has been explored extensively for coronary artery disease,[2–5] but has also been shown for a variety of other conditions.[6–8] This variability is not only due to chance. There may be genuine differences between test accuracy in different settings, such as primary care or hospital, different types of hospital, or the same type of hospital in different countries. As a consequence, the findings from a study may not be applicable to the specific decision problem for which the reader has turned to the literature.

We suggest that deciding whether the estimates of test accuracy from studies are transferable to other settings depends on an understanding of the possible reasons for variability in test discrimination and calibration across settings. Variability may be due to artefactual differences (for example different design features of studies in different settings) or true differences (such as different test types, or a different spectrum of disease). To decide on the transferability of test results, we are concerned with true differences, after artefactual differences have been addressed.[9–11]

This chapter is divided into two main sections. The first is concerned with the reasons for true variability in accuracy; it explores conceptual underpinnings. The second section is a pragmatic guide for those interpreting and designing studies of diagnostic tests. It is based on the view that value can be added to studies of diagnostic tests by exploring the extent to which we can characterise the reasons for variability in diagnostic performance between patients in different settings, and examining how much variability remains unexplained.

1. Reasons for true variability in test accuracy: conceptual underpinnings

Measures of diagnostic test performance: discrimination and calibration

There are many measures of test accuracy. Broadly speaking, we can think of them as falling into one of the following categories.

1 Global measures of test accuracy assess only discriminatory power. These measures assess the ability of the test to discriminate between diseased and non-diseased individuals. Common examples are the area under the receiver operating characteristic curve, and the odds ratio, sometimes also referred to as the diagnostic odds ratio. They may be sufficient for some broad health policy decisions, for example whether a new test is in general better than an existing test for that condition.

2 Measures of test performance to estimate the probability of disease in individuals require discrimination and calibration. These measures are used to estimate probabilities of the target condition in individuals who have a particular test result. An example is the predictive value: the proportion of people with a particular test result who have the disease of interest. To be useful for clinical practice, these estimates should be accompanied by other relevant information. For example, fracture rates in people with a particular result of a test for osteoporosis differ between people depending on their age, sex, and other characteristics. It is clumsy and difficult to estimate disease rates for all categories of patient who may have different prior probabilities. Therefore, the estimation is often done indirectly using Bayes' theorem, based on the patient-specific prior probability and some expression of the conditional distributions of test results: the distribution of test results in subjects with and without the target condition. Examples are the sensitivity and specificity of the test, and likelihood ratios for test results. These measures of test performance require more than the *discrimination* assessed by the global measures. They require tests to be *calibrated*. As an example of the difference between discrimination and calibration, consider two tests with identical odds ratios (and ROC curves) which therefore have the same discriminatory power. However, one test may operate at a threshold that gives a sensitivity of 90% and a specificity of 60%, whereas the other operates at a threshold that gives a sensitivity of 60% and a specificity of 90%. Therefore, they differ in the way they are calibrated.

Features that facilitate transferability of test results

The transferability of measures of test performance from one setting to another depends on which indicator of test performance is to be used. The possible assumptions involved in transferability are illustrated in Figure 6.1. Table 6.1 indicates the relationship between these assumptions and the transferability of the different measures of test performance.

The main assumptions in transferring tests across settings are:

1 *The definition of disease is constant.* Many diseases have ambiguous definitions. For example, there is no single reference standard for heart failure, Alzheimer's disease or diabetes. Reference standards may differ because conceptual frameworks differ between investigators, or because it is difficult to apply the same framework in a standardised way.

2 *The same test is used.* Although based on the same principle, tests may differ – for example over time, or if made by different manufacturers.

3 *The thresholds between categories of test result (for example positive and negative) are constant.* This is possible with a well standardised test that can be calibrated across different settings. However, there may be no accepted means of calibration: for example different observers of imaging tests may have different thresholds for calling an image "positive". The effect of different cut points is classically studied by the use of an ROC curve. In some cases calibration may be improved by using category specific likelihood ratios, rather than a single cut point.

4 *The distribution of test results in the disease group is constant in shape and location.* This assumption is likely to be violated if the spectrum of disease changes: for example, a screening setting is likely to include earlier disease, for which test results will be closer to a non-diseased group (hence a lower sensitivity).

5 *The distribution of test results in the non-disease group is constant in shape and location.* This assumption is likely to be violated if the spectrum of non-disease changes: for example the secondary care setting involves additional causes of false positives due to comorbidity, not seen in primary care.

6 *The ratio of disease to non-disease (pretest probability) is constant.* If this were the case, we could use the post-test probability ("predictive" values) directly. However, this assumption is likely to be frequently violated: for example, the pretest probability is likely to be lowest in screening and greatest in referral settings. This likely non-constancy is the reason for using Bayes' theorem to "adjust" the post-test probability for the pretest probability of each different setting.

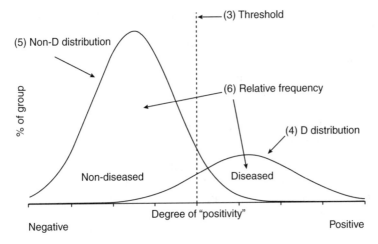

Figure 6.1 Distribution of test results in individuals with the disease of interest (D) and those without it (non-D). Numbers refer to assumptions for transferability of test results as explained in the text and Table 6.1.

Table 6.1 Assumptions for transferring different test performance characteristics. More important assumptions are marked **X** and those that are less crucial are marked *X*.

Measures of test discriminatory power	Assumption*				Comment
	3	4	5	6	
Odds ratio	**X**	**X**	**X**		Both of these measures are used for global assessment of discriminatory power and are transferable if the assumptions are met. Neither of them is concerned with calibration and therefore cannot be used for assessing the probability of disease in individuals
Area under ROC		**X**	**X**		
Measures of discriminatory power and calibration	3	4	5	6	
Predictive value	**X**	**X**	**X**	**X**	Directly estimates probability of disease in individuals
Sensitivity	**X**	**X**		*X*	
Specificity	**X**		**X**	*X*	These three measures can be used to estimate the probability of disease in individuals using Bayes' theorem
Likelihood ratios for a multicategory test	**X**	**X**	**X**		

*Assumptions are numbered as described in the text.

99

All the measures of test performance need the first two assumptions to be fulfilled. The extent to which the last four assumptions are sufficient is shown in Table 6.1, although they may not be necessary in every instance; occasionally the assumptions may be violated, but because of compensating differences transferability is still reasonable.

Lack of transferability and applicability of measures of test performance

We need first to distinguish artefactual variation from real variation in diagnostic performance. Artefactual variation arises when studies vary in the extent to which they incorporate study design features, such as whether consecutive patients were included, or whether the reference standard and the index test were read blind to each other. Once such artefactual sources of variation have been ruled out, we may explore the potential sources of true variation.[12] The issues to consider are similar to those for assessing interventions. For interventions, we consider patient, intervention, comparator, and outcome (PICO).[13,14] For tests the list is as follows, but with the target condition (equivalent to outcome in trials) shifted to the beginning of the list: (1) The target condition and reference standard used to assess it; (2) the population/clinical question; (3) the comparison; and (4) the index test. We now look at each of these in turn.

The target condition and the reference standard used to assess it

Test accuracy in any population will depend on how we define who has the target condition(s) that the test aims to detect. Clearly, the stage and spectrum of the target disease will influence the accuracy of the index test, as described later. However, even within a fixed spectrum and stage, there may be different definitions of who is "truly" diseased or not. Depending on the purpose of the study, the target conditions may be defined on grounds of clinical relevance, oriented to management decisions or prognosis, or defined on the grounds of pathological diagnosis. The definition of the target condition is therefore an active choice to be made by the investigator and its relevance interpreted by the reader of the study in the light of how they want to use the information. For example, should myocardial infarction include (a) "silent" myocardial infarction (with no chest pain)? (b) coronary thrombosis reversed by thrombolytic treatment, which then averts full infarction? This issue of the definition of the target condition and its method of ascertainment will clearly affect the apparent accuracy of the index test. For example, in parallel to considerations in clinical trials, the closer the reference standard is to a patient-relevant measure, the more this will help decisions about clinical applicability. Often reference standards that are considered objective and free of error are surrogates for (predictors of) natural history, which could be measured directly. Consider the reference standard for a test for appendicitis. The "objective" reference standard for a new test of appendicitis is often considered to be histology (arrow 2 on Figure 6.2.) In fact, conceptually, follow up of natural history is a far more useful reference standard than histology (Figure 6.2, arrow 1). It is patient-relevant: those people who would have been found to have abnormal histology but whose condition resolves without operation can be considered false positives of the histological reference standard (Figure 6.2, arrow 3). In practice, the data for arrow 3 cannot be established, and we need to use a combined reference standard that we would consider as natural history when available and histology when not, rather than (as it is usually conceptualised) histology when available and natural history when not.

The usual presentation deals with a dichotomous definition of the target condition: it is either present or absent. In most cases the possibility of multiple conditions is more plausible. If these are known in advance, the polytomous nature can be taken into account.[15–17]

Misclassification of the reference standard will tend to result in underestimation of test accuracy if the errors in the reference standard and test are uncorrelated. The degree of underestimation is prevalence dependent in a non-linear way. Estimation of sensitivity is underestimated most when the prevalence of the target condition is low, whereas specificity is underestimated most when the prevalence of the target condition is high.[18,19] The odds ratio is underestimated most when prevalence is at either extreme. Therefore, error in the reference standard may cause apparent (rather than real) effect modification of test discrimination in subgroups in which the target condition has different prevalences.[20,21] This is shown in Table 6.2 where the same hypothetical test and reference standard are applied to a population in which disease prevalence is 50%

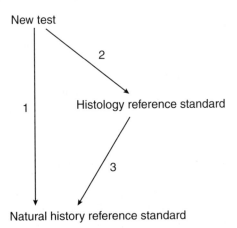

Figure 6.2 Choosing a relevant reference standard.

Table 6.2 Reference standard misclassification results in underestimation of test accuracy and apparent effect modification of different prevalences.

If reference standard has sensitivity = 0.9 and specificity = 0.8

Test	True disease			Test	Reference standard		
	Present	Absent	Total		Present	Absent	Total
Positive	80	30	110	Positive	78	32	110
Negative	20	70	90	Negative	32	58	90
Total	100	100	200	Total	110	90	200

Sensitivity = 0.80	OR = 9.3			Sensitivity = 0.71	OR = 4.4	
Specificity = 0.70				Specificity = 0.64		

If reference standard has sensitivity = 0.9 and specificity = 0.8

Test	True disease			Test	Reference standard		
	Present	Absent	Total		Present	Absent	Total
Positive	80	300	380	Positive	132	248	380
Negative	20	700	720	Negative	158	562	720
Total	100	1000	1100	Total	290	810	1100

Sensitivity = 0.80	OR = 9.3			Sensitivity = 0.46	OR = 1.9	
Specificity = 0.70				Specificity = 0.69		

(top half of table) and about 9% (bottom half). Sensitivity is reduced more in the population with 9% prevalence of disease, and specificity more in the population at 50% prevalence. The odds ratio is reduced most in the population at 9% prevalence. If errors in the reference standard are correlated with test errors, then the effect will be more difficult to predict. Correlated errors may result in overestimation of test accuracy.

The population and the clinical question

The population/clinical question are concerned not only with what disease is being tested for, but with what presentation of symptoms, signs and other information has prompted the use of the test. Test performance may vary in different populations and with minor changes in the clinical question. There are three critical concepts that help in understanding why this occurs. These are the spectrum of disease, the referral filter, and the incremental value of the test.

- *Spectrum of disease and non-disease.* Many diseases are not on/off states, but represent a spectrum ranging from mild to severe forms of disease.[22] Tumours, for example, start small, with a single cell, and then grow, leading eventually to symptoms. The ability of mammography, for example, to detect a breast tumour depends on its size. Therefore, test sensitivity will generally differ between asymptomatic and symptomatic persons. If previous tests have been carried out the spectrum of disease in tested patients may be limited, with patients who have very severe forms of disease or those with very mild forms being eliminated from the population. For example, in patients with more severe urinary tract infection, as judged by the presence of more severe symptoms and signs, the sensitivity of dipstick tests was much higher than in those with minor symptoms and signs.[6]

Likewise, patients without the target condition are not a homogeneous group. Even in the absence of disease, variability in results is the norm rather than the exception. For many laboratory tests, normal values in women differ from those in men. Similarly, values in children differ from those in adults, and values in young adults sometimes differ from those in the elderly.

Commonly, the "non-diseased" group consists of several different conditions, for each of which the test specificity may vary. The overall specificity will depend on the "mix" of alternative diagnoses: the proportion of people in each of the categories that constitute the non-diseased; for example, prostate specific antigen may have a lower specificity in older people or those with prostatic symptoms, as it is elevated in men with benign prostatic hypertrophy.[23] In principle, patients without that target condition could represent a wide range of other conditions. However, the decision to use a test is usually made because of the presenting problem of the patient and the route by which they reached the examining clinician. Hence, the actual range of variability in patients without the target condition will depend on the mechanism by which patients have ended up in that particular situation. As an example, consider a group of ambulant outpatients presenting with symptoms of venous thromboembolism without having this disease compared to a group of inpatients suspected of venous thromboembolism but actually having a malignancy. The specificity of a D-dimer test in outpatients will be lower than that in inpatients.[24]

• *Referral filter.* The discriminatory power of tests often varies across settings because patients presenting with a clinical problem in one setting – for example primary care – are very different from those presenting to a secondary care facility with that clinical problem.[25,26] Patients who are referred to secondary care may be those with a more difficult diagnostic problem, in whom the usual tests have not resolved the uncertainty. These patients have been through a referral filter to get to the tertiary care centre.

This concept can best be considered using the hypothetical results of a diagnostic test evaluation in primary care (Table 6.3). Imagine that patients are referred from this population to a source of secondary care, and that all the test positive patients are referred, but only a random half of the test negative patients. As shown in Table 6.4, the overall test discrimination, as reflected in the odds ratio, has not changed. However, there appears to be a shift in threshold, with an increased sensitivity and a decreased specificity.

Of course, it is unlikely that test negatives would be referred randomly; rather, it may be on the grounds of other clinical information that the practitioner is particularly concerned about those test negatives. If the practitioner is correct in identifying patients about whom there is an increased risk of disease, the table could well turn out like Table 6.5.

In this case, because of the clinician's skill and the use of other information, not only does the test threshold appear to be shifted, but the overall test performance of the test in secondary care has been eroded, as shown by the reduced odds ratio. The more successfully the primary care practitioner detects cases that are test negative but which nevertheless need

Table 6.3 Accuracy of a test in primary care.

Test	Disease		
	Present	Absent	Total
Positive	60	40	100
Negative	40	60	100
Total	100	100	200
Sensitivity = 0.60 OR = 2.25			
Specificity = 0.60			

Table 6.4 Test accuracy if a random sample of test negatives are referred for verification.

Test	Disease		
	Present	Absent	Total
Positive	60	40	100
Negative	20	30	50
Total	80	70	150
Sensitivity = 0.75 OR = 2.25			
Specificity = 0.43			

Table 6.5 Diagnostic performances vary by setting because of selective patient referral.

Test	Disease		
	Present	Absent	Total
Positive	60	40	100
Negative	25	25	50
Total	85	65	150
Sensitivity = 0.71 OR = 1.5			
Specificity = 0.38			

referral for management of the disease of interest, the more the performance of the test in secondary care is eroded.

- *To what prior tests is the incremental value of the new test being assessed?* In many situations several tests are being used and the value of a particular test may depend on what tests have been done before,[27] or simple prior clinical information.[28,29] In Table 6.6 two tests are cross-classified within diseased and non-diseased people. The sensitivity and specificity of each test is 0.6, and they remain 0.6 if test B is used after test A, that is, the test performance characteristics of B remain unaltered in categories of patients who are A positive and those who are A negative.

However, if the tests are conditionally dependent or associated with each other within diseased and non-diseased groups, for example because they both measure a similar metabolite, then the overall test performance of B is eroded, as judged by the OR changing from 2.25 to 2.00 (Table 6.7 and Figure 6.3). In addition, there appears to be a threshold shift: the test is more sensitive but less specific in patients for whom A is positive than in those for whom A is negative. In other words, not only is the *discrimination* of the new test (B) less if done after the existing test (A), as judged by the odds ratio, but the *calibration* appears to differ depending on the result of the prior test. In fact, the threshold has not altered but there has been a

Table 6.6 Incremental value when tests A and B are conditionally independent.

	Have disease			No disease		
	A+	A−	Total	A+	A−	Total
B+	36	24	60	16	24	40
B−	24	16	40	24	36	60
Total	60	40	100	40	60	100

"Crude" sensitivity and specificity of both A and B = 0.6 and odds ratio = 2.25.
If A is + or −, SnB = 0.6, SpB = 0.6 and OR = 2.25.

Table 6.7 Incremental value when tests A and B are conditionally dependent.

	Have disease			No disease		
	A+	A−	Total	A+	A−	Total
B+	40	20	60	20	20	40
B−	20	20	40	20	40	60
Total	60	40	100	40	60	100

"Crude" sensitivity and specificity of both A and B = 0.6.
Odds ratio = 2.25.
If A +, SnB = 0.67, SpB = 0.50 and OR = 2.00.
If A −, SnB = 0.50, SpB = 0.67 and OR = 2.00.

ROC curves for test B under different conditions

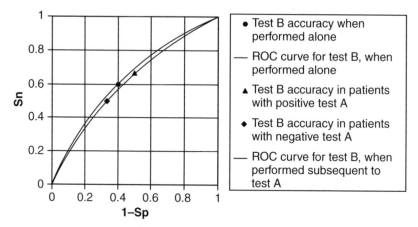

Figure 6.3 Test characteristics for test B alone and in those with positive and negative test A.

shift in the distribution of test results in diseased and non-diseased groups, conditional on the results of test A.

An example is provided by Mol and colleagues,[30] who evaluated the performance of serum hCG (human chorionic gonadotrophin) measurement in the diagnosis of women with suspected ectopic pregnancy. Several studies have reported an adequate sensitivity of this test.[30] However, the presence of an ectopic or intrauterine pregnancy can also be diagnosed with ultrasound. Mol et al. reported the sensitivity of hCG to be significantly different in patients with signs of an ectopic pregnancy (adnexal mass, or fluid in the pouch of Douglas) on ultrasound, compared to those without signs on ultrasound. As a consequence, an uncritical generalisation of the "unconditional" sensitivity will overestimate the diagnostic performance of this test if it is applied after an initial examination with ultrasound, as is the case in clinical practice.[30]

Categories of patients for whom new tests are most helpful are worth investigating. For example, whole-body positron emission tomography (PET) contributed most additional diagnostic information in the subgroup of patients in whom prior conventional diagnostic methods had been equivocal.[31]

The comparison: replacement or incremental test

Note that a new test may be evaluated as a *replacement* for the existing test, rather than being done after the existing test, in which case the *incremental* value is of interest. For assessment of replacement value, the cross-classification of the tests is not necessary to obtain unbiased estimates of how the diagnostic performance of the new test differs from that of the existing one. However, information about how they are associated from a cross-classification will provide extra useful information and improve precision.[32]

Readers may have noticed that the issue of incremental value and the decreased test performance if tests are conditionally dependent is related to the prior issue of decreased test performance if the primary care clinician is acting as an effective referral filter. In our previous example, imagine that the test being evaluated is B. The clinician may be using test A to alter the mix of A+ and A−s that get through to secondary care, and the test performance of B reflects the way in which this mix has occurred.

The test

- *Discriminatory power.* Information about the test is relevant to both discriminative power and calibration. Discrimination may differ between tests that bear the same generic name but which, for example, are made by different manufacturers. Tests may be less discriminatory when produced in "kit" form than in initial laboratory testing.[33] When tests require interpretative skill, they are often first evaluated in near-optimal situations. Special attention is usually devoted to the unambiguous and reproducible interpretation of test results. This has implications for the interpretation and generalisability of the results. If the readers of images are less than optimal in your own clinical setting, test accuracy will be affected downward.[34-36]

The usual presentation deals with a two-way definition of test results, into positive and negative. In many cases, *multiple categories of test results* is more plausible. In addition, there may be a category of uninterpretable test results that needs to be considered. The polytomous nature of tests should be taken into account, for which several methods are available. Rather than a simple positive–negative dichotomy and the associated characteristics sensitivity and specificity, likelihood ratios for the multiple categories and ROC curves can be calculated (see Chapter 7). In all cases, a more general $n \times n$ table can be used to describe test characteristics, and several likelihoods can be calculated.[16]

- *Calibration.* If the purpose of the study is clinical decision making, in which information is being derived to estimate probablilities of disease, then a second major issue is the calibration of test results. A continuous test may have equivalent ROCs and diagnostic ORs in two different settings, but very different likelihood ratios (LRs). For example, machine calibration may be different in the two settings, so that one machine may show results considerably higher than another. Likewise, even if two readers of radiographs have similar discriminative power, as shown by similar ROCs, the threshold they use to differentiate positive from negative tests (or adjacent categories of a multicategory test) may vary widely.[37-40]

In summary, variability in the discriminative power and calibration of the same test used in different places is the rule rather than the exception.

When we strive for parsimony in our descriptions, we run the risk of oversimplification. In the end, the researcher who reports a study, as well as the clinician searching the literature for help in interpreting test results, has to bear in mind that test performance characteristics are never just properties of the test itself: they depend on several factors, including prior clinical and test information, and the setting in which the test is done.

2. Implications of variation in discriminative power and calibration of tests: questions to ask yourself before you start designing the study

1 What is the target condition and the reference standard?
2 Is the objective to estimate test performance using a global measure, or a measure that will allow estimation of the probability of disease in individuals?
3 What is the population and clinical problem?
4 Is the test being considered as a replacement or incremental test?
5 To what extent do you want to study the reasons for variability of the results within your population?
6 To what extent do you want to study the transferability of the results to other settings?

In what follows, we assume that the usual criteria for adequate design of an evaluation of a diagnostic test have been fulfilled. The issue is then: How do we design a study which will also help to ensure that its transferability can be determined? Based on the concepts in the first part of this chapter, we suggest that investigators ask themselves the following questions to help ensure that readers have the necessary information to decide on the transferability of the study to their own setting.

1. What is the target condition and reference standard?

The target condition and reference standard need to be chosen to reflect the investigator's requirements. Is the choice appropriate to whether the investigator is doing the study to assist with predicting prognosis, deciding as the need for intervention, or researching pathological processes? For example, in a study of tests to assess stenosis of the carotid artery, it would be sensible to choose the reference standard as angiographic stenosis dichotomised around 70%, if this is the level of angiographic abnormality above which, on currently available evidence, the benefits of treatment outweigh the harm. On the other hand, if the study is being done by researchers whose interest is in basic science, they may wish to compare the test with stenosis assessed on surgically removed specimens at a different threshold, or across a range of thresholds.

Error in the reference standard is a major constraint on our ability to estimate test accuracy and explore reasons for variability of test characteristics.[18,19,41] Therefore, researchers should consider methods of minimising error in the reference standard, for example by using better methods or multiple assessments. Any information about the test performance characteristics of the reference standard will help interpretation, as will several different measures of the target condition, which can be combined. Multiple measures of the reference standard or multiple different tests also allow the use of more sophisticated analyses, such as latent class analysis, to minimise the potential for bias in estimates of test accuracy or factors that affect it.[21,42] Because the effects of misclassification in the reference standard have different effects in populations of different prevalence, as shown in Table 6.2, one may choose to assess a test in a population where any residual effects of error in the reference standard are minimised. For the odds ratio, this is at about 50% prevalence. For sensitivity it is when prevalence is high, and for specificity when prevalence is low. However, when using this strategy, consider whether the spectrum of disease may also vary with prevalence. If so, you will need to judge whether reference standard misclassification is a sufficiently important problem to outweigh the potential for spectrum bias induced by choosing a study in a population with specified prevalence.

2. Is the objective to estimate test performance using a global measure (discrimination) or a measure that will allow estimation of the probability of disease in individuals (discrimination and calibration)?

Global assessment of the discriminatory power of the test requires measures such as the area under the ROC curve, or the diagnostic odds ratio. These may be sufficient for some purposes, for example if a policy decision needs to be made about alternative tests of equivalent cost, or to decide whenever a test has sufficient accuracy to warrant further calibration. For estimating the probability of disease in individuals, likelihood ratios (or sensitivity and specificity) are needed, with additional information on how tests were calibrated. Information about calibration should be provided in papers for readers to be able to use the result of your study. Access to selected example material, such as radiographs of lesions, will help readers understand what thresholds have been used for reading in your study.

3. What is the population and clinical problem?

This question defines how the inception cohort should be selected for study, although the breadth of the group selected will also be determined by the extent to which you wish to address the following questions.

For example, a new test for carotid stenosis could be considered for all patients referred to a surgical unit. However, ultrasound is reasonably accurate at quantifying the extent of stenosis, and so investigators may choose to restrict the study of a more expensive or invasive test to patients in whom the ultrasound result is near the decision threshold for surgery. A useful planning tool is to draw a flow diagram of how patients reach the population/clinical problem of interest. This flow diagram includes what clinical information has been gathered and what tests have been done, and how the results of those tests determine entry into the population and clinical problem of interest. For example, in the flow diagram in Figure 6.4 the clinical problem is suspected appendicitis in children presenting to a hospital emergency service. The decisions based sequentially on clinical evidence and ultrasonography are shown. The flow diagram helps to clarify that computed tomography (CT) is being assessed only in patients in whom those prior tests had not resolved the clinical problem. Also as shown in the figure, in addition to being helpful at the design stage, publishing

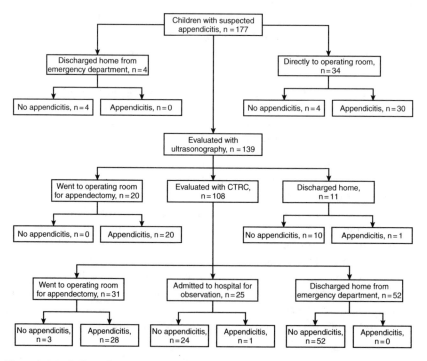

Figure 6.4 A flow diagram to formulate a diagnostic test research question. Study profile flow diagram of patients with suspected appendicitis. (From Garcia Pena BM *et al*. Ultrasonography and limited computed tomography in the diagnosis and management of appendicitis in children. *JAMA* 1999;**282**:1041–6. Reproduced with permission from the American Medical Association.[43])

such flow diagrams, with numbers of patients who follow each step, is very helpful to readers.[43]

4. Is the test being considered as a replacement or incremental test?

As outlined above, the population and the clinical problem define the initial presentation and referral filter. In addition, a key question is whether we are evaluating the test to assess whether it should replace an existing test (because it is better, or just as good and cheaper) or to assess whether it has value when used in addition to a particular existing test. This decision will also be a major determinant of how the data will be analysed.[44-46]

5. To what extent do you want to study the reasons for variability of the results within your population?

How much variability is there between readers/operators?

Data should be presented on the amount of variability between different readers or test types and tools to help calibration, such as standard radiographs,[39,40] or laboratory quality control measures. The extent to which other factors, such as experience or training, affect reading adequacy will also help guide readers of the study. Assessment of variability should include not only test discriminatory power but also calibration, if the objective is to provide study results that are useful for individual clinical decision making.

Do the findings vary in different (prespecified) subgroups within the study population?

Data should be analysed to determine the influence on test performance characteristics of the following variables, which should be available for each individual.

- The spectrum of disease and non-disease, for example by estimating "specificity" within each category of "non-disease". These can be considered separately by users or combined into a weighted specificity for different settings. The same approach can be used for levels (stage, grade) in the "diseased" group.
- The effect of other test results. This follows the approach often used in clinical prediction rules. It should take account of logical sequencing of tests (simplest, least invasive, and cheapest are generally first). It should also take account of possible effect modification by other tests. In some instances people would have been referred because of other tests being positive (or negative), so that the incremental value of the new test cannot be evaluated. In this case, knowing the referral filter and how tests have

been used in it (as in Figure 6.4) will help interpretation. For example, a study by Flamen[31] has shown that the major value of PET for recurrent colorectal adenocarcinoma is in the category of patients in whom prior (cheaper) tests gave inconclusive results. It would therefore be a useful incremental test in that category of patients, but would add little (except cost) if being considered as a replacement test for all patients, many of whom would have the diagnostic question resolved by the cheaper test. This suggests that PET is very helpful in this clinical situation.[31]

- Any other characteristics, such as age or gender.

There are often a vast number of characteristics that could be used to define subgroups in which one may wish to check whether there are differences in test performance. The essential descriptors of a clinical situation need to be decided by the researcher. As for subgroup analysis in randomised trials,[47] these characteristics should be prespecified, rather than decided at analysis stage. The decision is best made on the basis of an understanding of the pathophysiology of the disease, the mechanism by which the test assesses abnormality, an understanding of possible referral filters, and knowledge of which characteristics vary widely between centres. Remember that variability between test characteristics in subgroups may not be due to real subgroup differences if there is reference standard misclassification and the prevalence of disease differs between subgroups, as shown in Table 6.2. Modelling techniques can be used to assess the effect of several potential predictors of test accuracy simultaneously.[48–52]

6. To what extent do you want to study the transferability of the results to other settings?

To address this question, you need to perform the study in several populations or centres, and assess the extent to which test performance differs, as has been done for the General Health Questionnaire[53] and predictors of coma.[54] The extent to which observed variability is beyond that compatible with random sampling variability can be assessed using statistical tests for heterogeneity. Predictors (as discussed above) should also be measured to assess the extent to which within-population variables explain between-population variability. Because of the low power of tests of heterogeneity, this is worth doing even if tests for heterogeneity between centres or studies are not statistically significant. The more the measured variables explain between-population differences, the more they can be relied on when assessing the transferability of that study to the population in the reader's setting. Between-site variability can also be explored across different studies using meta-analytical techniques.[55,56]

Sites for inclusion in the multicentre comparison should be selected as being representative of the sorts of populations in which the results of the diagnostic study are likely to be used. The more the variability in site features can be characterised – and indeed taken account of in the sampling of sites for inclusion in studies – the more informative the study will be. Data should be analysed to determine the influence on results of the within-site (individually measured) patient characteristics mentioned above. They should also explore the following sources of between-site variability that are not accounted for by the within-site characteristics:

- Site characteristics, for example primary, secondary or tertiary care
- Other features, such as country
- Prevalence of the disease of interest.

Residual heterogeneity between sites should be explored to judge the extent to which there is inexplicable variability that may limit test applicability.

Explanatory note about prevalence

The inclusion of "prevalence" in the above list may seem unusual, as it is not obviously a predictor of test performance. However, there are many reasons why prevalence should be included in the list of potential predictors, in an analogous way to the exploration of trial result dependence on baseline risk.[57] First, many of the reasons for variation between centres may not be easy to characterise, and prevalence may contain some information about how centres differ that is not captured by other crude information, for example whether the test is evaluated in primary, secondary or tertiary care centres. Second, it is a direct test of the common assumption that test performance characteristics such as sensitivity and specificity are independent of prevalence. Third, non-linear prevalence dependence is an indication that there is misclassification of the reference standard.

In summary, there is merit in designing studies with heterogeneous study populations. This will allow exploration of the extent to which diagnostic performance depends on prespecified predictors, and how much residual

Table 6.8 The value of designing studies that enable the exploration of predictors of heterogeneity of diagnostic accuracy.

Heterogeneity in diagnostic accuracy	Heterogeneity in study population	
	Yes	No
Yes	To what extent is heterogeniety in accuracy explained by predictors? If not, transferability is limited	Transferability limited
No	Highly transferable	Design does not allow exploration of transferability

heterogeneity exists. The more heterogeneity there is in study populations, the greater the potential to explore the transferability of diagnostic performance to other settings, as shown in Table 6.8.

Concluding remarks

There is good evidence that measures of test accuracy are not as transferable across settings as is often assumed. This chapter outlines the conceptual underpinnings for this, and suggests some implications for how we should be designing studies that carry more information about the transferability of results. Major examples are examining the extent to which test discrimination and calibration depend on prespecified variables, and the extent to which there is residual variability between study populations which is not explained by these variables. This will require larger studies than have generally been done in the past for diagnostic tests. Improvements in study quality and designs to assess transferability are needed to ensure that the next generation of studies on test accuracy are more able to meet our needs.

Acknowledgement

We thank Petra Macaskill, Clement Loy, André Knottnerus, Margaret Pepe, Jonathan Craig, and Anthony Grabs for comments on earlier drafts. Clement Loy also provided Figure 6.3. We thank Barbara Garcia Pena for permission to use a figure from her paper as our Figure 6.4.

References

1 Begg C. Biases in the assessment of diagnostic tests. *Stat Med* 1987;**6**:411–23.
2 Moons K, van Es G, Deckers JW, Habbema JO, Grobbee DE. Limitations of sensitivity, specificity, likelihood ratio, and Bayes' theorem in assessing diagnostic probabilities: A clinical example. *Epidemiology* 1997; **8**:12–17.
3 Detrano R, Janosi A, Lyons KP *et al.* Factors affecting sensitivity and specificity of a diagnostic test: the exercise thallium scintigram. *Am J Med* 1988;**84**:699–710.
4 Hlatky M, Pryor D, Harrell FE Jr, Califf RM, Mark DB, Rosati RA. Factors affecting sensitivity and specificity of exercise electrocardiography. *Am J Med* 1984;**77**:64–71.
5 Rozanski ADG, Berman D, Forrester JS, Morris D, Swan HJC. The declining specificity of exercise radionuclide ventriculography. *N Engl J Med* 1983;**309**:518–22.
6 Lachs MS, Nachamkin I, Edelstein PH, Goldman J, Feinstein AR, Schwartz JS. Spectrum bias in the evaluation of diagnostic tests: lessons from the rapid dipstick test for urinary tract infection. *Ann Intern Med* 1992;**117**:135–40.
7 Molarius ASJ, Sans S, Tuomilehto J, Kuulasmaa K. Varying sensitivity of waist action levels to identify subjects with overweight or obesity in 19 populations of the WHO MONICA Project. *J Clin Epidemiol* 1999;**52**:1213–24.
8 Starmans R, Muris JW, Fijten GH, Schouten HJ, Pop P, Knottnerus JA. The diagnostic value of scoring models for organic and non-organic gastrointestinal disease, including the irritable-bowel syndrome. *Med Decision Making* 1994;**14**:208–16.

9 Glasziou P, Irwig L. An evidence-based approach to individualising treatment. *BMJ* 1995;**311**:1356–9.
10 National Health and Medical Research Council. How to use the evidence: assessment and application of scientific evidence. Handbook series on preparing clinical practice guidelines. Canberra, Commonwealth of Australia, 2000; (Website http://www.health.gov.au/nhmrc/publicat/synopses/cp65syn.htm)
11 Justice AC, Covinsky KE, Berlin JA. Assessing the generalizability of prognostic information. *Ann Intern Med* 1999;**130**:515–24.
12 Gatsonis C, McNeil BJ. Collaborative evaluations of diagnostic tests: experience of the Radiology Diagnostic Oncology Group. *Radiology* 1990;**175**:571–5.
13 Sackett D, Straus S, Richardson WS, Rosenberg W, Haynes RB. *Evidence-based Medicine: How to practice and teach EBM*. Edinburgh: Churchill Livingstone, 2000.
14 Richardson W, Wilson M, Nishikawa J, Hayward RS. The well-built clinical question: a key to evidence-based decisions. *ACP Journal Club* 1995;**123**:A12.
15 Brenner H. Measures of differential diagnostic value of diagnostic procedures. *J Clin Epidemiol* 1996;**49**:1435–9.
16 Sappenfield RW, Beeler MF, Catrou PG, Boudreau DA. Nine-cell diagnostic decision matrix. A model of the diagnostic process: a framework for evaluating diagnostic protocols. *Am J Clin Pathol* 1981;**75**:769–72.
17 Taube A, Tholander B. Over- and underestimation of the sensitivity of a diagnostic malignancy test due to various selections of the study population. *ACTA Oncol* 1990;**29**:1–5.
18 Buck A, Gart J. Comparison of a screening test and a reference test in epidemiologic studies. I. Indices of agreement and their relation to prevalence. *Am J Epidemiol* 1966;**83**:586–92.
19 Gart J, Buck A. Comparison of a screening test and a reference test in epidemiologic studies. II. A probabilistic model for the comparison of diagnostic tests. *Am J Epidemiol* 1966;**83**:593–602.
20 Kelsey JL, Whittemore AS, Evans AS, Thompson WD. *Methods in observational epidemiology*, 2nd edn. New York: Oxford University Press, 1996.
21 Walter SD, Irwig L, Glasziou PP. Meta-analysis of diagnostic tests with imperfect reference standards. *J Clin Epidemiol* 1999;**52**:943–51.
22 Ransohoff DF, Feinstein AR. Problems of spectrum and bias in evaluating the efficacy of diagnostic tests. *N Engl J Med* 1978;**299**:926–30.
23 Coley C, Barry M, Fleming C, Mulley AG. Early detection of prostate cancer. Part I: Prior probability and effectiveness of tests. *Ann Intern Med* 1997;**126**:394–406.
24 van Beek EJR, Schenk BE, Michel BC. The role of plasma D-dimer concentration in the exclusion of pulmonary embolism. *Br J Haematol* 1996;**92**:725–32.
25 Knottnerus J, Leffers P. The influence of referral patterns on the characteristics of diagnostic tests. *J Clin Epidemiol* 1992;**45**:1143–54.
26 van der Schouw YT, van Dijk R, Verbeek AL. Problems in selecting the adequate patient population from existing data files for assessment studies of new diagnostic tests. *J Clin Epidemiol* 1995;**48**:417–22.
27 Katz IA, Irwig L, Vinen JD, et al. Biochemical markers of acute myocardial infarction: strategies for improving their clinical usefulness. *Ann Clin Biochem* 1998;**35**:393–9.
28 Whitsel E, Boyko E, Siscovick DS. Reassessing the role of QT in the diagnosis of autonomic failure among patients with diabetes: a meta-analysis. *Arch Intern Med* 2000;**23**:241–7.
29 Conde-Agudelo A, Kafury-Goeta AC. Triple-marker test as screening for Down's syndrome: a meta-analysis. *Obstet Gynecol Surv* 1998;**53**:369–76.
30 Mol B, Hajenius P, Engelsbel S. Serum human chorionic gonadotrophin measurement in the diagnosis of ectopic pregnancy when transvaginal sonography is inconclusive. *Fertil Steril* 1995;**70**:972–81.
31 Flamen PSS, van Cutsem E, Dupont P, et al. Additional value of whole-body positron emission tomography with fluorine-18-2-fluoro-2-deoxy-D-glucose in recurrent colorectal cancer. *J Clin Oncol* 1999;**17**:894–901.
32 Decode Study Group. Glucose tolerance and mortality: comparison of WHO and American Diabetes Association diagnostic criteria. *Lancet* 1999;**354**:617–21.

33 Scouller K, Conigrave KM, Macaskill P, Irwig L, Whitfield JB. Should we use CDT instead of GGT for detecting problem drinkers? A systematic review and meta-analysis. *Clin Chem* 2000;**46**:1894–902.

34 West OC, Anbari MM, Pilgram TK, Wilson AJ. Acute cervical spine trauma: diagnostic performance of single-view versus three-view radiographic screening. *Radiology* 1997;**204**:819–23.

35 Scheiber CMM, Dumitresco B, Demangeat JL, *et al.* The pitfalls of planar three-phase bone scintigraphy in nontraumatic hip avascular osteonecrosis. *Clin Nucl Med* 1999;**24**:488–94.

36 Krupinski EA, Weinstein RS, Rozek LS. Experience-related differences in diagnosis from medical images displayed on monitors. *Telemed J* 1996;**2**:101–8.

37 Egglin TK, Feinstein AR. Context bias. A problem in diagnostic radiology. *JAMA* 1996;**276**:1752–5.

38 Irwig L, Groeneveld HT, Pretorius JP, Itnizdo E. Relative observer accuracy for dichotomized variables. *J Chronic Dis* 1985;**28**:899–906.

39 D'Orsi C, Swets J. Variability in the interpretation of mammograms. *N Engl J Med* 1995;**332**:1172.

40 Beam C, Layde P, Sullivan DC. Variability in the interpretation of screening mammograms by US radiologists. Findings from a national sample. *Arch Intern Med* 1996;**156**:209–13.

41 Valenstein PN. Evaluating diagnostic tests with imperfect standards. *Am J Clin Pathol* 1990;**93**:252–8.

42 Walter S, Irwig L. Estimation of test error rates, disease prevalence and relative risk from misclassified data: A review. *J Clin Epidemiol* 1988;**41**:923–37.

43 Garcia Pena BM, Mandl KD, Kraus SJ, *et al.* Ultrasonography and limited computed tomography in the diagnosis and management of appendicitis in children. *JAMA* 1999;**282**:1041–6.

44 Marshall R. The predictive value of simple rules for combining two diagnostic tests. *Biometrics* 1989;**45**:1213–22.

45 Biggerstaff B. Comparing diagnostic tests: a simple graphic using likelihood ratios. *Statistics Med* 2000;**19**:649–63.

46 Chock C, Irwig L, Berry G, Glaszion P. Comparing dichotomous screening tests when individuals negative on both tests are not verified. *J Clin Epidemiol* 1997;**50**:1211–17.

47 Oxman A, Guyatt G. A consumer guide to subgroup analyses. *Ann Intern Med* 1992;**116**:78–84.

48 Tosteson ANA, Weinstein MC, *et al.* ROC curve regression analysis: the use of ordinal regression models for diagnostic test assessment. *Environ Health Perspect* 1994;**102**(Suppl 8):73–8.

49 Toledano A, Gatsonis C. Ordinal regression methodology for ROC curves derived from correlated data. *Statistics Med* 1996;**15**:1807–26.

50 Pepe M. An interpretation for the ROC curve and inference using GLM procedures. *Biometrics* 2000;**56**:352–9.

51 Leisenring W, Pepe M. Regression modelling of diagnostic likelihood ratios for the evaluation of medical diagnostic tests. *Biometrics* 1998;**54**:444–52.

52 Leisenring W, Pepe M, Longton G. A marginal regression modelling framework for evaluating medical diagnostic tests. *Statistics Med* 1997;**16**:1263–81.

53 Furukawa T, Goldberg DP. Cultural invariance of likelihood ratios for the General Health Questionnaire. *Lancet* 1999;**353**:561–2.

54 Zandbergen EGJ, de Haan RJ, *et al.* Prognostic predictors of coma transferable from one setting to another in SR. *Lancet* 1998;**352**:1808–12.

55 Irwig L, Tosteson ANA, Gatsonis C, *et al.* Guidelines for meta-analyses evaluating diagnostic tests. *Ann Intern Med* 1994;**120**:667–76.

56 Rutter C, Gatsonis C. Regression methods for meta-analysis of diagnostic test data. *Acad Radiol* 1995;**2**(Suppl 1):S48–56.

57 Schmid C, Lau J, McIntosh MW, Cappelleri JC. An empirical study of the effect of the control rate as a predictor of treatment efficacy in meta-analysis of clinical trials. *Statistics Med* 1998;**17**:1923–42.

7 Analysis of data on the accuracy of diagnostic tests

J DIK F HABBEMA, RENÉ EIJKEMANS,
PIETA KRIJNEN, J ANDRÉ KNOTTNERUS

Summary box

- Neither sensitivity nor specificity is a measure of test performance on its own. It is the combination that matters.
- The statistical approach for analysing variability in probability estimates of test accuracy is the calculation of confidence intervals.
- The magnitude of the change from pretest to post-test probability (predictive value) reflects the informativeness of the diagnostic test result.
- The informative value of a test result is determined by the likelihood ratio: the ratio of the frequencies of occurrence of this result in patients with and patients without the disease.
- The odds ratio summarises the diagnostic value of a dichotomous test, but does not tell us the specific values of sensitivity and specificity and the likelihood ratios.
- A measure of performance for a continuous test is the area under the ROC curve. This varies between 0.5 for a totally uninformative test and 1.0 for a test perfectly separating diseased and non-diseased.
- Bayes' theorem implies that "post-test odds equals pretest odds times likelihood ratio".
- One can derive the optimal cut-off from the relative importance of false positives and false negatives.
- A sensitivity analysis is important for getting a feeling for the stability of our conclusions.

- From multiple logistic regression analysis one can not only learn about the predictive value of a combination of tests, but also what a certain test adds to other tests that have already been performed.
- When starting a data analysis one must be confident that the research data have been collected with avoidance of important bias and with acceptable generalisability to the target population.

Introduction

After the painstaking job of collecting, computerising and cleaning diagnostic data, we enter the exciting phase of analysing and interpreting these data and assessing the clinical implications of the results. It would be a pity if all the effort put into the research were not to be crowned with a sound analysis and interpretation. It is the purpose of this chapter to help readers to do so.

We will study the classic test performance measures introduced in Chapter 1: sensitivity, specificity, positive and negative predictive value, likelihood ratio, and error rate, first for dichotomous tests and later, for continuous tests, including the possibility of dichotomisation, with its quest for cut-off values. ROC curves are part of this.

Next, Bayes' theorem for the relationship between pretest and post-test probability of disease is discussed, followed by decision analytical considerations. For generalisation of the one-test situation to diagnostic conclusions based on many diagnostic test results, there will be a discussion on logistic regression and its link with Bayes' theorem.

The strengths and weaknesses of study designs, possible biases, and other methodological issues have been discussed in previous chapters and will not be repeated here, although the discussion will provide some links between biases and analysis results.

We will refer to software for performing the analysis. Also, we will include appendices with tables and graphs, which can support you in the analysis.

Clinical example

Renal artery stenosis in hypertension

We use data from a study on the diagnosis of renal artery stenosis. In about 1% of all hypertensive patients the hypertension is caused by a constriction (stenosis) of the renal artery. It is worth identifying these patients because their hypertension could be cured by surgery, and consequently their risk of myocardial infarction and stroke could be

Table 7.1 The first three and last three patients of 8×437 data array from a study on diagnostics in possible renal artery stenosis (RAS).

Patient code	Age	Gender	Atherosclerotic vascular disease	Abdominal bruit	Creatinine (micromol)	Abnormal renogram	RAS on angiography
1	62	F	No	Yes	87	No	Yes
2	52	M	No	No	146	Yes	Yes
3	49	F	No	No	77	No	No
...	...	...	...	...	...	...	...
...	...	...	...	...	...	...	...
435	36	M	No	No	84	No	No
436	51	M	Yes	No	74	No	No
437	55	M	No	No	83	No	No

reduced. Moreover, renal failure could be prevented by relieving the stenosis. The definitive diagnosis of renal artery stenosis is made by renal angiography. This diagnostic reference test should be used selectively, because it is a costly procedure that can involve serious complications. Thus, clinicians need a safe, reliable, and inexpensive screening test to help them select patients for angiography.

The diagnostic tests that we will use in this chapter are clinical characteristics suggestive of renal artery stenosis, and renography; angiography serves as the reference standard test for stenosis. The clinical characteristics used as examples are symptoms and signs of atherosclerotic vascular disease, the presence of an abdominal bruit and the serum creatinine concentration. Renography is a non-invasive test for detecting asymmetry in renal function between the kidneys, which also is suggestive of renal artery stenosis.

The data, listed as indicated in Table 7.1, are from a Dutch multicentre study aiming to optimise the diagnosis and treatment of renal artery stenosis (RAS). The study included 437 hypertensive patients aged 18–75 years, who had been referred for unsatisfactory blood pressure control or for analysis of possible secondary hypertension.

Diagnostic questions and concepts

One can ask a number of questions concerning this diagnostic problem. Some are mentioned below, with the diagnostic concept concerned in parentheses.

- How good is my diagnostic test in detecting patients with RAS (sensitivity)?
- How good is my diagnostic test in detecting patients without RAS (specificity)?
- How well does a positive/abnormal test result predict the presence of RAS (positive predictive value)?

119

- How well does a negative/normal test result predict the absence of RAS (negative predictive value)?
- What is a reasonable estimate for the pretest probability of RAS (prevalence of RAS)?
- How many false conclusions will I make when applying the diagnostic test (error rate)?
- How informative is my positive/negative test result (likelihood ratio)?
- How do I summarise the association between a dichotomous test and the standard diagnosis (diagnostic odds ratio)?
- What is an optimal cut-off level when I want to dichotomise a continuous test (ROC curve)?
- To what extent does the test result change my pretest belief/probability of RAS (Bayes' theorem)?
- How are the above concepts applied to a number of diagnostic tests simultaneously (logistic regression)?

Sensitivity and specificity for a dichotomous test

We will illustrate the dichotomous test situation by assessing how well renography is able to predict arterial stenosis. Therefore we construct from our database the 2×2 table with, as entries for renographic assessment, "abnormal/normal", and for angiography, "stenosis/no stenosis" (Table 7.2).

The generic table with the corresponding symbolism is given in Table 7.3, with N = total number of patients, N_{T+} = number of patients with positive test results, N_{T-} = number of patients with negative test results,

Table 7.2 2×2 table for analysing the diagnostic value of renographic assessment in predicting renal artery stenosis.

Renography	Angiography		
	Stenosis	No Stenosis	Total
Abnormal	71	33	104
Normal	29	304	333
	100	337	437

Table 7.3 Generic 2×2 table representing possible classifications for the relationship between a diagnostic test and a diagnosis (reference test).

Test	Diagnosis		
	+	−	
+	TP	FP	N_{T+}
−	FN	TN	N_{T-}
	N_{D+}	N_{D-}	N

N_{D-} = number of patients without the disease, N_{D+} = the number of patients with the disease, TP = number of true positives, TN = number of true negatives, FP = number of false positives, and FN = number of false negatives.

Together, *sensitivity* (the probability of a positive test result in diseased subjects, $P(T+|D+)$ and *specificity* (the probability of a negative test result in non-diseased subjects, $P(T-|D-)$, characterise the dichotomous test for the clinical situation at hand. Neither is a measure of test performance on its own: it is the combination that matters.[2]

For the example in Table 7.2 we can calculate:

Sensitivity = TP/N_{D+} = 71/100 = 71%
Specificity = TN/N_{D-} = 304/337 = 90%

In the next section we will see the degree of variability with which these estimates are associated.

Sampling variability and confidence intervals for probabilities

Confidence intervals

A main challenge in the analysis of diagnostic data is to assess how confident we can be about the test characteristics as observed in our patients. This may sound strange because an observed proportion, for example the sensitivity of renography in Table 7.2 of 71%, is a fact. However, it is unlikely that we will again find exactly 71% for sensitivity in a new series of 437 similar patients, and an indication of the limits of what can reasonably be expected is therefore important (even when the same patients would have been re-examined in the same or another setting, other data will be obtained because of inter- and intraobserver variability).

The statistical method for analysing the variability in estimates of sensitivity, and of all other probability estimates that we will discuss, is confidence intervals. The probability level of the confidence interval can be chosen. A higher level of confidence corresponds to a larger interval in terms of number of percentiles covered. Throughout the chapter, we will – conventionally – work with 95% confidence intervals. The interpretation of a *95% confidence interval* for an observed proportion, that is, a probability estimate, is as follows: when the data sampling is repeated many times, the 95% confidence interval calculated from each sample will, on average, contain the "true" value of the proportion in 95% of the samples. Variability in sensitivity estimates is illustrated in Table 7.4. In part(a) of this table, the 100 stenosis patients of our study are subdivided into four groups of 25 consecutive patients. It is seen that the four subgroup sensitivities range enormously, from 48% to 88% (tables and formulae for the confidence interval will be discussed later). Part(b) illustrates what sensitivities we would have obtained if we had finished the study earlier, that is, after observing the first 5, 10, 25, 50 and 100 stenosis patients of the present study.

As you see from Table 7.4(a), the 95% confidence intervals of the highest and lowest estimates of sensitivity of 0.88 and 0.48 just touch each other. Table 7.4(b) shows that the width and the confidence interval become smaller with increasing sample size, as you would expect. For confidence intervals, and more generally for the accuracy of statistical estimates, the square root rule applies: when one makes the sample size A times as large, the confidence interval will be a factor $\sqrt{A}$ smaller. For example, for a two-times smaller confidence interval one needs four times as many patients. You can check the (approximate) validity of the square root rule in Table 7.4(b).

The confidence interval for the 71% sensitivity estimate for the total study runs from 61% to 80% (bottom line in Table 7.4). Table 7.5 gives confidence intervals for a number of confidence levels, with wider intervals for higher levels.

For the specificity of renography in diagnosing RAS we get the following confidence interval around the 90% estimate for the total number of 337 non-diseased subjects: from 87% to 93%. As you can see, the confidence

Table 7.4 Analysis of diagnostic data of patients with possible renal artery stenosis (RAS): confidence intervals for sensitivity of renography in diagnosing RAS; (a) variability in sensitivity between equal numbers of RAS patients, and (b) smaller confidence intervals with larger sample size, as cumulated during the study.

	TP	N_{D+}	Sensitivity	95% Confidence interval
(a)	18	25	0.72	0.51–0.88
	22	25	0.88	0.69–0.97
	19	25	0.76	0.55–0.91
	12	25	0.48	0.28–0.69
(b)	3	5	0.60	0.15–0.95
	7	10	0.70	0.35–0.93
	18	25	0.72	0.51–0.88
	40	50	0.80	0.66–0.90
	71	100	0.71	0.61–0.80

Table 7.5 Confidence interval for the 71% (71 out of 100) sensitivity estimate of renography in diagnosing RAS, for different confidence levels.

Confidence level (%)	Confidence interval (%)
50	67–74
67	66–76
80	64–77
90	63–78
95	61–80
99	58–82
99.9	54–84

interval is roughly half the size of the confidence interval for the sensitivity, which reflects about four times as high the number of observations on which the estimate is based (square root rule!).

Some theory and a guide to the tables in the appendix

The theory of calculating confidence intervals for proportions is based on the binomial distribution and requires complicated calculations. In general, the confidence interval is asymmetrical around the point estimate of the sensitivity, because of the "floor" and "ceiling" effects implied by the limits of 0 and 1 to any probability.

Fortunately, when the numbers are not small the 95% confidence interval becomes approximately symmetrical and the upper, and lower limits can be calculated by adding or substracting $1.96 \times$ *standard error*, with the standard error calculated by:

$$\sqrt{\hat{p}(1 - \hat{p})/N}$$

where $\hat{p}$ stands for the proportion or probability estimate, and N for the number of observations on which the proportion is based (in practice, multiplication by 2 instead of the more tedious 1.96 works well).

For other confidence levels, the multiplication factor 1.96 should be replaced by other values (see Appendix A.3).

Appendix Tables A.1 and A.2 give confidence levels for situations with small sample sizes where you need the tedious binomial calculations. Table A.3 gives the confidence interval for a number of situations in which the above formula for the standard error works well. In cases not covered by the tables, the standard error can be calculated using the formula. The reader can now verify the correctness of the confidence intervals presented in this section.

Positive and negative predictive value: pre- and post-test probability of disease

The *positive predictive value* (PPV) is the probability that the patient has the disease when the test result is positive. This "post-test probability" is easily derived from Table 7.2. For the probability of RAS in case of abnormal renography, it is:

$$PPV = P(D+ \mid T+) = TP/N_{T+} = 71/104 = 68\%$$

The confidence interval (CI) can be estimated using the formula on page 137 or Table A.3.: the 95% confidence interval for PPV runs from 59% to 77%.

The *negative predictive value* (NPV), that is, the probability that the patient has the disease if the test result is negative, translates in our case to the probability of no stenosis in case of normal renography. We get:

$$NPV = P(D- \,|\, T-) = TN/N_{T-} = 304/333 = 91\%$$

with 95% CI from 88% to 94% (see Table A.3).

The probabilities of no stenosis for an abnormal renogram and of stenosis for a normal renogram, and their CIs, are obtained as 100% minus PPV and 100% minus NPV, respectively because the probabilities of stenosis and no stenosis have to add up to 100%:

$$P(D- \,|\, T+) = 1 - P(D+ \,|\, T+) = 32\% \ (95\% \ CI: 23\% \ to \ 41\%)$$
$$P(D+ \,|\, T-) = 1 - P(D- \,|\, T-) = 9\% \ (95\% \ CI: 6\% \ to \ 12\%)$$

The PPV and NPV are *post-test* probabilities, that is, they are the updated probabilities given the information provided by the positive and negative test results, respectively. Before the test, we have the *pretest* probabilities of presence and absence of disease, which for our RAS example are:

$$P(D+) = 100/437 = 23\% \ (95\% \ CI: 19\% \ to \ 27\%)$$
$$P(D-) = 337/437 = 77\% \ (95\% \ CI: 73\% \ to \ 81\%)$$

The magnitude of the change from pre- to post-test probability reflects the informativeness of the diagnostic test result. In our case, the pretest probability of stenosis of 23% changes to 68% in case of an abnormal renogram, and to 9% in case of a normal renogram.

Error rate

How well does our diagnostic test discriminate between patients with and without stenosis, or, more generally, how well does the test discriminate between the two disease categories? So far we have only looked at partial measures of performance, such as sensitivity, specificity, and predictive values. None of these concepts on its own gives an assessment of the performance of the test.

The most straightforward measure expresses how many errors we make when we diagnose patients with an abnormal test result as diseased, and those with a normal test result as non-diseased. This concept is known as the *error rate*. For our example, the error rate is easily calculated from Table 7.1. There are 29 false negative results, as the test was negative when stenosis was present, and 33 false positive results, with the test being abnormal when there was no stenosis. Thus, in total there are 62 errors, from a total of 437 patients.

This gives the following calculations for the error rate and its confidence interval, the latter being derived from Table A.3 (the closest entry is 60 out of 500, with a half-CI size of 0.028; interpolation to 70 and 300 shows that $\pm 3\%$ is indeed the correct CI):

Error rate(ER) = 62/437 = 14% (95% CI: 11% to 17%)

The error rate is a weighted average of errors among persons with the disease (the false negatives) and among those without the disease (the false positives), as is seen from the following equation:

$$ER = P(T- | D+) \times P(D+) + P(T+ | D-) \times P(D-)$$

For our stenosis example we can easily verify this expression for the error rate:

$$ER = (29/100) \times (100/437) + (33/337) \times (337/437) = 62/437 = 14\%$$

The weights in this formula are 23%, being the pretest probability of disease, and 77% for the probability of no disease.

This equation enables us to investigate what the error rate would be if the pretest probability of disease were different. For example, if the pretest probability of disease were 50% instead of 23%, the error rate would be calculated as:

$$ER = 29/100 \times 0.5 + 33/337 \times 0.5 = 19.4\%$$

Using this formula we can speculate about the performance of the test in situations that differ from the original context (the assumption is that false positive and false negative rates do not change. This is unfortunately not always valid; see Chapters 1, 2, and 6).

Information in a diagnostic test result: the likelihood ratio

The informative value, or weight of evidence, of a test result is determined by the frequency of occurrence of this result in patients with the disease compared to those without the disease. If, for example, a certain test result occurs twice as often in patients with the disease, this result gives an evidence factor of 2 in favour of the disease. If, on the other hand, a test result occurs twice as often in patients without the disease, it gives an evidence factor of 2 in favour of non-disease, that is, a factor 2 against the disease (or a factor 1/2 in favour of disease).

This important probability ratio is called the likelihood ratio (LR). Each test result X has its own likelihood ratio $LR(X) = P(X|D+)/P(X|D-)$.

For dichotomous tests, we have only two test results, T+ and T−, and therefore also only two likelihood ratios:

the LR of a positive test result: $LR(T+) = P(T+|D+)/P(T+|D-)$
$$= Se/(1-Sp)$$

125

the LR of a negative test result: $LR(T-) = P(T- \mid D+)/P(T- \mid D-)$
$$= (1-Se)/Sp$$

For our example of renal artery stenosis, we obtain the following values for the likelihood ratio of an abnormal and a normal renogram, respectively:

$LR(T+) = 0.71/0.10 = 7.1$ with 95% CI: 5.1 to 10.3
$LR(T-) = 0.29/0.90 = 0.32$ with 95% CI: 0.24 to 0.44.

Thus, an abnormal renogram provides a factor of 7 in favour of stenosis, whereas a normal renogram yields a factor of 3 (that is, $1/0.32$) in favour of no stenosis.

The following approximate formula has been used to calculate the 95% confidence interval for the likelihood ratio:

$$\exp\left(\ln\frac{p_1}{p_2} \pm 1.96\sqrt{\frac{1-p_1}{p_1 n_1} + \frac{1-p_2}{p_2 n_2}} \right)$$

in which $p_1 = P(X \mid D+)$ is based on sample size n_1 and $p_2 = P(X \mid D-)$ on sample size n_2.[3]

Diagnostic odds ratio

For a dichotomous test it is possible to summarise the association between the test and the diagnosis (reference standard) presented in the 2×2 table in one measure: the diagnostic odds ratio (OR), which is equivalent to the cross-product of the table. Looking at the example of renal artery stenosis (Table 7.2):

$OR = (71/33)/(29/304) = (71 \times 304)/(33 \times 29) = 22.6,$
   with 95% CI: 12.4 to 41.3

The OR is equivalent to the ratio of $LR(T+)$ and $LR(T-)$, as can be easily checked in the table. The 95% confidence interval of the OR is provided by the software recommended in the references with this chapter.

The advantage of the OR is that it summarises in one figure the diagnostic association in the whole table. However, this summary measure does not tell us the specific values of the likelihood ratios of the two test results, nor those of sensitivity and specificity. These measures have to be calculated as described earlier.

Continuous tests, and their dichotomisation and trichotomisation

Another test for investigating the presence or absence of renal artery stenosis is the serum creatinine concentration. This test has a continuous

126

range of possible test results. For analysis, results can best be grouped in classes of sufficient size (Table 7.6). Each class has its own evidence for and against stenosis, as expressed in the likelihood ratio.

The theory thus far has concerned only dichotomous tests, but the specific concepts for the dichotomous test situation can be translated into more general concepts for tests with more categories. The probabilities of observing a test result for stenosis and non-stenosis patients are given in Table 7.6. The likelihood ratio is a concept linked to a specific test result, and so also applies to multicategory tests. For example, the likelihood ratio for a test result in the category 61–70 micromol can be calculated as the ratio of the likelihood of this test result in diseased and the likelihood of this result in non-diseased, that is: $(4/100)/(36/337) = 0.37$. As expected, the likelihood ratio increases with higher serum creatinine levels. The irregularity in this increasing trend in the 81–90 class reflects sampling variation, and not an underlying biological phenomenon.

We will now analyse the relationship between the multicategory test of serum creatinine described in Table 7.6 and its possible simplification to a dichotomous test. *Dichotomisation* can take place at any category boundary. This is done in Table 7.7, which gives in each row the corresponding dichotomous test data. For example, based on a cut-off level of 80 the number of patients with and without stenosis over the value of 80 is 82 and 215, respectively, resulting in a sensitivity of 82% and a specificity of 36%. Likelihood ratios can again be calculated, now for the two results of the dichotomised test. As can be seen, much information is lost by the dichotomisation. All results above and below the threshold are aggregated, and the likelihood ratio after dichotomisation becomes an average of the likelihood ratios of the individual classes above and below this threshold. Also, the question of the choice of the cut-off value is a difficult one, especially

Table 7.6 Probability of test results and diagnostic information of serum creatinine concentration in relation to renal artery stenosis.

Serum creatinine (micromol/l)	Stenosis	No stenosis	All	Likelihood ratio (95% CI)
≤60	1 (1%)	19 (6%)	20 (5%)	0.18 (0.02–1.31)
61–70	4 (4%)	36 (11%)	40 (9%)	0.37 (0.14–1.03)
71–80	13 (13%)	67 (20%)	80 (18%)	0.65 (0.38–1.13)
81–90	12 (12%)	71 (21%)	83 (19%)	0.57 (0.32–1.01)
91–100	17 (17%)	71 (21%)	88 (20%)	0.81 (0.50–1.30)
101–110	15 (15%)	41 (12%)	56 (13%)	1.23 (0.71–2.13)
111–120	7 (7%)	10 (3%)	17 (4%)	2.33 (0.92–6.04)
121–130	9 (9%)	9 (3%)	18 (4%)	3.33 (1.37–8.26)
131–150	11 (11%)	8 (2%)	19 (4%)	4.58 (1.92–11.20)
>150	11 (11%)	5 (1%)	16 (4%)	7.33 (2.64–20.84)
All	100 (100%)	337 (100%)	437 (100%)	

Table 7.7 Probability of test results and diagnostic information of dichotomised serum creatinine concentration values for nine possible cut-offs between high and low values.

Serum creatinine (Micromol)	Stenosis Se	No stenosis 1 − Sp	All	LR+	LR−
>60	99 (99%)	318 (94%)	417 (95%)	1.05	0.18
>70	95 (95%)	282 (84%)	377 (81%)	1.14	0.31
>80	82 (82%)	215 (64%)	297 (68%)	1.29	0.50
>90	70 (70%)	144 (43%)	114 (49%)	1.64	0.52
>100	53 (53%)	73 (22%)	126 (29%)	2.44	0.60
>110	38 (38%)	32 (9%)	70 (16%)	4.00	0.69
>120	31 (31%)	22 (7%)	53 (12%)	4.77	0.74
>130	22 (22%)	13 (4%)	35 (8%)	5.64	0.81
>150	11 (11%)	5 (1%)	16 (4%)	7.33	0.90
Total	100 (100%)	337 (100%)	437 (100%)		

when patients require a different amount of evidence in deciding for or against a certain further action. In our case, it could well be that some patients with a history that more clearly corroborates renal artery stenosis only need limited further evidence in order to decide for surgical intervention, whereas others need high likelihood ratios for the same decision.

The sensitivity–specificity pairs obtained for different cut-off values can be connected in a graph, yielding the so-called *ROC curve* (Figure 7.1). The more the ROC curve moves toward the left upper corner, which represents a perfect dichotomous test with 100% sensitivity and 100% specificity, the better the test is. The steepness of the slope between two adjoining cut-off points represents the likelihood ratio of an observation falling in between these two points. This is shown in Figure 7.2. The likelihood ratios in Figure 7.2 are the same as those in Table 7.6.

A measure of performance for the test is the *area under the ROC curve*.[4] This varies between 0.5 for a totally uninformative test with a likelihood ratio of 1 for all its cut-off values (the diagonal of Figure 7.1), and 1 for a test that perfectly separates diseased and non-diseased (Se=Sp=1.0). The serum creatinine has an area under the curve of 0.70 for differentiating between stenosis and non-stenosis patients. The interpretation of the value of 0.70 is as follows. Consider the hypothetical situation that two patients, drawn randomly from the stenosis patients and the non-stenosis patients respectively, are subjected to the serum creatinine test. If the test results are used to guess which of the two is the stenosis patient, the test will be right 70% of the time. The confidence interval can be calculated using a computer program (see software references).

If a continuous test such as serum creatinine has to be summarised in a few classes for further condensation of the results or for further decision

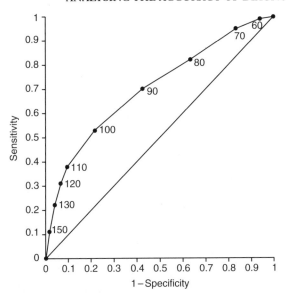

Figure 7.1 Receiver operating characteristic (ROC) curve for serum creatinine concentration in diagnosing renal artery stenosis. For each cut-off value of the serum creatinine, the probability of finding a higher value in stenosis (Se) and in non-stenosis patients (1−Sp) is plotted. The area under the ROC curve is 0.70 (95% CI 0.64–0.76).

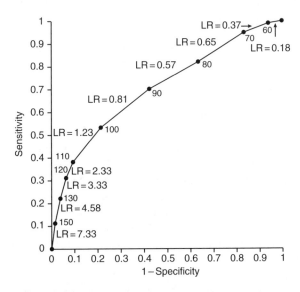

Figure 7.2 Receiver operating characteristic (ROC) curve for serum creatinine concentration in diagnosing renal artery stenosis, with the likelihood ratio for stenosis for each class of serum creatinine values.

129

Table 7.8 Probability of test results and diagnostic information of serum creatinine concentration for a trichotomisation of the test results.

Serum creatinine (Micromol/l)	Stenosis	No stenosis	All	Likelihood ratio
≤70	5 (5%)	55 (16%)	60 (14%)	0.31
71–110	57 (57%)	250 (74%)	307 (70%)	0.77
>110	38 (38%)	32 (10%)	70 (16%)	4.00
All	100 (100%)	337 (100%)	437 (100%)	

making, it is often more useful to consider a trichotomisation than a dichotomisation. In Table 7.8 we have divided the serum creatinine value into three classes, one for values giving a reasonable evidence for stenosis (likelihood ratio greater than 2.0), one for results giving reasonable evidence against stenosis (likelihood ratio smaller than 0.5), and an intermediate class for rather uninformative test results. It is seen that serum creatinine gives informative test results in about 30% of patients, whereas the test results are rather uninformative in the remaining 70%.

From pretest probability to post-test probability: Bayes' theorem

The formula for calculating how the pretest probability changes under the influence of diagnostic evidence into a post-test probability is known as Bayes' theorem. In words, this is as follows:

> "If disease was A times more probable than no disease before carrying out a certain test, and if the observed test result is B times as probable in diseased as in non-diseased subjects, then the disease is (A × B) as probable compared to no disease after the test."

A, B and A × B are respectively the pretest odds, the likelihood ratio, and the post-test odds, and a technical formulation of Bayes' theorem is therefore: "post-test odds equals pretest odds times likelihood ratio"; and in formula: $O(X) = O \times LR(X)$. An example: take the dichotomous renography test (Table 7.2). The pretest odds (A) are 100:337, or 0.30. Assuming a positive test result, the likelihood ratio B equals 7.1. Bayes' theorem tells us now that the post-test odds of disease are $0.30 \times 7.1 = 2.13$. This corresponds to a probability of $2.13/(2.13 + 1) = 0.68$, because of the relationship between probability P and odds O: $O = P/(1-P)$, and therefore $P = O/(1 + O)$.

Another example: take the category 61–70 for serum creatinine (Table 7.6) with a likelihood ratio of 0.37. In the post-test situation, stenosis is $0.30 \times 0.37 = 0.11$ times as probable as no disease. This yields a probability of stenosis of $0.11/1.11 = 0.10$.

130

It is best seen as a generalised form of Bayes' theorem, using a ...ic transformation, in order to have an additive instead of a ...ative formula. Thus "post-test odds equals pretest odds times ...d ratio", becomes, after taking the logarithm, "log post-test odds ...g pretest odds *plus* log likelihood ratio". Or, in formula form, with ...dicating "logarithm":

$$O \times LR \text{ becomes } LO(X) = LO + LLR(X)$$

...imilar generalised *formula of logistic regression* is as follows: the log ...disease, (also called logit (LO)), given test results $X_1, X_2, \ldots X_k$, is ...function of the test results:

$$\ldots, X_2, \cdots X_k) = b_0 + b_1X_1 + b_2X_2 + \cdots + b_kX_k$$

...lly, the natural logarithm (Ln) is used, as we will do in the ...der of this section. We will illustrate logistic regression by applying it ...ngle dichotomous test, because in such a case calculations are easily ...y hand. We take again the renography test for renal artery stenosis, ...ults of which were depicted in Table 7.2.

...start with the situation prior to performing the test: our best estimate ...nosis is then the prior or pretest probability, based on the observation ...ve have 100 patients with and 337 patients without stenosis. The ...c formula in this case $LnO = b_0$, and contains only a constant b_0, ...se no tests have been performed yet. Thus b_0, the Ln pretest odds, ...in this case is Ln $(100/337) = -1.21$.

...xt the renography test is performed. The test result is coded as $X_1 = 0$ ...nal) or $X_1 = 1$ (abnormal), and the logistic formula is $LnO(X_1) = b_0 +$ ...We will derive the coefficients b_0 and b_1 by applying the log odds ...of Bayes' theorem to both the normal and the abnormal test results. ...logistic formula follows immediately from the results.

...case of a normal renogram ($X_1 = 0$) there are 29 patients with and 304 ...ents without stenosis in Table 7.2. Bayes' theorem tells that the log odds ...stenosis for result $X_1 = 0$, $LnO(X_1 = 0) = Ln(29/304) = -2.35$, equals ...Ln pretest odds of -1.21 plus the Ln likelihood ratio of a normal ...ogram, which is -1.14.

...case of an abnormal renogram ($X_1 = 1$) there are 71 patients with and ...patients without stenosis, and $LnO(X_1 = 1) = Ln(71/33) = 0.77$, being ...Ln pretest odds of -1.21 plus the Ln likelihood ratio 1.98 of an ...ormal renogram. Combining the two applications of Bayes' theorem, ...get:

$$O(X_1) = -1.21 - 1.14 \text{ (when } X_1 = 0) + 1.98 \text{ (when } X_1 = 1).$$

...is can be simplified to the logistic formula:

$$nO(X_1) = b_0 + b_1X_1 = -2.35 + 3.12 \, X_1.$$

4

The formula of Bayes' theorem for directly calculating the post-test probability is as follows:

$$P(D+ \,|\, X) = \frac{P(D+) \times P(X\,|\,D+)}{P(D+) \times P(X\,|\,D+) + P(D-) \times P(X\,|\,D-)}$$

For dichotomous test we can express this formula in terms of sensitivity (Se) and specificity (Sp), and positive and negative predictive values (PPV and NPV), as can also be easily derived from the (2×2) Tables 7.2 and 7.3:

$$PPV = \frac{P(D+) \times Se}{P(D+) \times Se + P(D-) \times (1 - Sp)} \quad \text{and}$$

$$NPV = \frac{P(D-) \times Sp}{P(D-) \times Sp + P(D+) \times (1 - Se)}$$

Figure 7.3 gives a graphical presentation of Bayes' theorem and enables you to directly calculate the post-test probability from pretest probability and likelihood ratio. The two examples described earlier can be graphically

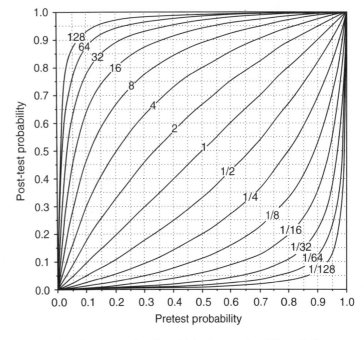

Figure 7.3 Graphical presentation in which the result of Bayes' theorem can be read for a number of likelihood ratios. Each curve represents one likelihood ratio. For example, a pretest probability of 0.7 and a likelihood ratio of 4 give rise to a post-test probability of about 0.90.

131

verified with a pretest probability of stenosis of 23%: a likelihood ratio of 7.1 gives a post-test probability of 68%, and a likelihood ratio of 0.37 gives a post-test probability of 10% (these post-test probabilities can only be read approximately in the figure). For an alternative, nomogram type of representation of Bayes' theorem, see Chapter 2, Figure 2.1.

Decision analytical approach of the optimal cut-off value

The error rate is a good measure of test performance, as it gives the number of false positives and false negatives in relation to the total number of diagnostic judgements made. It should be realised that the error rate implicitly assumes that false positives and false negatives have an equal weight. This may not be reasonable: for example a missed stenosis may be judged as much more serious than a missed non-stenosis. Here we enter the realm of decision science, where the loss of wrong decisions is explicitly taken into account. As an appetiser to decision analysis, look at Table 7.9. This is based on Table 7.7, but now with an indication of how many false positives are additionally avoided and how many additional false negatives are induced by increasing the threshold between positive and negative ("cut-off") with one class of serum creatinine values at a time.

With the (uninteresting) cut-off value of 0, we would have 337 false positives (FP) and 0 false negatives (FN). Increasing the threshold from 0 to 60 would decrease the FP by 19 and increase the FN by 1. A shift from 60 to 70 would decrease the FP by 36 and increase the FN by four, and so on, until the last step in cut-off from 150 to "very high" serum creatinine

Table 7.9 Decrease in false positives and increase in false negatives when increasing the cut-off between high and low serum creatinine values by one class at a time. Eleven possible cut-offs are considered.

Serum creatinine (micromol/l)	No stenosis	Stenosis	FP decrease: FN increase per step	Approximate trade-off
>0	337	100	337:0	
>60	318	99	19:1	20:1
>70	282	95	36:4	10:1
>80	215	82	67:13	5:1
>90	144	70	71:12	5:1
>100	73	53	71:17	5:1
>110	32	38	41:15	3:1
>120	22	31	10:7	1:1
>130	13	22	9:9	1:1
>150	5	11	8:11	1:1
"Very high"	0	0	5:11	1:2
Total	337	100		

values, by which the last five FP are preven patients are turned into FN.

One can derive the optimal cut-off from positives and false negatives. For example, i be four times more serious than a false neg 100, because all shifts in cut-off between 0 ar least five FN to one FP, which is better tha relative seriousness of the two types of error. A is not indicated because the associated trade- FP or more, which is worse than the 4:1 judge pretest values of stenosis the FN:FP trade-of also the optimal threshold. For example, if the times higher, the threshold would shift to 60 (c

For a further study of decision analytical co referred to Sox et al.[5]

Sensitivity analysis

In a sensitivity analysis we look at what woul conclusions in case of other, but plausible, assum for getting a feeling for the stability of the conclus

We saw an example of a sensitivity analysis in ou rate, when we looked what the error rate would probability of stenosis had been different from the

Sensitivity analysis could also be conducted graphical representation of Bayes' theorem. Using t for the pretest probability and for the likelihood r associated uncertainty in the post-test probability. I have a confidence interval for the pretest probability and a confidence interval for the likelihood ratio of ou 4 and 8, Figure 7.3 tells us that values for the post-tes 0.8 and 0.95 are possible.

A third type of sensitivity analysis could be dor seriousness of false positive and false negative results i threshold between positive and negative test results will values for this relative seriousness are considered.

"Many" diagnostic tests: logistic regressio

The analysis of many diagnostic tests is more complicate of a single diagnostic test. There is, however, a standard logistic regression, that can be applied in this situatio method for the analysis of binary data, such as the prese

Two remarks can be made: the coefficient b_1 (3.12) is precisely the Ln of the diagnostic odds ratio (22.6) of renography discussed earlier. And b_0 in the logistic formula can no longer be interpreted as a pretest log odds of stenosis, but as the $LnO(X_1=0)$. This completes the logistic regression analysis of one dichotomous test.

When more than one test is involved the calculations are extensions of the described single test situation, using the multiple logistic regression formula:

$$Ln(X_1, X_2, \cdots X_k) = b_0 + b_1X_1 + b_2X_2 + \cdots + b_kX_k$$

Using this approach, the investigator can account for dependency and interaction between the various tests.[7] However, such multivariate calculations are very troublesome to do by hand. In general, when many tests, including continuous tests, are involved, standard statistical software such as SPSS, SAS or BMDP will have to be used. This software also provides 95% confidence intervals for b_0, b_1, b_2, ... b_k, and the corresponding odds ratios (e^b).

From multiple logistic regression analysis one can not only learn about the predictive value of a combination of tests, but also what a certain test adds to other tests that have already been performed.

Concluding remarks

In this chapter we have given an overview of the most important performance measures of diagnostic tests, illustrated with a clinical example. Also, the estimation of confidence intervals to account for sampling variability has been explained. Furthermore, decision analytical considerations and sensitivity analysis, as methods to deal with value judgements and uncertainties, have been introduced. Finally, the principles of logistic regression to analyse the predictive value of multiple tests, when applied simultaneously, have been outlined.

In applying the presented analysis techniques it is presupposed that the research data have been collected with the avoidance of important bias (affecting internal validity) and with acceptable generalisability to the target population where the diagnostic test(s) are to be applied (external validity). These issues regarding the validity of the study design are dealt with in Chapters 1–6. As a general rule, in the analysis phase one cannot correct for shortcomings of the validity of the study design, such as bias resulting from an unclear or inappropriate process of selection of study subjects, or from an inadequate reference standard. However, if potential factors that may affect test performance are measured during the study, these can be included as independent covariables in the analysis. An example may be age as a potential effect modifier of the performance of renography. The potential influence of other possible biases can be explored using sensitivity analysis.

In the past decade, new data analytical challenges have resulted from the need to synthesise a number of studies and to analyse the pooled data of those studies (meta-analysis). Also, in such a pooled analysis the usual performance measures of diagnostic tests can be assessed, as is shown in Chapter 8. Finally, although it is always the aim to minimise the number of lost outcomes or not-performed tests, in most studies these will not be totally avoided. Although associated methodological problems are discussed in Chapter 2, there are various options for the analytical approach to such "missing values" on which professional biostatisticians can give advice.

References

1 Altman DG, Machin D, Bryant TN, Gardner MJ. *Statistics with confidence*, 2nd edn. London: BMJ Books, 2000 (includes software).
2 Sackett DL, Haynes PB, Tugwell P. *Clinical epidemiology: a basic science for clinical medicine.* Boston: Little, Brown and Co, 1985.
3 Simel DL, Samsa GP, Matchar DB. Likelihood ratios with confidence: sample size estimation for diagnostic test studies. *J Clin Epidemiol* 1991;**44**:763–70.
4 Hanley JA, McNeil BJ. The meaning and use of the area under a receiver operating characteristic (ROC) curve. *Radiology* 1982;**143**:29–36.
5 Sox HC Jr, Blatt MA, Higgins MC, Marton KI. *Medical decision making.* Stoneham, MA: Butterworths, 1988.
6 Hosmer DW, Lemeshow S. *Applied logistic regression.* New York: Wiley, 1989.
7 Knottnerus JA. Application of logistic regression to the analysis of diagnostic data: exact modeling of a probability tree of multiple binary variables. *Med Decision Making* 1992;**12**:93–108.

Software

- For the analysis of test results, including logistic regression for single and multiple tests and confidence intervals for the diagnostic odds ratio, standard statistical software such as SPSS, SAS or BMDP may be used. In SPSS and SAS analysis of the area under the ROC curve (plus confidence intervals) can be performed.
- Visual Bayes is a freely available program introducing basic methods for the interpretation and validation of diagnostic tests in an intuitive way. It may be downloaded from http://www.imbi.uni-freiburg.de/medinf.
- Treeage-DATA is a decision analysis program in which diagnostic tests and subsequent treatment decisions can be represented. Good opportunities for sensitivity analysis.

Appendix: Tables for confidence intervals for proportions

Table A.1–A.2 Exact confidence intervals for proportions based on small N (**Table A.1**) or on small n (**Table A.2**).

Table A.3 Half 95% confidence intervals for proportions.

For all tables N = number of observations (denominator), n = number of successes (numerator).

Table A.1 Example: In a group of five patients with renal artery stenosis, three were positive on diagnostic renography. The estimated sensitivity of renography is therefore 3/5, that is, 0.6 with 95% confidence interval (0.15–0.95).

Table A.2 Exact confidence intervals for small n. Because the binomial distribution is symmetric around $p = 0.5$, the table can also be used for small values of N-n: when using N-n instead of n the resulting confidence interval changes to $(1 - \text{upper limit}, 1 - \text{lower limit})$.

Example for small n: A new screening test for a disease is required to have a very low false positive rate that is, high specificity. In a sample of 200 proven non-diseased subjects only one had a positive test result. The false positive rate is estimated at $1/200 = 0.005$ and the exact 95% confidence interval is (0.000–0.028)

Example for small N-n: In the previous example we can estimate the specificity as $199/200 = 0.995$, with 95% confidence interval (0.972–1.000).

Table A.3 The half 95% confidence interval for proportions, based on the normal approximation to the binomial distribution for large numbers of observations. With this approximation, the half 95% confidence interval for a proportion $\hat{p} = n/N$ is $1.96 \times SE$, with SE being the standard error. The 95% confidence interval is constructed by subtracting (lower confidence limit) or adding (upper confidence limit) the number from the table to the estimate p. By symmetry the values for n and for N-n are the same. When the values of n and N are not given directly in the table, linear interpolation for n and/or N may be used.

Example

In a group of 333 patients with a negative renography, 29 nevertheless appeared to suffer from renal artery stenosis. The estimated negative predictive value (NPV) of renography is therefore (333–29)/333, that is, 0.91.

The value from the table is required for $N = 333$ and N-$n = 29$. We use linear interpolation for N. At $N = 300$, the table gives a value of 0.0335 and at $N = 500$ the value is 0.0205, for $n = 29$, taking the averages of the values for $n = 28$ and 30.

Linear interpolation at $N = 333$ requires:
({Value at $N = 333$} $- 0.0355) : (0.0205 - 0.0335) = (333 - 300) : (500 - 300)$. Thus {Value at $N = 333$} $= 0.03$.
The 95% confidence interval becomes $(0.91 - 0.03, 0.91 + 0.03) = (0.88 - 0.94)$.

Note 1

Instead of interpolation, the formula for SE could have been used directly:

$$SE = \sqrt{\frac{\hat{p}(1 - \hat{p})}{N}}, \text{ giving SE} = \sqrt{\frac{\frac{304}{333}\left(1 - \frac{29}{333}\right)}{333}} = 0.0154$$

Multiplying by 1.96 gives a value of 0.03 for the half 95% confidence interval.

Note 2

For other levels of confidence the numbers in Table A.3 have to be multiplied by a factor. The following table gives multiplication factors for a few commonly used levels of confidence:

Confidence level (%)	Multiplication factor
50	0.34
67	0.49
80	0.65
90	0.84
95	1
99	1.31
99.9	1.68

Table A.1 Exact 95% confidence intervals for proportions n/N for N from 2 to 25

n	p	95% CI		n	p	95% CI		n	p	95% CI	

n	p	95% CI		n	p	95% CI		n	p	95% CI	
	$N=2$				$N=8$(cont'd)				$N=12$(cont'd)		
0	0	0.00	0.78	3	0.38	0.09	0.76	2	0.17	0.02	0.48
1	0.5	0.01	0.99	4	0.5	0.16	0.84	3	0.25	0.05	0.57
2	1	0.22	1.00	5	0.63	0.24	0.91	4	0.33	0.10	0.65
				6	0.75	0.35	0.97	5	0.42	0.15	0.72
[$N=3$]				7	0.88	0.47	1.00	6	0.5	0.21	0.79
				8	1	0.69	1.00	7	0.58	0.28	0.85
0	0	0.00	0.63					8	0.67	0.35	0.90
1	0.33	0.01	0.91					9	0.75	0.43	0.95
2	0.67	0.09	0.99		$N=9$			10	0.83	0.52	0.98
3	1	0.37	1.00	0	0	0.00	0.28	11	0.92	0.62	1.00
				1	0.11	0.00	0.48	12	1	0.78	1.00
[$N=4$]				2	0.22	0.03	0.60				
				3	0.33	0.07	0.70		$N=13$		
0	0	0.00	0.53	4	0.44	0.14	0.79				
1	0.25	0.01	0.81	5	0.56	0.21	0.86	0	0	0.00	0.21
2	0.5	0.07	0.93	6	0.67	0.30	0.93	1	0.08	0.00	0.36
3	0.75	0.19	0.99	7	0.78	0.40	0.97	2	0.15	0.02	0.45
4	1	0.47	1.00	8	0.89	0.52	1.00	3	0.23	0.05	0.54
				9	1	0.72	1.00	4	0.31	0.09	0.61
[$N=5$]								5	0.38	0.14	0.68
					$N=10$			6	0.46	0.19	0.75
0	0	0.00	0.45					7	0.54	0.25	0.81
1	0.2	0.01	0.72	0	0	0.00	0.26	8	0.62	0.32	0.86
2	0.4	0.05	0.85	1	0.1	0.00	0.45	9	0.69	0.39	0.91
3	0.6	0.15	0.95	2	0.2	0.03	0.56	10	0.77	0.46	0.95
4	0.8	0.28	0.99	3	0.3	0.07	0.65	11	0.85	0.55	0.98
5	1	0.55	1.00	4	0.4	0.12	0.74	12	0.92	0.64	1.00
				5	0.5	0.19	0.81	13	1	0.79	1.00
[$N=6$]				6	0.6	0.26	0.88				
				7	0.7	0.35	0.93		$N=14$		
0	0	0.00	0.39	8	0.8	0.44	0.97				
1	0.17	0.00	0.64	9	0.9	0.55	1.00	0	0	0.00	0.19
2	0.33	0.04	0.78	10	1	0.74	1.00	1	0.07	0.00	0.34
3	0.5	0.12	0.88					2	0.14	0.02	0.43
4	0.67	0.22	0.96		$N=11$			3	0.21	0.05	0.51
5	0.83	0.36	1.00					4	0.29	0.08	0.58
6	1	0.61	1.00	0	0	0.00	0.24	5	0.36	0.13	0.65
				1	0.09	0.00	0.41	6	0.43	0.18	0.71
[$N=7$]				2	0.18	0.02	0.52	7	0.5	0.23	0.77
				3	0.27	0.06	0.61	8	0.57	0.29	0.82
0	0	0.00	0.35	4	0.36	0.11	0.69	9	0.64	0.35	0.87
1	0.14	0.00	0.58	5	0.45	0.17	0.77	10	0.71	0.42	0.92
2	0.29	0.04	0.71	6	0.55	0.23	0.83	11	0.79	0.49	0.95
3	0.43	0.10	0.82	7	0.64	0.31	0.89	12	0.86	0.57	0.98
4	0.57	0.18	0.90	8	0.73	0.39	0.94	13	0.93	0.66	1.00
5	0.71	0.29	0.96	9	0.82	0.48	0.98	14	1	0.81	1.00
6	0.86	0.42	1.00	10	0.91	0.59	1.00				
7	1	0.65	1.00	11	1	0.76	1.00		$N=15$		
								0	0	0.00	0.18
[$N=8$]					$N=12$			1	0.07	0.00	0.32
								2	0.13	0.02	0.40
0	0	0.00	0.31	0	0	0.00	0.22	3	0.2	0.04	0.48
1	0.13	0.00	0.53	1	0.08	0.00	0.38				
2	0.25	0.03	0.65								

Table A.1 Continued

n	p	95% CI		n	p	95% CI		n	p	95% CI	
N=15(cont'd)				**N=18**				**N=20(cont'd)**			
4	0.27	0.08	0.55	0	0	0.00	0.15	7	0.35	0.15	0.59
5	0.33	0.12	0.62	1	0.06	0.00	0.27	8	0.4	0.19	0.64
6	0.4	0.16	0.68	2	0.11	0.01	0.35	9	0.45	0.23	0.68
7	0.47	0.21	0.73	3	0.17	0.04	0.41	10	0.5	0.27	0.73
8	0.53	0.27	0.79	4	0.22	0.06	0.48	11	0.55	0.32	0.77
9	0.6	0.32	0.84	5	0.28	0.10	0.53	12	0.6	0.36	0.81
10	0.67	0.38	0.88	6	0.33	0.13	0.59	13	0.65	0.41	0.85
11	0.73	0.45	0.92	7	0.39	0.17	0.64	14	0.7	0.46	0.88
12	0.8	0.52	0.96	8	0.44	0.22	0.69	15	0.75	0.51	0.91
13	0.87	0.60	0.98	9	0.5	0.26	0.74	16	0.8	0.56	0.94
14	0.93	0.68	1.00	10	0.56	0.31	0.78	17	0.85	0.62	0.97
15	1	0.82	1.00	11	0.61	0.36	0.83	18	0.9	0.68	0.99
				12	0.67	0.41	0.87	19	0.95	0.75	1.00
[N = 16]				13	0.72	0.47	0.90	20	1	0.86	1.00
0	0	0.00	0.17	14	0.78	0.52	0.94				
1	0.06	0.00	0.30	15	0.83	0.59	0.96	**N = 21**			
2	0.13	0.02	0.38	16	0.89	0.65	0.99				
3	0.19	0.04	0.46	17	0.94	0.73	1.00	0	0	0.00	0.13
4	0.25	0.07	0.52	18	1	0.85	1.00	1	0.05	0.00	0.24
5	0.31	0.11	0.59					2	0.1	0.01	0.30
6	0.38	0.15	0.65					3	0.14	0.03	0.36
7	0.44	0.20	0.70	**N = 19**				4	0.19	0.05	0.42
8	0.5	0.25	0.75	0	0	0.00	0.15	5	0.24	0.08	0.47
9	0.56	0.30	0.80	1	0.05	0.00	0.26	6	0.29	0.11	0.52
10	0.63	0.35	0.85	2	0.11	0.01	0.33	7	0.33	0.15	0.57
11	0.69	0.41	0.89	3	0.16	0.03	0.40	8	0.38	0.18	0.62
12	0.75	0.48	0.93	4	0.21	0.06	0.46	9	0.43	0.22	0.66
13	0.81	0.54	0.96	5	0.26	0.09	0.51	10	0.48	0.26	0.70
14	0.88	0.62	0.98	6	0.32	0.13	0.57	11	0.52	0.30	0.74
15	0.94	0.70	1.00	7	0.37	0.16	0.62	12	0.57	0.34	0.78
16	1	0.83	1.00	8	0.42	0.20	0.67	13	0.62	0.38	0.82
				9	0.47	0.24	0.71	14	0.67	0.43	0.85
				10	0.53	0.29	0.76	15	0.71	0.48	0.89
[N = 17]				11	0.58	0.33	0.80	16	0.76	0.53	0.92
0	0	0.00	0.16	12	0.63	0.38	0.84	17	0.81	0.58	0.95
1	0.06	0.00	0.29	13	0.68	0.43	0.87	18	0.86	0.64	0.97
2	0.12	0.01	0.36	14	0.74	0.49	0.91	19	0.9	0.70	0.99
3	0.18	0.04	0.43	15	0.79	0.54	0.94	20	0.95	0.76	1.00
4	0.24	0.07	0.50	16	0.84	0.60	0.97	21	1	0.87	1.00
5	0.29	0.10	0.56	17	0.89	0.67	0.99				
6	0.35	0.14	0.62	18	0.95	0.74	1.00	**N = 22**			
7	0.41	0.18	0.67	19	1	0.85	1.00				
8	0.47	0.23	0.72					0	0	0.00	0.13
9	0.53	0.28	0.77					1	0.05	0.00	0.23
10	0.59	0.33	0.82	**N = 20**				2	0.09	0.01	0.29
11	0.65	0.38	0.86	0	0	0.00	0.14	3	0.14	0.03	0.35
12	0.71	0.44	0.90	1	0.05	0.00	0.25	4	0.18	0.05	0.40
13	0.76	0.50	0.93	2	0.1	0.01	0.32	5	0.23	0.08	0.45
14	0.82	0.57	0.96	3	0.15	0.03	0.38	6	0.27	0.11	0.50
15	0.88	0.64	0.99	4	0.2	0.06	0.44	7	0.32	0.14	0.55
16	0.94	0.71	1.00	5	0.25	0.09	0.49	8	0.36	0.17	0.59
17	1	0.84	1.00	6	0.3	0.12	0.54	9	0.41	0.21	0.64
								10	0.45	0.24	0.68

Table A.1 Continued

n	p	95% CI		n	p	95% CI		n	p	95% CI	
	N=22(cont'd)				*N*=23(cont'd)				*N*=24(cont'd)		
11	0.5	0.28	0.72	17	0.74	0.52	0.90	22	0.92	0.73	0.99
12	0.55	0.32	0.76	18	0.78	0.56	0.93	23	0.96	0.79	1.00
13	0.59	0.36	0.79	19	0.83	0.61	0.95	24	1	0.88	1.00
14	0.64	0.41	0.83	20	0.87	0.66	0.97				
15	0.68	0.45	0.86	21	0.91	0.72	0.99				
16	0.73	0.50	0.89	22	0.96	0.78	1.00		*N* = 25		
17	0.77	0.55	0.92	23	1	0.88	1.00	0	0	0.00	0.11
18	0.82	0.60	0.95					1	0.04	0.00	0.20
19	0.86	0.65	0.97					2	0.08	0.01	0.26
20	0.91	0.71	0.99		*N* = 24			3	0.12	0.03	0.31
21	0.95	0.77	1.00	0	0	0.00	0.12	4	0.16	0.05	0.36
22	1	0.87	1.00	1	0.04	0.00	0.21	5	0.2	0.07	0.41
				2	0.08	0.01	0.27	6	0.24	0.09	0.45
				3	0.13	0.03	0.32	7	0.28	0.12	0.49
[*N* = 23]				4	0.17	0.05	0.37	8	0.32	0.15	0.54
0	0	0.00	0.12	5	0.21	0.07	0.42	9	0.36	0.18	0.57
1	0.04	0.00	0.22	6	0.25	0.10	0.47	10	0.4	0.21	0.61
2	0.09	0.01	0.28	7	0.29	0.13	0.51	11	0.44	0.24	0.65
3	0.13	0.03	0.34	8	0.33	0.16	0.55	12	0.48	0.28	0.69
4	0.17	0.05	0.39	9	0.38	0.19	0.59	13	0.52	0.31	0.72
5	0.22	0.07	0.44	10	0.42	0.22	0.63	14	0.56	0.35	0.76
6	0.26	0.10	0.48	11	0.46	0.26	0.67	15	0.6	0.39	0.79
7	0.3	0.13	0.53	12	0.5	0.29	0.71	16	0.64	0.43	0.82
8	0.35	0.16	0.57	13	0.54	0.33	0.74	17	0.68	0.46	0.85
9	0.39	0.20	0.61	14	0.58	0.37	0.78	18	0.72	0.51	0.88
10	0.43	0.23	0.66	15	0.63	0.41	0.81	19	0.76	0.55	0.91
11	0.48	0.27	0.69	16	0.67	0.45	0.84	20	0.8	0.59	0.93
12	0.52	0.31	0.73	17	0.71	0.49	0.87	21	0.84	0.64	0.95
13	0.57	0.34	0.77	18	0.75	0.53	0.90	22	0.88	0.69	0.97
14	0.61	0.39	0.80	19	0.79	0.58	0.93	23	0.92	0.74	0.99
15	0.65	0.43	0.84	20	0.83	0.63	0.95	24	0.96	0.80	1.00
16	0.7	0.47	0.87	21	0.88	0.68	0.97	25	1	0.89	1.00

Table A.2 Exact 95% confidence intervals for proportions n/N for small n (0–7) and $N = 30, 35, \ldots, 70, 80, 90, 100, 120, 150, 200, 300, 500, 1000, 2000$.

N	n = 0	1	2	3	4	5	6	7
30	0.000 0.095	0.001 0.172	0.008 0.221	0.021 0.265	0.038 0.307	0.056 0.347	0.077 0.386	0.099 0.423
35	0.000 0.082	0.001 0.149	0.007 0.192	0.018 0.231	0.032 0.267	0.048 0.303	0.066 0.336	0.084 0.369
40	0.000 0.072	0.001 0.132	0.006 0.169	0.016 0.204	0.028 0.237	0.042 0.268	0.057 0.298	0.073 0.328
45	0.000 0.064	0.001 0.118	0.005 0.151	0.014 0.183	0.025 0.212	0.037 0.241	0.051 0.268	0.065 0.295
50	0.000 0.058	0.001 0.106	0.005 0.137	0.013 0.165	0.022 0.192	0.033 0.218	0.045 0.243	0.058 0.267
55	0.000 0.053	0.000 0.097	0.004 0.125	0.011 0.151	0.020 0.176	0.030 0.200	0.041 0.222	0.053 0.245
60	0.000 0.049	0.000 0.089	0.004 0.115	0.010 0.139	0.018 0.162	0.028 0.184	0.038 0.205	0.048 0.226
65	0.000 0.045	0.000 0.083	0.004 0.107	0.010 0.129	0.017 0.150	0.025 0.170	0.035 0.190	0.044 0.209
70	0.000 0.042	0.000 0.077	0.003 0.099	0.009 0.120	0.016 0.140	0.024 0.159	0.032 0.177	0.041 0.195
80	0.000 0.037	0.000 0.068	0.003 0.087	0.008 0.106	0.014 0.123	0.021 0.140	0.028 0.156	0.036 0.172
90	0.000 0.033	0.000 0.060	0.003 0.078	0.007 0.094	0.012 0.110	0.018 0.125	0.025 0.139	0.032 0.154
100	0.000 0.030	0.000 0.054	0.002 0.070	0.006 0.085	0.011 0.099	0.016 0.113	0.022 0.126	0.029 0.139
120	0.000 0.025	0.000 0.046	0.002 0.059	0.005 0.071	0.009 0.083	0.014 0.095	0.019 0.106	0.024 0.116
150	0.000 0.020	0.000 0.037	0.002 0.047	0.004 0.057	0.007 0.067	0.011 0.076	0.015 0.085	0.019 0.094
200	0.000 0.015	0.000 0.028	0.001 0.036	0.003 0.043	0.005 0.050	0.008 0.057	0.011 0.064	0.014 0.071
300	0.000 0.010	0.000 0.018	0.001 0.024	0.002 0.029	0.004 0.034	0.005 0.038	0.007 0.043	0.009 0.047
500	0.000 0.006	0.000 0.011	0.000 0.014	0.001 0.017	0.002 0.020	0.003 0.023	0.004 0.026	0.006 0.029
1000	0.000 0.003	0.000 0.006	0.000 0.007	0.001 0.009	0.001 0.010	0.002 0.012	0.002 0.013	0.003 0.014
2000	0.000 0.001	0.000 0.003	0.000 0.004	0.000 0.004	0.001 0.005	0.001 0.006	0.001 0.007	0.001 0.007

Table A.3 Half 95% confidence intervals ($=1.96 \times$ SE) of proportions n/N for $N = 30,35,\dots, 70, 80, 90, 100, 120, 150, 200, 300, 500, 1000, 2000$.

$N-n$										N									
	30	35	40	45	50	55	60	65	70	80	90	100	120	150	200	300	500	1000	2000
8	0.158	0.139	0.124	0.112	0.102	0.093	0.086	0.080	0.075	0.066	0.059	0.053	0.045	0.036	0.027	0.018	0.011	0.006	0.003
9	0.164	0.145	0.129	0.117	0.106	0.098	0.090	0.084	0.078	0.069	0.062	0.056	0.047	0.038	0.029	0.019	0.012	0.006	0.003
10	0.169	0.150	0.134	0.121	0.111	0.102	0.094	0.088	0.082	0.072	0.065	0.059	0.049	0.040	0.030	0.020	0.012	0.006	0.003
11	0.172	0.154	0.138	0.126	0.115	0.106	0.098	0.091	0.085	0.075	0.068	0.061	0.052	0.042	0.032	0.021	0.013	0.006	0.003
12	0.175	0.157	0.142	0.129	0.118	0.109	0.101	0.094	0.088	0.078	0.070	0.064	0.054	0.043	0.033	0.022	0.013	0.007	0.003
13	0.177	0.160	0.145	0.132	0.122	0.112	0.104	0.097	0.091	0.081	0.073	0.066	0.056	0.045	0.034	0.023	0.014	0.007	0.004
14	0.179	0.162	0.148	0.135	0.124	0.115	0.107	0.100	0.094	0.083	0.075	0.068	0.057	0.047	0.035	0.024	0.014	0.007	0.004
15	0.179	0.164	0.150	0.138	0.127	0.118	0.110	0.102	0.096	0.086	0.077	0.070	0.059	0.048	0.037	0.025	0.015	0.008	0.004
16		0.165	0.152	0.140	0.129	0.120	0.112	0.105	0.098	0.088	0.079	0.072	0.061	0.049	0.038	0.025	0.015	0.008	0.004
17		0.166	0.153	0.142	0.131	0.122	0.114	0.107	0.100	0.090	0.081	0.074	0.062	0.051	0.039	0.026	0.016	0.008	0.004
18		0.166	0.154	0.143	0.133	0.124	0.116	0.109	0.102	0.092	0.083	0.075	0.064	0.052	0.040	0.027	0.016	0.008	0.004
19			0.155	0.144	0.135	0.126	0.118	0.111	0.104	0.093	0.084	0.077	0.065	0.053	0.041	0.028	0.017	0.008	0.004
20			0.155	0.145	0.136	0.127	0.119	0.112	0.106	0.095	0.086	0.078	0.067	0.054	0.042	0.028	0.017	0.009	0.004
22				0.146	0.138	0.129	0.122	0.115	0.109	0.098	0.089	0.081	0.069	0.057	0.043	0.029	0.018	0.009	0.005
24					0.138	0.131	0.124	0.117	0.111	0.100	0.091	0.084	0.072	0.059	0.045	0.031	0.019	0.009	0.005
26						0.132	0.125	0.119	0.113	0.103	0.094	0.086	0.074	0.061	0.047	0.032	0.019	0.010	0.005
28							0.126	0.120	0.115	0.105	0.096	0.088	0.076	0.062	0.048	0.033	0.020	0.010	0.005
30							0.127	0.121	0.116	0.106	0.097	0.090	0.077	0.064	0.049	0.034	0.021	0.010	0.005
32								0.122	0.117	0.107	0.099	0.091	0.079	0.066	0.051	0.035	0.021	0.011	0.005
34									0.117	0.108	0.100	0.093	0.081	0.067	0.052	0.036	0.022	0.011	0.006
36										0.109	0.101	0.094	0.082	0.068	0.053	0.037	0.023	0.012	0.006

38	0.109	0.102	0.095	0.083	0.070	0.054	0.038	0.023	0.012	0.006
40	0.110	0.103	0.096	0.084	0.071	0.055	0.038	0.024	0.012	0.006
45		0.103	0.098	0.087	0.073	0.058	0.040	0.025	0.013	0.006
50			0.098	0.088	0.075	0.060	0.042	0.026	0.014	0.007
55				0.089	0.077	0.062	0.044	0.027	0.015	0.007
60				0.089	0.078	0.064	0.045	0.028	0.016	0.007
70					0.080	0.066	0.048	0.030	0.017	0.008
80						0.068	0.050	0.032	0.018	0.009
90						0.069	0.052	0.034	0.019	0.009
100						0.069	0.053	0.035	0.020	0.010
120							0.055	0.037	0.022	0.010
140							0.056	0.039	0.023	0.011
160							0.056	0.041	0.024	0.012
180								0.042	0.025	0.013
200								0.043	0.028	0.013
300									0.030	0.016
400									0.031	0.018
500										0.019
1000										0.022

8 Guidelines for conducting systematic reviews of studies evaluating the accuracy of diagnostic tests

WALTER L DEVILLÉ, FRANK BUNTINX
On behalf of an ad hoc working group of the Cochrane
Methods Group on Screening and Diagnostic Tests[*]

Summary box

- A systematic review should include all available evidence, and so a systematic and comprehensive search of the literature is needed in computerised databases and other sources.
- The search strategy must be based on an explicit description of the subjects receiving the test of interest, the diagnostic test and its accuracy estimates, the target disease, and the study design. These elements can be specified in the criteria for inclusion of primary studies in the review.
- Two independent reviewers should screen the titles and abstracts of the identified citations using specific prespecified inclusion criteria. In case of disagreement or insufficient information, a third reviewer and/or the full papers should be consulted. The publications to be evaluated should provide sufficient information on the reference standard, the study population, and the setting(s) studied.

[*]Riekie de Vet, Jeroen Lijmer, Victor Montori

- The methodological quality of each selected paper should be assessed independently by at least two reviewers. Chance-adjusted agreement should be reported and disagreement solved by consensus or arbitration. Internal and external validity criteria, describing participants, diagnostic test, and target disease of interest, and study methods can be used in meta-analysis to assess the overall "level of evidence", and in sensitivity and subgroup analyses.
- Two reviewers should independently extract the required information from the primary studies, about the participants, the testing procedure, the cut-off points used, exclusions, and indeterminate results.
- To be able to carry out subgroup analyses, sources of heterogeneity should be defined based on *a priori* existing hypotheses.
- Whether meta-analysis with statistical pooling can be conducted depends on the number and methodological quality of the primary studies.
- In view of the low methodological quality of most published diagnostic studies, the use of random effect models for pooling may be useful, even if there is no apparent heterogeneity.
- Methods for statistical pooling of proportions, likelihood ratios, and ROC curves are provided.

Introduction

Systematic reviews and meta-analyses of studies evaluating the accuracy of diagnostic tests (we will refer to them generically as diagnostic systematic reviews) are appearing more often in the medical literature.[1,2] Of the 26 reviews on diagnostic tests published between 1996 and 1997, 19 were systematic reviews or meta-analyses.[2] In the field of clinical chemistry and haematology, 23 of 45 reviews published between 1985 and 1998 were systematic reviews.[3] Although guidelines for the critical appraisal of diagnostic research and meta-analyses have already been published,[1,4–7] these may be difficult for clinical researchers to understand.

We here present a set of practical guidelines, based on evidence and the expertise of the Cochrane Collaboration, to facilitate the understanding of and appropriate adherence to methodological principles when conducting diagnostic systematic reviews. We reviewed reports of systematic searches of the literature for diagnostic research,[8–11] methodological criteria to evaluate diagnostic research,[1,4–7] methods for statistical pooling of data on diagnostic accuracy,[12–20] and methods for exploring heterogeneity.[21–25]

Guidelines for conducting diagnostic systematic reviews are presented in a stepwise fashion and are followed by comments providing further information. Examples are given using the results of two systematic reviews on the accuracy of the urine dipstick in the diagnosis of urinary tract infections,[26] and on the accuracy of the straight-leg raising test in the diagnosis of intervertebral disc hernia.[27]

The guidelines

How to search the literature for studies evaluating the accuracy of diagnostic tests

A systematic review should include all available evidence, and so a systematic and comprehensive search of the literature is needed. The reviewer has to design a search strategy based on a clear and explicit description of the subjects receiving the test of interest, the diagnostic test and its accuracy estimates, the target disease, and the study design. These elements are usually specified in the criteria for inclusion of primary studies in the review. The search will include electronic literature databases. However, because computerised databases only index a subset of all the available literature, the search should be extended using other sources.[9] The search to identify primary studies may take the following basic but labour intensive steps:

1. A computer aided search of MEDLINE (PubMed website (http://www.ncbi.nlm.nih.gov/PUBMED), EMBASE and other databases. A search strategy begins by creating a list of database specific keywords and text words that describe the diagnostic test and the target disease of interest (subject specific strategy). Because the number of diagnostic accuracy studies is often small, the subject specific strategy usually yields a limited number of publications to be screened.[10] An accurate search strategy for diagnostic publications (generic strategy) was recently published[11] and can be combined with the subject specific strategy if the number of publications resulting from the latter is large. We found a combination of two published generic strategies adapted for use in PubMed (MEDLINE) to be more sensitive and precise than previously published strategies[8,10] (Box 8.1). Each electronic database will need to be searched using a specially designed search strategy.

2. The reference section of primary studies, narrative reviews, and systematic reviews should be checked to search for additional primary studies that could have been missed by the electronic search. Identification methods for systematic reviews have also been published.[28] The MEDION database, available at the University of

Maastricht, the Netherlands, collects some 250 published reviews of diagnostic and screening studies. It is available through berna.schouten@hag.unimaas.nl and will shortly be published on the internet.

3. Consultation of experts in the disease of interest to identify further published and unpublished primary studies. As diagnostic accuracy studies are often based on routinely collected data, publication bias may be more prevalent in diagnostic than in therapeutic research.[17]

Box 8.1 Search strategy in PubMed (MEDLINE) for publications about the evaluation of diagnostic accuracy

((((((((((((("sensitivity and specificity"[All Fields] OR "sensitivity and specificity/standards"[All Fields]) OR "specificity"[All Fields]) OR "screening"[All Fields]) OR "false positive"[All Fields]) OR "false negative"[All Fields]) OR "accuracy"[All Fields]) OR (((("predictive value"[All Fields] OR "predictive value of tests"[All Fields]) OR "predictive value of tests/standards"[All Fields]) OR "predictive values"[All Fields]) OR "predictive values of tests"[All Fields])) OR (("reference value"[All Fields] OR "reference values"[All Fields]) OR "reference values/standards"[All Fields])) OR (((((((((("roc"[All Fields] OR "roc analyses"[All Fields]) OR "roc analysis"[All Fields]) OR "roc and"[All Fields]) OR "roc area"[All Fields]) OR "roc auc"[All Fields]) OR "roc characteristics"[All Fields]) OR "roc curve"[All Fields]) OR "roc curve method" [All Fields]) OR "roc curves"[All Fields]) OR "roc estimated"[All Fields]) OR "roc evaluation"[All Fields])) OR "likelihood ratio"[All Fields]) AND notpubref[sb]) AND "human"[MeSH Terms])

Comments

The first step in a literature search is the identification of relevant publications. Diagnostic research reports – older publications in particular – are often poorly indexed in the electronic databases. It is often fruitful to conduct pilot searches using the subject specific strategy. This process is repeated after identifying and incorporating additional keywords and text words to describe and index the retrieved reports. Studies found only in the reference sections of the retrieved reports but missed by the search strategy should be searched for in the database, using the article title or the first author's name. If a study is found in the database, its keywords should be noted and added to the strategy. Citation tracking may provide additional studies. The Science Citation Index could be searched forward in time to identify articles citing relevant publications.[29] Once the search is completed, two independent reviewers should screen the titles and abstracts of the identified citations using specific prespecified inclusion criteria. These can be pilot tested on a sample of articles. If disagreements cannot be resolved by consensus, or if insufficient information is available, a third reviewer and/or the full papers should be consulted.

Inclusion criteria

• *Reference test* The accuracy of a diagnostic or screening test should be evaluated by comparing its results with a "gold standard", criterion standard, or reference test accepted as the best available by content experts. The reference test may be a single test, a combination of different tests, or the clinical follow up of patients.[20] The publication should describe the reference test, as it is an essential prerequisite for the evaluation of a diagnostic test.

• *Population* Detailed information about the participants in diagnostic research is often lacking. Participants should be defined explicitly in terms of age, gender, complaints, signs, and symptoms, and their duration. At least a definition of participants with and without the disease, as determined by the reference test, should be available. The minimal number of participants needed with and without the disease depends on the type of study, the estimates of diagnostic accuracy, and the precision used to estimate these parameters.[30]

• *Outcome data* Information should be available to allow the construction of the diagnostic 2×2 table with its four cells: true positives, false negatives, false positives and true negatives.

• *Language* If a review is limited to publications in certain languages, this should be reported.

Comments

As the patient mix (spectrum of disease severity) is different at different levels of care, a diagnostic review may focus on a specific setting (primary care, etc.) or include all levels. This information may be important for subgroup analyses in case of heterogeneity. All evidence available should be reviewed, regardless of the language of publication. It is not easy to identify non-English publications, as they are often not indexed in computerised databases. In the field of intervention research there is some evidence of bias when excluding non-English publications.[31] Our research on the accuracy of the urine dipstick revealed differences in methodological validity between European and American studies, but these differences had no effect on accuracy.

Although large samples are no guarantee against selection bias, small samples seldom result from a consecutive series of patients or a random sample. Small studies are very vulnerable to selection bias.

Methodological quality

The methodological quality of each selected paper should be assessed independently by at least two reviewers. Chance-adjusted agreement should be reported, and disagreements solved by consensus or arbitration. To improve agreement, reviewers should pilot their quality assessment tools in a subset of included studies or studies evaluating a different diagnostic test.

Validity criteria for diagnostic research have been published by the Cochrane Methods Group on Screening and Diagnostic Tests[32] (http://www.som.fmc.flinders.edu.au/fusa/cochrane), and by other authors.[4–6] Criteria assessing internal and external validity should be coded and described explicitly in the review (Table 8.1). The internal validity criteria refer to study characteristics that safeguard against the intrusion of systematic error or bias. External validity criteria provide insight into the generalisability of the study and judge whether the test under evaluation was performed according to accepted standards. Internal and external validity criteria, describing participants, diagnostic test and target disease of interest, and study methods may be used in meta-analysis to assess the overall "level of evidence" and in sensitivity and subgroup analyses (see Data extraction and Data analysis sections).

It is important to remember that studies may appear to be of poor methodological quality because they were either poorly conducted or poorly reported. Methodological appraisal of the primary studies is frequently hindered by lack of information. In these instances reviewers may choose to contact the studies' authors, or to score items as "don't know" or "unclear".

Example A urine dipstick is usually read before the material is cultured. So, it can be interpreted that the dipstick was read without awareness of the results of the culture. However, the culture (reference test) may be interpreted with full awareness of the results of the dipstick. If blinding is not explicitly mentioned, reviewers may choose to score this item as "don't know" or "diagnostic test blinded for reference test" (implicitly scoring the reference test as not blinded). Or, the authors may be contacted for clarification.

A survey of the diagnostic literature from 1990 to 1993 in a number of peer-reviewed journals showed that only a minority of the studies satisfied methodological standards.[7] There is some evidence that inadequate methods may have an impact on the reported accuracy of a diagnostic test: Lijmer[2] screened diagnostic meta-analyses published in 1996 and 1997, and showed that the diagnostic accuracy of a test was overestimated in studies (1) with a case–control design; (2) using different reference tests for

Table 8.1 Validity criteria operationalised for papers reporting on the accuracy of urine dipsticks in the diagnosis of urinary tract infections (UTI) or bacteriuria.

	Positive score
Criteria of internal validity (IV)	
1 Valid reference standard	(Semi-)quantitative (2 points) to dipslide culture (1 point)
2 Definition of cut-off point for reference standard	Definition of urinary tract infection/ bacteriuria by colony forming units per ml (1 point)
3 Blind measurement of index test and reference test	In both directions (2 points) or only index or reference test
4 Avoidance of verification bias	Assessment by reference standard independent from index test results (1 point)
5 Index test interpreted independently of all clinical information	Explicitly mentioned in the publication, or urine samples from mixed outpatient populations examined in a general laboratory (1 point)
6 Design	Prospective (consecutive series) (1 point) or retrospective collection of data (0 points)
Criteria of external validity (EV)	
1 Spectrum of disease	In- and/or exclusion criteria mentioned (1 point)
2 Setting	Enough information to identify setting (1 point)(community through tertiary care)
3 Previous tests/referral filter	Details given about clinical and other diagnostic information as to which index test is being evaluated (symptomatic or asymptomatic patients (1 point)
4 Duration of illness before diagnosis	Duration mentioned (1 point)
5 Comorbid conditions	Details given (type of population) (1 point)
6 Demographic information	Age (1 point) and/or gender (1 point) data provided
7 Execution of index test	Information about standard procedure directly or indirectly available, urine collection procedure, first voided urine, distribution of microorganisms, procedure of contaminated urine samples, time of transportation of urine sample, way of reading index test, persons reading index test (1 point each)
8 Explanation of cut-off point of index test	Trace, 2 or more + (1 point if applicable)
9 Percentage missing	If appropriate: missings mentioned (1 point)
10 Reproducibility of index test	Reproducibility studied or reference mentioned (1 point)

Blinding (IV3): When information about *blinding* of measurements was not given and the dipstick was performed in setting other than the culture, we assumed blind assessment of the index test versus the reference test, but not vice versa.
Explanation of the cut-off point (EV8) was only necessary for the leukocyte esterase measurement.

positive and negative results of the index test; (3) accepting the results of observers who were unblinded to the index test results when performing the reference test; (4) that did not describe diagnostic criteria for the index test; and (5) where participants were inadequately described.

Comments

Ideally, all participants should be submitted to the same reference test. Sometimes different groups of patients are submitted to different reference tests, but details are not given. In this case it is important to assess whether the different reference tests are recognised by experts as being adequate. Verification or work-up bias may be present if not all participants who received the index test are referred to the reference test(s). Verification bias is present if the participants are referred according to the index test results. This is usually the case in screening studies where only subjects with positive index test results receive the reference test, so that only a positive predictive value can be calculated. Estimation of accuracy will not be possible in these studies unless complete follow up registries are available. This is the case if, for example, cancer screening registries and cancer diagnosis registries are coupled.

Data extraction

Two reviewers should independently extract the required information from the primary studies. Detailed information must be extracted about the participants included in the study and about the testing procedures. The cut-off point used in dichotomous testing, and the reasons and the number of participants excluded because of indeterminate results or infeasibility, are always required.

Example Detailed information extracted in the case of the dipstick meta-analysis: mean age, male/female ratio, different cut-off points for leukocyte esterase (trace, 2+, 3+), time needed for transportation, whether indeterminate results were excluded, included as negative, or repeated.

As the information extracted may be used in subgroup analyses and statistical pooling of the validity, possible sources of heterogeneity should be defined based on existing evidence or hypotheses.

Example In the dipstick meta-analysis we hypothesised that the following factors may explain heterogeneity if present: procedures of collection of test material (method of urine collection, delay between urine collection and culture), who was executing the test and how (manually or automatic), and different brands of commercial products.

Accuracy may be presented in different ways. For the meta-analysis of dichotomous tests (see below) it is necessary to construct the diagnostic

2×2 table: absolute numbers in the four cells are needed. Totals of "diseased" and "non-diseased" participants are needed to calculate prior probability (pretest probability), and to reconstruct the 2×2 table from sensitivity, specificity, likelihood ratios, predictive values or receiver operator characteristic (ROC) curves. If possible, the 2×2 table should be generated for all relevant subgroups. Further information to extract includes year of publication, language of publication, and country or region of the world where the study was performed.

Comments

A standardised data extraction form may be used simultaneously with but separately from the quality assessment form. This approach facilitates data extraction and comparison between reviewers. The form has to be piloted to ensure that all reviewers interpret data in the same way. As in other steps of the review where judgements are made, disagreements should be recorded and resolved by consensus or arbitration. Lack of details about test results or cut-off points, inconsequential rounding off of percentages, and data errors require common sense and careful data handling when reconstructing 2×2 tables. If predictive values are presented with sensitivity and specificity in "diseased" and "non-diseased" individuals, the calculation of the four cells from sensitivity and specificity can be confirmed by using the predictive values. Details can be requested from the authors of the studies, but these attempts are often unsuccessful, as the raw data may no longer be available.

Example In a review of the accuracy of the CAGE questionnaire for the diagnosis of alcohol abuse, sufficient data were made available in only nine of the 22 studies selected, although the authors of the review tried to contact the original authors by all means.[33]

Data analysis

Whether or not a meta-analysis – statistical analysis and calculation of a summary diagnostic accuracy estimate – can be conducted depends on the number and methodological quality of primary studies included and the degree of heterogeneity of their estimates of diagnostic accuracy. Because diagnostic accuracy studies are often heterogeneous and present limited information it is typically difficult to complete a meta-analysis. If heterogeneity is identified, important information is obtained from attempts to explain it. For instance, the effect that each validity criterion has on the estimates of diagnostic accuracy and the influence of previously defined study characteristics should be explored as potential explanations of the observed study to study variation.[21–25] If meta-analysis is not possible

153

or advisable, the review can be limited to a qualitative descriptive analysis of the diagnostic research available (best evidence synthesis).[34]

Several meta-analytical methods for diagnostic research have been published in the last decade.[12-20] For the analysis we recommend the following steps: (1) presentation of the results of individual studies; (2) searching for the presence of heterogeneity; (3) testing for the presence of an (implicit) cut-point effect; (4) dealing with heterogeneity; (5) deciding which model should be used if statistical pooling is appropriate; and (6) statistical pooling.

Describing the results of individual studies

Reporting the main results of all included studies is an essential part of each review. It provides the reader with the outcome measures and gives an insight into their heterogeneity. Each study is presented with some background information (year of publication, geographical region, number of diseased and non-diseased patients, selection of the patients, methodological characteristics) and a summary of the results. In view of the asymmetrical nature of most diagnostic tests (some tests are good to exclude a disease, others to confirm it), it is important to report pairs of complementary outcome measures, that is, both sensitivity and specificity, positive and negative predictive value, likelihood ratio of a positive and of a negative test, or a combination of these. The diagnostic odds ratio (DOR) can be added, but better not alone, as a same odds ratio can relate to different combinations of sensitivity and specificity. Main outcome measures should be reported with their 95% confidence intervals (CI).

$$DOR = \frac{sensitivity/(1-sensitivity)}{(1-specificity)/specificity}$$

Searching for heterogeneity

Basically, heterogeneity relates to the input characteristics of each study (study population, test methods, etc.). When setting inclusion criteria, most reviewers will try to define a more or less homogeneous set of studies. The reality, however, is that even then most diagnostic reviews suffer from considerable heterogeneity. When different studies have largely different results, this can be because of either random error or heterogeneity. To test for homogeneity of sensitivity and specificity, a χ^2 test or an extension of Fisher's exact test for small studies[35] can be used. This may offer some guidance, although the power of this test tends to be low. A basic but very informative method when searching for heterogeneity is to produce a graph in which the individual study outcomes are plotted, together with their 95% confidence intervals (Figure 8.1).

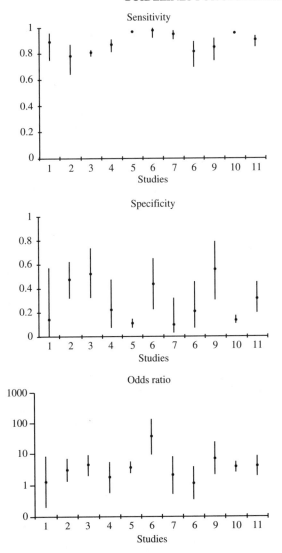

Figure 8.1 Point estimates (with confidence limits) of, respectively, sensitivity, specificity, and diagnostic odds ratio of 11 studies on the validity of the test of Lasègue for the diagnosis of disc hernia in low back pain. Study 6 is an outlier.

Searching for the presence of an (implicit) cut-off point effect

Estimates of diagnostic accuracy differ if not all studies use the same cut-off point for a positive test result or for the reference standard. The interpretation of test results often depends on human factors (for example radiology, pathology, etc.) or on the process of testing (for example clinical examination). In such cases different studies may use a different implicit cut-off point. Variation in the parameters of accuracy may be partly due to variation in cut-off points. One can test for the presence of a cut-off point effect between studies by calculating a Spearman correlation coefficient between the sensitivity and the specificity of all included studies. If strongly negatively correlated ($\rho > -0.4$), pairs of parameters represent the same DOR. A strong correlation between both parameters will usually result in a homogeneous logarithmic transformed DOR (lnDOR). The test for homogeneity of the lnDOR is described by Fleiss.[35] If the LnDORs of the included studies are homogeneous, a summary ROC curve can be fitted based on the pairs of sensitivity and specificity of the individual studies (see page 159). If sufficient information is available, the pooling of ROC curves of individual studies will also be possible.

Dealing with heterogeneity

In many cases the interpretation of present heterogeneity is the most fascinating and productive part of a meta-analysis. The inspection of the plot of all outcome parameters with their 95% CI may indicate the presence of outliers. In such cases the reason for this situation should be carefully examined.

Example In a review of the diagnostic value of macroscopic haematuria for the diagnosis of urological cancers in primary care, the positive predictive values (PPV) indicated a homogeneous series of five studies with a pooled PPV of 0.19 (95% CI = 0.17–0.23) and one other with a PPV of 0.40.[36] The reason for this high PPV was mentioned in the original study: "GPs' services in the region are extremely good and cases of less serious conditions are probably adequately shifted out and treated without referral", leading to a highly selected study population with a high prior probability.

In such cases an outlier can be excluded and the analysis continued with the homogeneous group of remaining studies. Deviant results should be explored and explained. The decision to exclude outliers is complex and should be handled in the same way as in other fields of research.

Outliers can also be searched by using a Galbraith plot.[37] To construct this plot, the standardised lnDOR = lnDOR/se is plotted (*y* axis) against the inverse of the se (1/se) (*x* axis). A regression line that goes through the origin is calculated, together with 95% boundaries (starting at +2 and −2 on the *y* axis). Studies outside these 95% boundaries may be considered as outliers (Figure 8.2).

Subgroup analyses defined in the protocol could be conducted to detect homogeneous subgroups. Analysis of variance, with the lnDOR as a dependent variable and categorical variables for subgroups as factors, can be used to look for differences among subgroups.

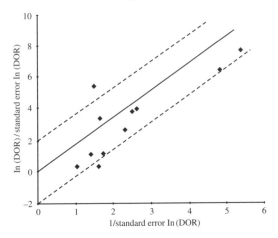

Figure 8.2 Galbraith plot of 11 studies on the validity of the Lasègue test for the diagnosis of disc hernia in low back pain. Study 6 is an outlier.

Example In the dipstick review, sensitivity and specificity were weakly associated ($\rho = -0.227$) and very heterogeneous. Subgroup analysis showed significant differences of the lnDOR between six different populations of participants. In three populations there was a strong negative association between sensitivity and specificity ($\rho = -0.539$, -0.559, and -1.00, respectively), yielding homogeneous lnDOR in the three subgroups. Different SROC curves for each subgroup could be fitted (see section on statistical pooling) (Figure 8.3).

If many studies are available, a more complex multivariate model can be built in which a number of study characteristics are entered as possible covariates. Multivariate models search for the independent effect of study characteristics, adjusted for the influence of other, more powerful ones.

Deciding on the model to be used for statistical pooling

Models

There are two underlying models that can be used when pooling the results of individual studies.

A *fixed effect model* assumes that all studies are a certain random sample of one large common study, and that differences between study outcomes only result from random error. Pooling is simple. It consists essentially of calculating a weighted average of the individual study results. Studies are weighted by the inverse of the variance of the parameter of test accuracy, or by the number of participants.

157

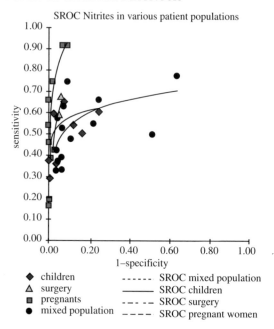

Figure 8.3 Summary ROC curves of nitrites in urine dipsticks for the diagnosis of bacteriuria and urinary tract infections in various homogeneous subgroups of patient populations.

A *random effect model* assumes that in addition to the presence of random error, differences between studies can also result from real differences between study populations and procedures. The weighting factor is mathematically more complex, and is based on the work of Der Simonian and Laird, initially performed and published for the meta-analysis of trials.[38] It includes both within-study and between-study variation.

Homogeneous studies

If the parameters are homogeneous, and if they show no (implicit) cut-off effect, their results can be pooled and a fixed effect model can be used. If there is evidence of a cut-off effect, SROC curves can be constructed or ROC curves can be pooled.

Heterogeneous studies

If heterogeneity is present, the reviewer has the following options:

1. Refrain from pooling and restrict the analysis to a qualitative overview.
2. Subgroup analysis if possible, on prior factors and pooling within homogeneous subgroups.

3. As a last resort pooling can be performed, using methods that are based on a random effect model.

In view of the poor methodological quality of most of the diagnostic studies that have been carried out, there is a tendency to advise using random effect models for the pooling of all diagnostic studies, even if there is no apparent heterogeneity.

Statistical pooling

Pooling of proportions

- *Homogeneous sensitivity and/or specificity*

If *fixed effect* pooling can be used, pooled proportions are the average of all individual study results, weighted for the sample sizes. This is easily done by adding together all numerators and dividing the total by the sum of all denominators[14] (see Appendix to this chapter).

- *Cut-off point effect: SROC curve*

The SROC curve is presented with sensitivity on the y axis and $1 -$ specificity on the x axis (ROC plot), where each study provides one value of sensitivity and one value of specificity (Figure 8.3). If a SROC curve can be fitted, a regression model (metaregression) is used, with the natural logarithm of the DOR (lnDOR) of the studies as dependent variable and two parameters as independent variables: one for the intercept (to be interpreted as the mean lnDOR) and one for the slope of the curve (as an estimate of the variation of the lnDOR across the studies due to threshold differences). Details and formulae for fitting the curve can be found in the paper presented by Littenberg and Moses[13] (see Appendix). Covariates representing different study characteristics or pretest probabilities can be added to the model to examine any possible association of the diagnostic odds ratio with these variables.[39] The pooled lnDOR and confidence limits have to be back-transformed into a diagnostic odds ratio and its confidence intervals. Metaregression can be unweighted or weighted, using the inverse of the variance as the weighting factor. A problem that is encountered in diagnostic research is the often negative association of the weighting factor with the lnDOR, giving studies with lower discriminative diagnostic odds ratios – because of lower sensitivity and/or specificity – a larger weight. This problem has not yet been resolved.[17,19]

Pooling of likelihood ratios

Continuous test results can be transformed into likelihood ratios, obtained by using different cut-off points. Individual data points from the selected studies can be used to calculate result specific likelihood ratios,[40] which can be obtained by logistic modelling. The natural log posterior odds are converted into a log likelihood ratio by adding a constant to the regression equation. The constant adjusts for the ratio of the number of "non-diseased" to "diseased" participants in the respective studies[17] (see Appendix).

Pooling of the ROC curves

The results of diagnostic studies with a dichotomous gold standard outcome, and a test result that is reported on a continuous scale, are generally presented as an ROC curve with or without the related area under the curve (AUC) and its 95% CI. To pool such results, the reviewer has three options: to pool sensitivities and specificities for all relevant cut-off points; to pool the AUCs; or to model and pool the ROC curves themselves.

- A pooled ROC curve and its confidence interval can be constructed on the basis of the pooled sensitivity/specificity values per cut-off point. To make this possible, sufficient raw data have to be available, which is seldom the case.
- The AUC, like all one-dimensional measures, provides no information about the asymmetrical nature of a diagnostic test. It cannot distinguish between curves with a high sensitivity at moderate values of the specificity and those with a high specificity at moderate values of the sensitivity.
- As ROC curves are based on ranking, they are robust with respect to interstudy shifts in the value or meaning of cut-off points. They also provide information about the asymmetrical nature of the test information. To enable direct pooling of ROC curves, a method has been developed that requires only the published curves and the number of positive and negative participants on the gold standard test as input.[41] The ROC curve is scanned into a graphic computer file and then converted into a series of sensitivity versus specificity data, using appropiate software or, ultimately, by hand. Subsequently, a model is fitted for each study, similar to that used for producing SROC curves.

For continuous scale tests, weighted linear regression is used to estimate the parameters for each curve, including a bootstrap method to estimate the standard errors. For ordinal tests, maximum likelihood estimation yields the parameters and their standard errors. The resulting estimates are pooled separately, using a random effect model, and the resulting model is back-transformed into a new pooled curve with its 95% confidence band. In addition to causing calculation problems in specific situations, pooling published ROC curves also hides the test values from the picture. Although this is not a problem when evaluating a test method, or when comparing different methods, it limits the possible use of the pooled curve for evaluating the diagnostic value of each specific test result. Moreover, a published curve can be a fitted estimate of the real curve based on the initial values, and any bias resulting from this estimation will be included in the pooled estimates.

Data presentation

A DOR is difficult to interpret because it is a combination of sensitivity and specificity. However, it is useful to present pooled sensitivity and specificity estimates, together with the relevant diagnostic odds ratios for different study characteristics or subgroups. To make this information accessible to clinicians, the predictive values could be obtained by using the mean prior (pretest) probabilities of each subgroup. Alternatively, likelihood ratios could be reported so that users can calculate post-test probabilities based on the pretest probabilities applicable to their patients.

Pooled DOR (and confidence intervals) of different subgroups can also be presented graphically on a logarithmic scale to give symmetrical confidence intervals and to reduce the width of confidence intervals.

Example taken from the straight-leg raising test review. In Figure 8.4 the DOR and confidence boundaries are plotted on the *y* axis on a logarithmic scale. Relevant study characteristics (that is, double blind versus single

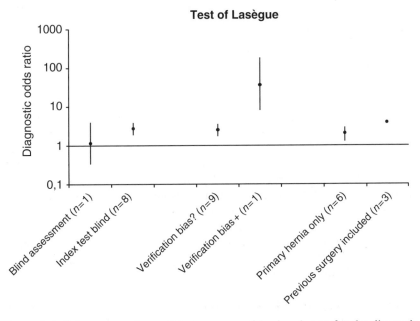

Figure 8.4 Subgroup analyses of the accuracy of Lasègue's test for the diagnosis of disc hernia in low back pain. Odds ratios are pooled per subgroup.

161

Example taken from the dipstick review:

Factor	DOR (95% CI)	Sensitivity (95% CI)	Specificity (95% CI)	Prior probability	PPV	NPV
Mixed population	11 (6–21)	0.50 (0.44–0.58)	0.82 (0.71–0.95)	0.32	0.57	0.78
Surgery	34 (25–47)	0.54 (0.39–0.74)	0.96 (0.93–0.99)	0.20	0.76	0.89

blind studies, studies with or without verification bias) are plotted on the *x* axis.

Discussion

Although the methodology to conduct a systematic review and meta-analysis of diagnostic research is developed to a certain extent, at least for dichotomised tests, the exercise itself remains quite a challenge. Systematic reviews have to meet high methodological standards and the results should always be interpreted with caution. Several complicating issues need careful consideration: (1) it is difficult to discover all published evidence, as diagnostic research is often inadequately indexed in electronic databases; (2) the studies are often poorly reported and a set of minimal reporting standards for diagnostic research has only recently been discussed; (3) the methodological quality and validity of diagnostic research reports is often limited (that is, no clear definition of "diseased" participants, no blinding, no independent interpretation of test results, insufficient description of participants); (4) accuracy estimates are often very heterogeneous, yet examining heterogeneity is cumbersome and the process is full of pitfalls; (5) results have to be translated into information that is clinically relevant, taking into account the clinical reality at different levels of health care (prevalence of disease, spectrum of disease, available clinical and other diagnostic information). Even in a state of the art systematic review, the reviewers have to make many subjective decisions when deciding on the inclusion or exclusion of studies, on quality assessment and the interpretation of limited information, on the exclusion of outliers, and on choosing and conducting subgroup analyses. Subjective aspects have to be assessed independently by more than one reviewer, with tracking of disagreements and resolution by consensus or arbitration. These subjective decisions should be explicitly acknowledged in the report to allow the readers some insight into the possible consequences of these decisions on the outcomes of the review and the strength of inference derived from it.

Whereas some researchers question the usefulness of pooling the results of poorly designed research or meta-analyses based on limited information,[42–43] we think that examining the effects of validity criteria on the diagnostic accuracy measures and the analysis of subgroups adds valuable evidence to the field of diagnostic accuracy studies. The generation of a pooled estimate – the most likely estimate of the test's accuracy – provides clinicians with useful information until better-conducted studies are published. The reader should remember that evidence about the influence of validity of studies on diagnostic accuracy is still limited.[2,3,6] Consequently, it is difficult to recommend a strict set of methodological criteria, recognising that any minimum set of methodological criteria is largely arbitrary. Although we have discussed some practical approaches to statistical pooling, other methods are available in the literature.[18,19] Experience with these methods, however, is limited. The development of guidelines for systematic reviews of tests with continuous or ordinal outcomes, reviews of diagnostic strategies of more than one test, and reviews of the reproducibility of diagnostic tests, remains another challenge, as the methodology is still limited[1] or even non-existent.

References

1 Irwig L, Tosteson ANA, Gatsonis C, *et al*. Guidelines for meta-analyses evaluating diagnostic tests. *Ann Intern Med* 1994;**120**:667–76.

2 Lijmer JG, Mol BW, Heisterkamp S, *et al*. Empirical evidence of design-related bias in studies of diagnostic tests. *JAMA* 1999;**282**:1061–6.

3 Oosterhuis WP, Niessen RWLM, Bossuyt PMM. The science of systematic reviewing studies of diagnostic tests. *Clin Chem Lab Med* 2000;**38**:577–88.

4 Jeaschke R, Guyatt GH, Sackett DL. User's guidelines to the medical literature, III: how to use an article about a diagnostic test, A: are the results of the study valid? *JAMA* 1994;**271**:389–91.

5 Jeaschke R, Guyatt GH, Sackett DL. User's guidelines to the medical literature, III: how to use an article about a diagnostic test, B: what are the results and will they help me in caring for my patients? *JAMA* 1994;**271**:703–7.

6 Greenhalgh T. How to read a paper: papers that report diagnostic or screening tests. *BMJ* 1997;**315**:540–3.

7 Reid MC, Lachs MS, Feinstein AR. Use of methodological standards in diagnostic test research: getting better but still not good. *JAMA* 1995;**274**:645–51.

8 Haynes RB, Wilczynski N, McKibbon KA, Walker CJ, Sinclair JC. Developing optimal search strategies for detecting clinically sound studies in Medline. *J Am Med Informatics Assoc* 1994;**1**:447–58.

9 Dickersin K, Scherer R, Lefebvre C. Identifying relevant studies for systematic reviews. *BMJ* 1994;**309**:1286–91.

10 van der Weijden T, IJzermans CJ, Dinant GJ, van Duijn NP, de Vet R, Buntinx F. Identifying relevant diagnostic studies in MEDLINE. The diagnostic value of the erythrocyte sedimentation rate (ESR) and dipstick as an example. *Fam Pract* 1997; **14**:204–8.

11 Deville WLJM, Bezemer PD, Bouter LM. Publications on diagnostic test evaluation in family medicine journals: an optimal search strategy. *J Clin Epidemiol* 2000;**53**:65–9.

12 McClish DK. Combining and comparing area estimates across studies or strata. *Med Decision Making* 1992;**12**:274–9.

13 Littenberg B, Moses LE. Estimating diagnostic accuracy from multiple conflicting reports: a new meta-analytic method. *Med Decision Making* 1993;**13**:313–21.

14 Midgette AS, Stukel TA, Littenberg B. A meta-analytic method for summarising diagnostic test performances: receiver-operating-characteristic-summary point estimates. *Med Decision Making* 1993;**13**:253–7.

163

15 Moses LE, Shapiro D, Littenberg B. Combining independent studies of a diagnostic test into a summary ROC curve: data-analytic approaches and some additional considerations. *Stat Med* 1993;**12**:1293–316.

16 Hasselblad V, Hedges LV. Meta-analysis of screening and diagnostic tests. *Psych Bull* 1995; **117**:167–78.

17 Irwig L, Macaskill P, Glasziou P, Fahey M. Meta-analytic methods for diagnostic accuracy. *J Clin Epidemiol* 1995;**48**:119–30.

18 Rutter CM, Gatsonis CA. Regression methods for meta-analysis of diagnostic test data. *Acad Radiol* 1995; **2**:S48–S56.

19 Shapiro DE. Issues in combining independent estimates of the sensitivity and specificity of a diagnostic test. *Acad Radiol* 1995;**2**:S37–S47.

20 Walter SD, Irwig L, Glasziou PP. Meta-analysis of diagnostic tests with imperfect reference standards. *J Clin Epidemiol* 1999;**52**:943–51.

21 Yusuf S, Wittes J, Probsfield J, Tyroler HA. Analysis and interpretation of treatment effects in subgroups of patients in randomised clinical trials. *JAMA* 1991;**266**:93–8.

22 Oxman A, Guyatt G. A consumer's guide to subgroup analysis. *Ann Intern Med* 1992; **116**:78–84.

23 Thompson SG. Why sources of heterogeneity in meta-analysis should be investigated. *BMJ* 1994;**309**:1351–5.

24 Colditz GA, Burdick E, Mosteller F. Heterogeneity in meta-analysis of data from epidemiologic studies: a commentary. *Am J Epidemiol* 1995;**142**:371–82.

25 Mulrow C, Langhorne P, Grimshaw J. Integrating heterogeneous pieces of evidence in systematic reviews. *Ann Intern Med* 1997;**127**:989–95.

26 Deville WLJM, Yzermans JC, van Duin NP, van der Windt DAWM, Bezemer PD, Bouter LM. Which factors affect the accuracy of the urine dipstick for the detection of bacteriuria or urinary tract infections? A meta-analysis. In: *Evidence in diagnostic research. Reviewing diagnostic accuracy: from search to guidelines.* PhD thesis, Amsterdam: Vrije Universiteit, pp 39–73.

27 Deville WLJM, van der Windt DAWM, Dzaferagic A, Bezemer PD, Bouter LM. The test of Lasègue: systematic review of the accuracy in diagnosing herniated discs. *Spine* 2000;**25**:1140–7.

28 Hunt DL, McKibbon KA. Locating and appraising systematic reviews. *Ann Intern Med* 1997;**126**:532–8.

29 van Tulder MW, Assendelft WJJ, Koes BW, Bouter LM and the Editorial Board of the Cochrane Collaboration Back Review Group. Method guidelines for systematic reviews in the Cochrane Collaboration Back Review Group for spinal disorders. *Spine* 1997;**22**:2323–30.

30 Obuchowski NA. Sample size calculations in studies of test accuracy. *Stat Meth Med Res* 1998;**7**:371–92.

31 Grégoire G, Derderian F, Le Lorier J. Selecting the language of the publications included in a meta-analysis: is there a Tower of Babel bias? *J Clin Epidemiol* 1995;**48**:159–63.

32 Cochrane Methods Group on Screening and Diagnostic Tests. Recommended methods. http://www.som.fmc.flinders.edu.au/fusa/cochrane

33 Aertgeerts B, Buntinx F, Kester A, Fevery J. Diagnostic value of the CAGE questionnaire in screening for alcohol abuse and alcohol dependence: a meta-analysis. In: *Screening for alcohol abuse or dependence.* PhD thesis, Leuven: Katholieke Universiteit 2000, Appendix 3.

34 Centre for Evidence Based Medicine. Levels of Evidence and Grades of Recommendations. http://cebm.jr2.ox.ac.uk/docs/levels.html

35 Fleiss Jl. The statistical basis of meta-analysis. *Stat Meth Med Res* 1993;**2**:121–45.

36 Buntinx F, Wauters H. The diagnostic value of macroscopic haematuria in diagnosing urological cancers. A meta-analysis. *Fam Pract* 1997;**14**:63–8.

37 Galbraith RF. A note on graphical presentation of estimated odds ratios from several clinical trials. *Stat Med* 1988;**7**:889–94.

38 DerSimonian R, Laird N. Meta-analysis in clinical trials. *Controlled Clin Trials* 1986;**7**:177–88.

39 Greenland S. Invited commentary: a critical look at some popular meta-analytic methods. *Am J Epidemiol* 1994;**140**:290–6.

40 Irwig L. Modelling result-specific likelihood ratios. *J Clin Epidemiol* 1989;**42**:1021–4.

41 Kester A, Buntinx F. Meta-analysis of ROC-curves. *Med Decision Making* 2000;**20**:430–9.
42 Greenland S. A critical look at some popular meta-analytic methods. *Am J Epidemiol* 1994;**140**:290–301.
43 Shapiro S. Meta-analysis/Shmeta-analysis. *Am J Epidemiol* 1994;**140**:771–7.

Appendix: statistical formulae

Pooling of proportions

Homogeneous sensitivity and/or specificity

For example, for the sensitivity:

$$\text{Sensitivity}_{\text{pooled}} = \sum_{i=1}^{k} a_i / \sum (a_i + c_i)$$

where a = true positives, c = false negatives, i = study number, and, k = total number of studies, with standard error:

$$SE = \sqrt{\frac{p(1-p)}{n}}$$

where $p = \text{sensitivity}_{\text{pooled}}$, and

$$n = \sum_{i=1}^{k} (a_i + c_i)$$

Cut-off point effect: SROC curve

Basic meta-regression formula:

$$\ln(DOR)_{\text{pooled}} = \alpha + \beta S$$

where α = intercept, β = regression coefficient, and

$$S = \text{estimate of cut-off point} = \ln\left[\frac{\text{sensitivity}}{(1-\text{sensitivity})}\right] + \ln\left[\frac{(1-\text{specificity})}{\text{specificity}}\right]$$

With standard error:

$$SE_{\ln(DOR)} = \sqrt{\frac{1}{a} + \frac{1}{b} + \frac{1}{c} + \frac{1}{d}}$$

Pooling of likelihood ratios

$$\log(LR)_{\text{pooled}} = \log\left[\frac{N_{\bar{D}}}{N_D}\right] + \alpha + \beta x$$

where LR = likelihood ratio

$$\log\left[\frac{N_{\bar{D}}}{N_D}\right] = \text{correction factor}$$

$$= \log(\text{number non-diseased/number diseased})$$

$\alpha = $ i ntercept in logistic regression, β = regression coefficient, and x = test measurement.

9 Diagnostic decision support: contributions from medical informatics

JOHAN VAN DER LEI, JAN H VAN BEMMEL

Summary box

- Applying information and communication technology (ICT) to a given medical domain is not merely adding a new technique, but has the potential to radically change processes in that domain.
- When introduced into an environment, ICT will initially often emulate or resemble the existing processes. When workers and researchers in that domain begin to appreciate the potential of ICT, this initial stage is followed by more fundamental changes in that domain that take advantage of the potential of ICT.
- Many researchers argue that the fundamental enabling technology is the introduction of electronic medical records. The explicit purpose of automating medical records is to use the data in those records to support not only the care of individual patients, but also applications such as decision support, quality control, cost control, or epidemiology.
- To understand the scope of the potential changes enabled by electronic records, three principal changes need to be understood. First, data recorded on computer can readily be retrieved and reused for a variety of purposes. Second, once data are available on computer, they can easily be transported. Third, as clinicians (and patients) are using computers to record medical data, the same electronic record can be used to introduce other computer programs that interact with the user.

- As electronic medical records are becoming available, researchers use them to change medical practice by providing decision support, and to analyse observational databases to study the delivery of care. New usage of data, however, generates additional requirements. Thus the experience in developing decision support systems and analysing observational databases feeds back into the requirements for electronic medical records.
- Each patient–doctor encounter, each investigation, each laboratory test, and each treatment in medical practice constitutes, in principle, an experiment. Ideally, we learn from each experiment. Paper as a medium to record data limits our ability to exploit that potential. Electronic medical records will facilitate research that relies on data recorded in routine medical practice. The potential of ICT, however, lies in its ability to close the loop between clinical practice, research, and education.

Introduction

The term medical informatics dates from the second half of the 1970s and is based on the French term *informatique médicale*. Although the term is now widely used, other names, such as medical computer science, medical information sciences, or computers in medicine, are sometimes used. Research in informatics ranges from fundamental computer science to applied informatics. Several definitions of medical informatics take both the scientific, fundamental aspect and the applied, pragmatic aspect into account. Shortliffe, for example, provides the following definition:

"Medical Information Science is the science of using system-analytic tools … to develop procedures (algorithms) for management, process control, decision-making and scientific analysis of medical knowledge."[1] and Van Bemmel defines the field as: "Medical Informatics comprises the theoretical and practical aspects of information processing and communication, based on knowledge and experience derived from processes in medicine and health care."[1]

Medical informatics is determined by the intersection of the terms medicine and informatics. Medicine identifies the area of research; informatics identifies the methodology used. In medical informatics, we develop and assess methods and systems for the acquisition, processing, and interpretation of patient data. Computers are the vehicles to realise these goals. The role of computers in medical informatics, however, varies. If the medical informatics research is applied, the objective is to develop a computer system that will be used by healthcare professionals, for example research aimed at the development of electronic medical records. If the research is more fundamental, the computer plays a role as an experimental environment for models that are developed; the objective is not to build a system, but to verify a hypothesis or to investigate the limitations of models. Some research in the area of artificial intelligence in medicine, for example, fits this last category.

Applying ICT to a given medical domain is not merely adding a new technique: ICT has the potential to radically change processes in that domain. Such change, however, may not be apparent at the beginning. When introduced into an environment, ICT will initially often emulate or resemble the already existing processes. Typically, this is only a temporary stage. When workers and researchers in that domain begin to appreciate the potential of ICT, this initial stage is followed by more fundamental changes in that domain that take advantage of the potential of ICT.

Electronic communication, for example, is a relatively simple technology. The contents of a message may be structured (that is, contain a predefined set of data) or free text. When introduced into the healthcare process, electronic communication is used to replace existing paper documents. The names of the first electronic messages often even carry the names of their paper counterpart: electronic discharge letter, electronic prescription, etc. At first glance, little has changed compared to the previous paper based communication, except the speed of delivery. At this stage, the infrastructure (for example computers, lines) required for ICT has been installed, but its impact on the processes is still very limited. Subsequently, however, the ability to send data using electronic communication is used to support new forms of collaboration between healthcare professionals. At present, the emphasis has shifted from replacing paper documents to sharing data between colleagues. As clinicians increasingly share data, issues such as the standardisation of the content of medical records are becoming important areas of research. In addition, the fact that data can be transferred easily over distances enables clinicians to interpret data while the patient is located miles away (resulting in, for example, the so-called "telediagnosis"), or to communicate with patients over longer distances using, for example, the internet.

In this chapter we will focus on the contribution of medical informatics to diagnostic decision support. We believe that the use of ICT in the domain of diagnostic decision support is still in an early stage. Although in a few specialties (for example radiology), ICT is used extensively for decision support, most clinicians have little or no experience with decision support systems. Many researchers argue that the fundamental enabling technology is the introduction of electronic medical records. Once electronic medical records are available, they argue, we will witness a rapid increase in the use of diagnostic decision support systems.[2] We will first discuss the developments with respect to electronic medical records.

Electronic medical records

In its early stages, the written medical record had the purpose of documenting the care given to a patient, and thus to facilitate continuity of that care. The entries in the record enabled the clinician to recall previous episodes of illness and treatment. In recent years, however, medical records have been used increasingly for other purposes: they are used as a data source for purposes ranging from billing the patient to performing epidemiological studies, and from performing quality control to defending oneself against legal claims. One of the major barriers for using the data in such ways is the inaccessible and often unstructured nature of the paper record. The introduction of computer based medical records to a large degree, removes that barrier.

Recent decades have seen a rapid increase in the role of computers in medical record keeping, and professional organisations have started to play an active role in the introduction of electronic records. For example, in 1978 the first Dutch general practitioners started using personal computers in their practices. Five years later, in 1983, 35 general practitioners (that is, 0.6% of all Dutch GPs) were using a computer. In 1990, 35% of Dutch GPs were using one or more computer applications; although the majority of these are administrative, an increasing number of clinicians use computer stored medical records.[3] Now the electronic medical record has replaced paper records as the dominant form of record in Dutch primary care. Other countries, such as the United Kingdom, have also witnessed a rapid introduction of electronic records into primary care. In secondary care, although progress has been made, the introduction of electronic records is slower.

The explicit purpose of automating medical records is to use the data in those records to support not only the care of individual patients, but also applications such as decision support, quality control, cost control, or epidemiology.[2] The quality of medical record data, however, has often been lamentable. The reliability of clinical data, for example, has long been questioned, and tensions between reimbursement schemes and coding schemes have been discussed. Some researchers argue that the process of automation may further reduce the reliability of data. Burnum,[4] for example, states: "With the advent of the information era in medicine, we are pouring out a torrent of medical record misinformation". Although we disagree with this pessimistic view, we acknowledge that medical data are recorded for a specific purpose and that this purpose has an influence on what data are recorded and how. In developing systems that record medical data, designers make decisions about how to model those data in order to perform a given task. For example, in designing the computer based medical record system Elias,[3] the designers focused on issues such as ease of data entry and emulating existing paper records. The same designers subsequently discovered significant limitations in the Elias records when they developed a decision support system that uses these records as a data source.[5]

Despite the limitations of the current computer based medical records and the data contained in them, many researchers believe electronic medical records will significantly change medical practice.[2,6] To understand the scope of these potential changes, three principles need to be understood. First, data recorded on computer can be readily retrieved and reused for a variety of purposes. As a result, databases containing data on millions of patients are available. Although the subsequent analysis of the data may prove difficult, both clinicians and researchers are moving from a period of "data starvation" to "data overload". Second, once data are available in this way, they can easily be transported. The result is that processes that interpret the data (for example diagnosis or consultation) are no longer closely associated with the physical location where they were collected. Data can be collected in one place and processed in another (for example telediagnosis). Third, as clinicians (and patients) are using computers to record medical data, the same electronic record can be used to introduce other computer programs that interact with the user. Electronic medical records require both an extensive ICT infrastructure and clinicians experienced in using that infrastructure. Once that infrastructure is operational, other applications (such as decision support or access to literature) are much easier to introduce.

Electronic medical records will stimulate and enable other developments. We will discuss two of them: the development and use of integrated decision support systems, and the creation of observational databases.

Clinical decision support systems

A number of definitions for clinical decision support systems have been proposed. Shortliffe,[1] for example, defines a clinical decision support system as: "any computer program designed to help health professionals make clinical decisions".

The disadvantage of such a broad definition is that it includes any program that stores, retrieves or displays medical data or knowledge. To further specify what we mean by the term clinical decision support system, we use the definition proposed by Wyatt and Spiegelhalter[1]: "active knowledge systems that use two or more items of patient data to generate case specific advice". This definition captures the main components of a clinical decision support system: medical knowledge, patient data, and patient specific advice.

In a clinical decision support system, medical knowledge is modelled. That is, the designers of the system encode in a formalism the medical knowledge that is required to make decisions. Such formalisms or models have traditionally been divided into two main groups: quantitative and qualitative. The quantitative models are based on well defined statistical methods and may rely on training sets of patient data to "train" the model. Examples of such models are neural networks, fuzzy sets, bayesian models, or belief nets. Qualitative models are typically less formal and are often based on perceptions of human reasoning. Examples are truth tables, decision trees, or clinical algorithms. Increasingly, however, builders of decision support systems will combine different models in a given system: a bayesian network may be used to model the diagnostic knowledge and a decision tree may be used to model treatment decisions, and a pharmacokinetic model may be used to calculate dosage regimens.

Clinical decision support systems require patient data. Without them, patient-specific advice cannot be generated. Some systems may require interaction between the system and the clinician. The clinician initiates a dialogue with the system and provides it with data by entering symptoms or answering questions. Experience has shown that the acceptance of this type of system by clinicians is relatively low. Other systems are integrated with electronic medical records, and use the data in them as input. In such settings, receiving decision support requires little or no additional data input on the part of the clinician. Finally, some systems are directly connected to the devices that generate the data, for example systems that interpret ECGs or laboratory data.

By applying the medical knowledge to the patient data, the system generates patient-specific advice. Some systems, especially those integrated with electronic medical records, provide advice independent of a clinician's request for it – unsolicited advice. Examples are reminding systems that continuously screen patient data for conditions that should be brought to the clinician's attention (for example the patient's kidney function is decreasing, or the patient is eligible for preventive screening). Other systems, such as critiquing systems, may monitor the decisions of the clinician and report deviations from guidelines.

Although hundreds of clinical decision support systems have been reported in the literature, only a few have been the subject of a rigorous clinical evaluation. Of those that have been evaluated, however, the majority of the studies showed an impact on clinician performance.[7] In particular, systems integrated with electronic medical records have been demonstrated to improve the quality of care. In light of the currently available evidence, clinical decision support systems constitute a possible method to support the implementation of clinical guidelines in practice.

Observational databases

As a result of the increased use of electronic medical records, large observational databases containing data on millions of patients have become available for researchers. The data contained in these databases is not of the same quality as the data collected in, for example, a clinical trial. They are collected in routine practice, and, although most observational databases attempt to standardise the recording of data and to monitor their quality, only a few observational databases require the clinician to record additional information.[8]

In the absence of a clear study design (for example a randomised controlled trial to compare the effectiveness of possible treatment regimens) and specification of the data required for that study, the data in observational databases are difficult to interpret because of possible confounding. The advantage of observational databases, however, is that they reflect current clinical practice. Moreover, the data are readily available and the costs are not prohibitive. In settings where all the medical data are recorded electronically, the opportunities for research are similar to studies carried out using paper charts. Compared to paper charts, these observational databases provide an environment where the analysis can be performed faster, the data are legible, "normal" practice can be studied, rare events can be studied, longitudinal follow up of patients is possible, and subgroups for further study (such as additional data collection, or patients eligible for prospective trails) can be identified. In cases where a rapid analysis is required (for example a suspected side effect of a drug), observational databases provide a setting for a quick assessment of the question.

Researchers in medical informatics use these observational databases to assess the behaviour of a decision support system prior to introducing that system into clinical practice. Such an analysis allows the researchers to determine, for example, the frequency of advice (for example the frequency of reminders) and to study the trade off between false positive and false negative alerts. When the clinical decision support system relies on a model that uses patient data to train that model, observational databases allow the tuning of that model to the population in which it will be used.

Observational databases that rely on electronic records have limitations. Analysis of the contents of the records shows that information important for a researcher is often not recorded. Medical records typically contain data describing the patient's state (for example the results of laboratory tests) and the actions of the clinician (such as prescribing medication). Relationships between data are often not recorded. The medical record mainly reflects what is done, rather than why. A further complicating factor is that when data in the medical record describe the relationship between observations (or findings) and actions (for example treatment), the information is often recorded in the form of free text. The clinician's first and most important objective in keeping automated medical records is to document with the purpose of ensuring the quality and continuity of medical care. From the clinician's perspective, free text is often an ideal method for expressing the patient's condition. Researchers, on the other hand, prefer coded data to facilitate the automatic processing of large numbers of patients. It is unrealistic, however, to expect clinicians to code all relevant data: the time required to do so would render it impractical. In addition, coding is in essence a process of reducing the rich presentation of the patient–doctor encounter to a limited set of predefined terms. The data available in an observational database may therefore not be sufficient to answer a specific research question validly. The completeness of data can only be discussed in the context of a specific study. It is not possible to predict all possible data that would be required for all possible studies. As a result, data in observational databases will be incomplete. Depending on the study question and the impact of incomplete information, additional data may need to be collected.

Confounding by indication

To illustrate the caveats when analysing observational databases, we discuss the problem of confounding by indication. In essence, confounding by indication is often "confounding by diagnosis", since diagnostic assessment is the starting point for any treatment. As an example we will use an observational database used by Dutch GPs: the so-called IPCI database.[8] In this database, we will study the use of long-acting β agonists (LBA). LBA, introduced into the Dutch market in 1992, are long-acting bronchodilators that are used in the treatment of asthma. Dutch guidelines emphasise that LBA are primarily a chronic medication and should be combined with inhaled corticosteroids (IC). We focus on the use of long-acting β_2 agonists and their concomitant use with corticosteroids in general practice.

We conducted a retrospective cohort study during the period 1992–1999 among patients in the Netherlands receiving at least one prescription for one of the long-acting β_2 agonists (LBA) or the short-acting inhaled β_2 agonists. We assessed the indication for the prescription, the characteristics of recipients, the daily dose, and the treatment duration of long-acting β_2 agonists. In addition, we assessed the concomitant use of inhaled corticosteroids, and the incidence of episodes of oral corticosteroid use prior to and during treatment. In the setting of this study, we used the oral corticosteroids as a marker for exacerbations.

We found that the use of LBA among all inhaled β_2 agonist users increased from 3.0% in 1992 to 14.4% in 1999. Of the users, 61% were treated exclusively by the GP and not referred to a specialist. The most common indication for use of LBA was asthma (44%), followed by emphysema (36%) and chronic bronchitis (7%). Only 1.5% of the LBA prescriptions were issued on an "if needed" basis; the most frequent dosing regimen was two puffs per day (78%). Only 67% of the LBA users received inhaled corticosteroids concomitantly. LBA were used for short periods: 32% of the users received only a single prescription, and 49% were treated for less than 90 days.

Table 9.1 For different durations of treatment of patients with asthma with long-acting β_2 agonists (LBA), the frequency of oral corticosteroid use (in prescriptions per 1000 person-days) in the 12 months before the start of the treatment with LBA and during the treatment with LBA.

Duration of treatment with LBA	Corticosteroids 12 months before LBA treatment	Corticosteroids during LBA treatment
From 90 to 180 days	1.3	1.8
From 180 days to 1 year	1.5	1.3
The full year	1.6	0.9

As shown in Table 9.1, among asthma patients who received LBA for at least 1 year the episodes of oral corticosteroid use decreased from 1.6 prescriptions/1000 patient-days (PD) prior to starting LBA, to 0.9/1000 PD during the use of LBA. The rate of corticosteroid use prior to and during LBA use increased in patients with a duration of LBA treatment from 90 to 180 days (from 1.3 to 1.8 per 1000 person-days).

We conclude that the short duration of use of LBAs, and the fact that 33% of patients do not use LBA and IC concomitantly, shows that the use of LBA by Dutch GPs is not in agreement with Dutch guidelines for the treatment of asthma. The interpretation of the use of oral corticosteroids, however, is difficult. The fact that oral corticosteroid use in the patients treated continuously with LBA decreased during treatment, seems to indicate that use of LBA has a positive effect in reducing the number of exacerbations. On the other hand, a comparison of the incidence of exacerbations prior to and during treatment among patients treated with LBA from 90 to 180 days shows that the incidence increases during treatment. It would be dangerous to conclude, based on these crude data, that LBA treatment causes exacerbations in this group of patients. Patients who receive short-term LBA may be different from those with strong fluctuations in asthma severity, for example. The reason (indication) for prescription in this group of patients may be a diagnosed temporary worsening of asthma (increasing severity) that in itself would lead to a higher incidence of exacerbations. Diagnosing severity of the underlying disease that changes over time may therefore, have caused this result: confounded by indication.

In order to be able to adjust for confounding during the analysis of observational studies, we would need an accurate indicator of the severity of the disease over time. For diseases such as asthma it is difficult reliably to assess changing severity by using data collected during routine care. In the absence of a reliable severity indicator any interpretation can be flawed by the potential (residual) confounding. In case of inability to assess severity, the only method to counter confounding would be the randomisation of patients to different treatment arms in order to make both arms similar as to the spectrum of severity. Currently, however, this option is not feasible in "naturalistic" circumstances.

Closing the loop

One of the fundamental changes when conventional paper based medical records are replaced with computerised records involves the ability to process the data in those records for different purposes. As electronic medical records are becoming available, researchers use them to change medical practice by providing decision support, and analyse observational databases to study the delivery of care. New usage of data, however, generates additional requirements. Thus the experience in developing decision support systems and analysing observational databases feeds back into the requirements for electronic medical records. And as new requirements for the electronic record are formulated, the record itself begins to change.

In the area of decision support systems, researchers are combining reminder systems that rely solely on recorded data with systems that request additional information from clinicians. The resulting systems rely on the one hand on data already available in the electronic record to determine eligible patients, and subsequently interact with the clinician to assess, for example, whether the patient should be treated according to a certain protocol. The results of that interaction are recorded in the medical record. Researchers working on the development of observational databases are beginning to combine retrospective research with prospective research. Trials are translated into software, distributed electronically, and added to an electronic medical record. Based on the data in that record, the system automatically detects patients eligible for a trial. It then informs the clinician that the patient is eligible, and requests permission to include them in the trial. The system subsequently performs the randomisation between treatment arms during patient consultation, and the electronic record supports subsequent data collection. As a result, the boundaries between an electronic record, a decision support system, and systems for clinical trials are beginning to fade.

Each patient–doctor encounter, each investigation, each laboratory test, and each treatment in medical practice constitutes, in principle, an experiment. Ideally, we learn from each experiment. Paper as a medium to record data limits our ability to exploit that potential. Electronic medical records will facilitate research that relies on data recorded in routine medical practice. The potential of ICT, however, lies in its ability to close the loop between clinical practice, research, and education.

References

1 van Bemmel JH, Musen MA, eds. *Handbook of Medical Informatics*. Heidelberg: Springer Verlag, 1997.
2 Institute of Medicine, Committee on Improving the Patient Record. *The Computer-Based Patient Record: An Essential Technology for Health Care* (revised edn). Washington DC: National Academy Press, 1997.

3 van der Lei J, Duisterhout JS, Westerhof HP, *et al*. The introduction of computer-based patient records in the Netherlands. *Ann Intern Med* 1993;**119**:1036–41.

4 Burnum JF. The misinformation era: the fall of the medical record. *Ann Intern Med* 1989;**110**:482–4.

5 van der Lei J, Musen MA, van der Does E, Man in't veld AJ, van Bemmel JH. Comparison of computer-aided and human review of general practitioners' management of hypertension. *Lancet* 1991;**338**:1505–8.

6 Knottnerus JA. The role of electronic patient records in the development of general practice in the Netherlands. *Meth Inform Med* 1999;**38**:350–5.

7 Hunt DL, Haynes RB, Hanna SE, Smith K. Effects of computer-based decision support systems on clinician performance and patient outcomes: a systematic review. *JAMA* 1998;**280**:1339–46.

8 Vlug AE, van der Lei J, Mosseveld BMT, *et al*. Postmarketing surveillance based on electronic patient records: the IPCI project. *Meth Inform Med* 1999;**38**:339–44.

10 Clinical problem solving and diagnostic decision making: a selective review of the cognitive research literature

ARTHUR S ELSTEIN, ALAN SCHWARTZ

Summary box

- Research on clinical diagnostic reasoning has been conducted chiefly within two research paradigms, problem solving and decision making.
- The key steps in the problem solving paradigm are hypothesis generation, the interpretation of clinical data to test hypotheses, pattern recognition, and categorisation.
- The controversy about whether rapid pattern recognition is accomplished via retrieval of specific instances or by matching to a more abstract prototype can be resolved by recognising that the method selected depends upon the characteristics of the problem.
- Diagnostic performance can be influenced by errors in hypothesis generation and restructuring.
- The decision making paradigm views diagnosis as updating opinion with imperfect information; the normative rule for this process is Bayes' theorem.
- Well documented errors in probability estimation and revision include acquiring redundant evidence, neglecting the role of

disease prevalence in estimating a post-test probability, under-estimating the strength of the evidence, the effect of order of presentation of clinical information on final diagnostic conclusions, and the tendency to overestimate the probability of serious but treatable diseases to avoid missing them.

- Problem based learning and ambulatory clinical experiences make sense from the viewpoint of cognitive theory because students generalise less from specific clinical experiences than educators have traditionally hoped.

- A formal quantitative approach to the evidence might have greater generalisability. In residency training, both practice guidelines and evidence-based medicine are seen as responses to the psychological limitations of unaided clinical judgement.

Introduction

This chapter reviews the cognitive processes involved in diagnostic reasoning in clinical medicine and sketches our current understanding of these principles. It describes and analyses the psychological processes and mental structures employed in identifying and solving diagnostic problems of varying degrees of complexity, and reviews common errors and pitfalls in diagnostic reasoning. It does not consider a parallel set of issues in selecting a treatment or developing a management plan. For theoretical background we draw upon two approaches that have been particularly influential in research in this field: problem solving[1-6] and decision making.[7-11]

Problem-solving research has usually focused on how an ill-structured problem situation is defined and structured (as by generating a set of diagnostic hypotheses). Psychological decision research has typically looked at factors affecting diagnosis or treatment choice in well defined, tightly controlled problems. Despite a common theme of limited rationality, the problem-solving paradigm focuses on the wisdom of practice by concentrating on identifying the strategies of experts in a field to help learners acquire them more efficiently. Research in this tradition has aimed at providing students with some guidelines on how to develop their skills in clinical reasoning. Consequently, it has emphasised how experts generally function effectively despite limits on their rational capacities. Behavioural decision research, on the other hand, contrasts human performance with a normative statistical model of reasoning under uncertainty, Bayes' theorem. This research tradition emphasises positive standards for reasoning about uncertainty, demonstrates that even experts in a domain do not always meet these standards, and thus raises the case for some type of decision support. Behavioural decision research implies that contrasting intuitive diagnostic conclusions with those that would be reached by the formal application of Bayes' theorem would give us greater insight into both clinical reasoning and the probable underlying state of the patient.

Problem solving: diagnosis as hypothesis selection

To solve a clinical diagnostic problem means, first, to recognise a malfunction and then to set about tracing or identifying its causes. The diagnosis is ideally an explanation of disordered function – where possible, a causal explanation. The level of causal explanation changes as fundamental scientific understanding of disease mechanisms evolves. In many instances a diagnosis is a category for which no causal explanation has yet been found.

In most cases, not all of the information needed to identify and explain the situation is available early in the clinical encounter, and so the clinician must decide what information to collect, what aspects of the situation need attention, and what can be safely set aside. Thus, data collection is both sequential and selective. Experienced clinicians execute this task rapidly, almost automatically; novices struggle to develop a plan.

The hypothetico-deductive method

Early hypothesis generation and selective data collection

Difficult diagnostic problems are solved by a process of generating a limited number of hypotheses or problem formulations early in the work up and using them to guide subsequent data collection.[2] Each hypothesis can be used to predict what additional findings ought to be present, if it were true, and then the work up is a guided search for these findings; hence, the method is hypothetico-deductive. The process of problem structuring via hypothesis generation begins with a very limited dataset and occurs rapidly and automatically, even when clinicians are explicitly instructed not to generate hypotheses. Given the complexity of the clinical situation and the limited capacity of working memory, hypothesis generation is a psychological necessity. It structures the problem by generating a small set of possible solutions – a very efficient way to solve diagnostic problems. The content of experienced clinicians' hypotheses are of higher quality; some novices have difficulty in moving beyond data collection to considering possibilities.[3]

Data interpretation

To what extent do the data strengthen or weaken belief in the correctness of a particular diagnostic hypothesis? A bayesian approach to answering these questions is strongly advocated in much recent writing (for example [12,13]), and is clearly a pillar of the decision making approach to interpreting clinical findings. Yet it is likely that only a minority of clinicians employ it in daily practice, and that informal methods of opinion revision still predominate. In our experience, clinicians trained in methods of evidence-based medicine[14] are more likely to use a bayesian approach to interpreting findings than are other clinicians.

Accuracy of data interpretation and thoroughness of data collection are separate issues. A clinician could collect data thoroughly but nevertheless ignore, misunderstand, or misinterpret some findings. In contrast, a clinician might be overly economical in data collection, but could interpret whatever is available accurately. Elstein et al.[2] found no significant association between thoroughness of data collection and accuracy of data interpretation. This finding led to an increased emphasis upon data interpretation in research and education, and argued for studying clinical judgement while controlling the database. This strategy is currently the most widely used in research on clinical reasoning. Sometimes clinical information is presented sequentially: the case unfolds in a simulation of real time, but the subject is given few or no options in data collection (for example[15–17]). The analysis may focus on memory organisation, knowledge utilisation, data interpretation, or problem representation (for example[3,17,18]). In other studies, clinicians are given all the data simultaneously and asked to make a diagnosis.[19,20]

Pattern recognition or categorisation

Problem-solving expertise varies greatly across cases and is highly dependent on the clinician's mastery of the particular domain. Clinicians differ more in their understanding of problems and their problem representations than in the reasoning strategies employed.[2] From this point of view, it makes more sense to consider reasons for success and failure in a particular case, than generic traits or strategies of expert diagnosticians.

This finding of case specificity challenged the hypothetico-deductive model of clinical reasoning for several reasons: both successful and unsuccessful diagnosticians used hypothesis testing, and so it was argued that diagnostic accuracy did not depend as much on strategy as on mastery of domain content. The clinical reasoning of experts in familiar situations frequently does not display explicit hypothesis testing,[5,21–23] but is instead rapid, automatic, and often non-verbal. The speed, efficiency, and accuracy of experienced clinicians suggests that they might not even use the same reasoning processes as novices, and that experience itself might make hypothesis testing unnecessary.[5] It is likely that experienced clinicians use a hypothetico-deductive strategy only with difficult cases.[24,25] Much of the daily practice of experienced clinicians consists of seeing new cases that strongly resemble those seen previously, and their reasoning in these situations looks more like pattern recognition or direct automatic retrieval. The question then becomes, what is retrieved? What are the patterns?

Pattern recognition implies that clinical reasoning is rapid, difficult to verbalise, and has a perceptual component. Thinking of diagnosis as fitting a case into a category brings some other issues into clearer view. How is a new case categorised? Two somewhat competing accounts have been offered, and research evidence supports both. Category assignment can be based on matching the case either to a specific instance – so-called instance based or exemplar based recognition – or to a more abstract prototype. In instance based recognition a new case is categorised by its resemblance to memories of instances previously seen.[5,22,26,27] For example, acute myocardial infarction (AMI) is rapidly hypothesised in a 50-year-old male heavy smoker with severe crushing, substernal chest pain because the clinician has seen previous instances of similar men with very similar symptoms who proved to have AMI. This model is supported by the fact that clinical diagnosis is strongly affected by context (for example the location of a skin rash on the body), even when this context is normatively irrelevant.[27] These context effects suggest that clinicians are matching a new case to a previous one, not to an abstraction from several cases, because an abstraction should not include irrelevant features.

The prototype model holds that clinical experience – augmented by teaching, discussion, and the entire round of training – facilitates the construction of abstractions or prototypes.[4,28] Differences between stronger and weaker diagnosticians are explained by variations in the content and complexity of their prototypes. Better diagnosticians have constructed more diversified and abstract sets of semantic relations to represent the links between clinical features or aspects of the problem.[3,29] Support for this view is found in the fact that experts in a domain are more able to relate findings to each other and to potential diagnoses, and to identify the additional findings needed to complete a picture.[24] These capabilities suggest that experts utilise abstract representations and do not merely match a new case to a previous instance.

The controversy about the methods used in diagnostic reasoning can be resolved by recognising that clinicians, like people generally, are flexible in approaching problems: the method selected depends upon the perceived characteristics of the problem. There is an interaction between the clinician's level of skill and the perceived difficulty of the task.[30] Easy cases can be solved by pattern recognition or by going directly from data to diagnostic classification (forward reasoning).[21] Difficult cases need systematic hypothesis generation and testing. Whether a diagnostic problem is easy or difficult is a function of the knowledge and experience of the clinician who is trying to solve it. When we say that a diagnostic problem is difficult, we really mean that a significant fraction of the clinicians who encounter this problem will find it difficult, although for some it may be quite easy.

183

Errors in hypothesis generation and restructuring

Neither pattern recognition nor hypothesis testing is an error-proof strategy, nor are they always consistent with statistical rules of inference. Errors that can occur in difficult cases in internal medicine are illustrated and discussed by Kassirer and Kopelman.[17] Another classification of diagnostic errors is found in Bordage.[31] The frequency of errors in actual practice is unknown, and studies to better establish the prevalence of various errors are much needed.

Many diagnostic problems are so complex that the correct solution is not contained within the initial set of hypotheses. Restructuring and reformulating occur as data are obtained and the clinical picture evolves. However, as any problem solver works with a particular set of hypotheses, psychological commitment takes place and it becomes more difficult to restructure the problem.[32]

A related problem is that knowledge stored in long-term memory may not be activated unless triggered by a hypothesis or some other cognitive structure that provides an access channel to the contents of memory. This phenomenon has been demonstrated experimentally in a non-clinical context: recall of the details of the layout of a house varies depending on whether one takes the perspective of a burglar or a potential buyer.[33] We are unaware of an experimental demonstration of this effect in medical education, presumably because of the difficulty of ensuring that an experimental trigger has been effective. However, the complaint of many medical educators that students who can solve problems in the classroom setting appear to be unable to do so in the clinic with real patients, illustrates the role of social context in facilitating or hampering access to the memory store. On the other side of this equation there are students who struggle academically but are competent clinicians, presumably because the clinical context facilitates their thinking. These observations are all consistent with Bartlett's[34] classic proposal that memory is organised schematically, not in the storage of unconnected bits. Stories help us to remember the details and also provide guidance as to what details "must be there". This phenomenon has been demonstrated in medical students.[6]

Decision making: diagnosis as opinion revision

Bayes' theorem

From the point of view of decision theory, reaching a diagnosis involves updating an opinion with imperfect information (the clinical evidence).[10–12,35] The normative mathematical rule for this task is Bayes' theorem. The pretest probability is either the known prevalence of the disease or the clinician's subjective probability of disease before new information is acquired. As new information is obtained, the probability of each diagnostic possibility is continuously revised. The post-test probability – the probability of each disease given the information – is a function of two variables, pretest probability and the strength of the evidence. The latter is measured by a "likelihood ratio", the ratio of the probabilities of observing a particular finding in patients with and without the disease of interest.[*]

If the data are conditionally independent[†] each post-test probability becomes the pretest probability for the next stage of the inference process. Using Bayes' theorem becomes hopelessly complicated and impractical when this assumption is violated and more than two correlated cues are involved in a diagnostic judgement, as is often the case in clinical medicine. In these situations, linear and logistic regression techniques are commonly used to derive an equation or clinical prediction rule. A review of these methods is beyond the scope of this chapter. We simply point out that the coefficients (weights) in a regression equation depend on the composition of the derivation sample. Bayes' theorem distinguishes the effect of disease prevalence and the strength of the evidence on the diagnostic judgement, but ordinary regression analytical methods confound these variables in the regression coefficients. (For alternative regression approaches that address this problem, see[36]). If the index disease is overrepresented in the derivation sample, a prediction rule should be applied cautiously to populations where the prevalence of that disease is different. Despite this limitation, these rules are useful. Clinical applications of statistically derived prediction rules can outperform human judgement[37]; this is the rationale for a range of clinical prediction rules that have been developed during the past two decades. Reports of the accuracy of such rules and the reasons for their success have been available in the psychological literature on judgement for over 40 years,[38] but application in clinical practice has been slow because of continuing concerns about:

- whether a rule derived from a particular population generalises accurately to another
- eroding the professional authority and responsibility of clinicians, and
- whether guidelines (at least in the United States) are intended more to ration care and contain costs than to improve quality.[39]

Both evidence-based medicine (EBM) and decision analysis are efforts to introduce quantification into the diagnostic process and still leave a

---

[*] Formally, $LR+ = $ Sensitivity/$(1-$Specificity$)$ and $LR- = (1-$Sensitivity$)$/Specificity.
[†] Two tests are conditionally independent if the sensitivity and specificity of each test is the same whether the other is positive or negative. Formally, if T_1 and T_2 are conditionally independent tests for a disease D, then:
$p(T_2+ \,|\, D+ \text{ and } T_1+) = p(T_2+ \,|\, D+)$ and
$p(T_2- \,|\, D- \text{ and } T_1-) = p(T_2- \,|\, D-)$

substantial role for clinical judgement.[40,41] EBM leaves the application of research results, including a clinical guideline, up to the clinical judgement of the clinician, who should be guided by canons for interpreting the literature. Decision analysis proposes to offer the clinician insight into the crucial variables in a decision problem, together with a recommended strategy that maximises expected utility (for example, see[42]). Both attempt to avoid quasimandatory prescriptive guidelines and to leave room for professional discretion.

Bayes' theorem is a normative rule for diagnostic reasoning: it tells us how we *should* reason, but it does not claim that we use it to revise opinion. It directs attention to two major classes of error in clinical reasoning: in the assessment of either pretest probability or the strength of the evidence. The psychological study of diagnostic reasoning from the bayesian viewpoint has focused on errors in both components.

Errors in probability estimation

Availability

People are prone to overestimate the frequency of vivid or easily recalled events and to underestimate the frequency of events that are either very ordinary or difficult to recall.[43,44] Diseases or injuries that receive considerable media attention (for example injuries due to shark attacks) are often considered more probable than their true prevalence. This psychological principle is exemplified clinically in *overemphasising rare conditions*. Unusual cases are more memorable than routine problems. The clinical aphorism "When you hear hoofbeats, think horses, not zebras" calls attention to this bias.

Representativeness

Earlier, clinical diagnosis was viewed as a categorisation process. The strategy of estimating the probability of disease by judging how similar a case is to a diagnostic category or prototype can lead to an overestimation of the probability of a disease in two ways. First, post-test probability can be confused with test sensitivity.[45,46] For example, although fever is a typical finding in meningitis, the probability of meningitis given fever alone as a symptom is quite low. Second, representativeness neglects base rates and implicitly considers all hypotheses as equally likely. This is an error, because if a case resembles disease A and disease B equally well, and there are 10 times as many cases of A as of B, then the case is more likely an instance of A. This heuristic drives the "conjunction fallacy": incorrectly concluding that the probability of a joint event (such as the combination of multiple symptoms to form a typical clinical picture) is greater than the probability of any one of those events alone. The joint event may be more representative (typical) of the diagnostic category, but it cannot be more probable than a single component.

Probability distortions

Normative decision theory assumes that probabilities are mentally processed linearly, that is, they are not transformed from the ordinary probability scale. Because behavioural decision research has demonstrated several violations of this principle, it has been necessary to formulate descriptive theories of risky choice that will better account for choice behaviour in a wide range of situations involving uncertainty. One of the earliest of these theories is prospect theory (PT),[47] which was formulated explicitly to account for choices involving two-outcome gambles (or one two-outcome gamble and a certain outcome). Cumulative prospect theory (CPT)[48] extends the theory to the multioutcome case. Both PT and CPT propose that decision makers first edit the decision stimulus in some way, and then evaluate the edited stimulus. Options are evaluated by using an expected-utility-like rule, except that a transformation of the probabilities, called decision weights, are multiplied by subjective values and summed to yield the valuation of a lottery. Probabilities are transformed by a function that is sensitive to both the magnitude of each probability and its rank in the cumulative probability distribution. Hence, it is a *rank-dependent* utility theory. In general, small probabilities are overweighted and large probabilities underweighted. This "compression error"[49] results in discontinuities at probabilities of 0 and 1, and permits this model to predict "certainty effect" violations of expected utility theory (in which the difference between 99% and 100% is psychologically much greater than the difference between, say, 60% and 61%). Cumulative prospect theory and similar rank-dependent utility theories provide formal descriptions of how probabilities are distorted in risky decision making. The distortions are exacerbated when the probabilities are not precisely known,[50] a situation that is fairly common in clinical medicine. It should be stressed that cumulative prospect theory does not assert that individuals are in fact carrying out mentally a set of calculations which are even more complex than those required to calculate expected utility. Rather, the theory claims that observed choices (that is, behaviour) can be better modelled by this complex function than by the simpler expected-utility rule.

Support theory

Several probability estimation biases are captured by support theory,[51–53] which posits that subjective estimates of the frequency or probability of an event are influenced by how detailed the description is. More explicit descriptions yield higher probability estimates than compact, condensed descriptions, even when the two refer to exactly the same events (such as "probability of death due to a car accident, train accident, plane accident, or other moving vehicle accident" versus "probability of death due to a moving vehicle accident"). This theory can explain availability (when memories of an available event include more detailed descriptions than those of less available events) and representativeness (when a typical case description includes a cluster of details that "fit", whereas a less typical case lacks some of these features). Clinically, support theory implies that a longer, more detailed case description will be assigned a higher subjective probability of the index disease than a brief abstract of the same case, even if they contain the same information about that disease. Thus, subjective assessments of events, although often necessary in clinical practice, can be affected by factors unrelated to true prevalence.[53]

Errors in probability revision

Errors in interpreting the diagnostic value of clinical information have been found by several research teams.[2,6,54,55]

Conservatism

In clinical case discussions data are commonly presented sequentially, and diagnostic probabilities are not revised as much as is implied by Bayes' theorem. This "stickiness" has been called "conservatism", and was one of the earliest cognitive biases identified.[56]

Anchoring and adjustment

One explanation of conservatism is that diagnostic opinions are revised up or down from an initial anchor, which is either given in the problem or formed subjectively. Anchoring and adjustment means that final opinions are sensitive to the starting point (the "anchor"), that the shift ("adjustment") from it is typically insufficient, and so the final judgement is closer to the anchor than is implied by Bayes' theorem.[43] Both of these biases will lead to the collection of more information than is normatively necessary to reach a desired level of diagnostic certainty. The common complaint that clinicians overuse laboratory tests is indirect evidence that these biases operate in clinical practice.

Confounding the probability and value of an outcome

It is difficult for everyday judgement to keep separate accounts of the probability of a particular disease and the benefits that accrue from detecting it. Probability revision errors that are systematically linked to the perceived cost of mistakes demonstrate the difficulties experienced in separating assessments of probability from values.[57,58] For example, there is a tendency to overestimate the probability of more serious but treatable diseases, because a clinician would hate to miss one.[57]

188

Acquiring redundant evidence

"Pseudodiagnosticity"[59] or "confirmation bias"[54] is the tendency to seek information that confirms a hypothesis rather than the data that facilitate efficient testing of competing hypotheses. For example, in one study, residents in internal medicine preferred about 25% of the time to order findings that would give a more detailed clinical picture of one disease, rather than findings that would allow them to test between two potential diagnoses.[54] Here, the problem is knowing what information would be useful, rather than overestimating the value (likelihood ratio) of the information, or failing to combine it optimally with other data.[55]

Incorrect interpretation

A common error is interpreting findings as consistent with hypotheses already under consideration.[2,6,60] Where findings are distorted in recall, it is generally in the direction of making the facts more consistent with typical clinical pictures.[2] Positive findings are overemphasised and negative findings tend to be discounted.[2,61] From a bayesian standpoint these are all errors in assessing the diagnostic value of information, that is, errors in subjectively assessing the likelihood ratio. Even when clinicians agree on the presence of certain clinical findings, wide variations have been found in the weights assigned in interpreting cues,[20] and this variation may be due partly to the effect of the hypotheses being considered.[60]

Order effects

Bayes' theorem implies that clinicians given identical information should reach the same diagnostic opinion, regardless of the order in which the information is presented. However, final opinions are also affected by the order of presentation: information presented later in a case is given more weight than that presented earlier.[15,62] This may partly explain why it is difficult to get medical students to pay as much attention to history and the physical examination as their teachers would wish. Modern diagnostic studies tend to have very high likelihood ratios, and they also are obtained late in the diagnostic work up.

Educational implications

Two recent innovations in undergraduate medical education and residency training, problem based learning and evidence-based medicine, are consistent with the educational implications of this research.

Problem based learning (PBL)[63–65] can be understood as an effort to introduce formulating and testing clinical hypotheses into a preclinical curriculum dominated by biological sciences. The cognitive–instructional theory behind this reform was that, because experienced clinicians use this strategy with difficult problems, and as practically any clinical situation selected for instructional purposes will be difficult for students, it makes sense to call this strategy to their attention and to provide opportunities to practise it, first using case simulations and then with real patients.

The finding of case specificity showed the limits of a focus on teaching a general problem solving strategy. Problem solving expertise can be separated from content analytically, but not in practice. This realisation shifted the emphasis toward helping students acquire a functional organisation of content with clinically usable schemata. This became the new rationale for problem based learning.[66,67]

Because transfer from one context to another is limited, clinical experience is needed in contexts closely related to future practice. The instance-based model of problem solving supports providing more experience in outpatient care because it implies that students do not generalise as much from one training setting to another as has traditionally been thought. But a clinician overly dependent on context sees every case as unique, as all of the circumstances are never exactly replicated. The unwanted intrusion of irrelevant context effects implies that an important educational goal is to reduce inappropriate dependence on context. In our opinion, there are two ways to do this:

1. Emphasise that students should strive to develop prototypes and abstractions from their clinical experience. Clinical experience that is not subject to reflection and review is not enough. It must be reviewed and analysed so that the correct general models and principles are abstracted. Most students do this, but some struggle, and medical educators ought not to count upon its spontaneous occurrence. Well designed educational experiences to facilitate the development of the desired cognitive structures should include extensive focused practice and feedback with a variety of problems.[5,68] The current climate, with its emphasis on seeing more patients to compensate for declining patient care revenues, threatens medical education at this level because it makes it more difficult for clinical preceptors to provide the needed critique and feedback, and for students to have time for the necessary reflection.[69]

2. A practical bayesian approach to diagnosis can be introduced. EBM[14,70] may be viewed as the most recent – and, by most standards, the most successful – effort to date to apply these methods to clinical diagnosis. EBM uses likelihood ratios to quantify the strength of the clinical evidence, and shows how this measure should be combined with disease prevalence (or prior probability) to yield a post-test probability. This is Bayes' theorem offered to clinicians in a practical, useful format! Its strengths are in stressing the role of data in clinical reasoning, and in

encouraging clinicians to rely on their judgement to apply the results of a particular study to their patients. Its weaknesses, in our view, are that it does not deal systematically with the role of patient preferences in these decisions, or with methods for quantifying preferences, and that it blurs the distinction between probability driven and utility driven decisions.

In our experience teaching EBM, residents soon learn how to interpret studies of diagnostic tests and how to use a nomogram[70,71] to compute post-test probabilities. The nomogram, or a 2×2 table, combines their prior index of suspicion (a subjective probability) and the test characteristics reported in the clinical literature. It has been more difficult to introduce concepts of decision thresholds (at what probability should management change?) and the expected value of information (should a test that cannot result in a change in action be performed at all?).

Methodological guidelines

1. Psychological research on clinical reasoning began in a thinking-aloud tradition, which remains attractive to many investigators. It seems quite natural to ask a clinician to articulate and discuss the reasoning involved in a particular case, and to record these verbalisations for later analysis. Whatever its shortcomings, this research strategy has high face validity. Because the clinicians involved in these studies frequently discuss real cases (for example[2,17]), content validity on the clinical side is not a problem.

The problems of this approach are easily summarised: first, it is labour intensive, and therefore most studies have used small samples of both clinicians and cases. Therefore, they lack statistical power and are best suited for exploratory analysis. But to demonstrate statistically significant differences between experts (senior attending clinicians) and novices (medical students or junior house officers), researchers must take into account two facts: (1) within any group of clinicians at any level of clinical experience, or within any speciality, there is a great amount of variation, both in reasoning and in practice. With small samples, within-group variance will make it difficult to demonstrate significant between-group differences; and (2) the performance of clinicians varies considerably across cases. These two features imply that research on diagnostic reasoning must use adequate samples of both clinicians and cases if there is to be any hope of reaching generalisable conclusions. Most research to date has not paid adequate attention to issues of sample size (of both cases and research participants) and statistical power.

2. Many important cognitive processes are not available to consciousness and are not verbalised. Indeed, the more automatic and overlearned a mental process is, the less likely is it that one can verbalise

how the process works. Once a person has lived for some time at a given address, it becomes impossible to tell how one knows that address: it is simply "known". Closer to our concerns, participants do not report that a subjective probability is overestimated because of the availability bias: the existence of the bias is inferred by comparing estimates with known frequencies. For these reasons, much recent work has shifted toward a research paradigm that owes much to experimental cognitive psychology: research participants are presented with a task and their responses are recorded. Their verbalisations are one more source of data, but are not treated as a true account of internal mental processes. This research has yielded many of the findings summarised in this chapter, but it is at times criticised for using artificial tasks (lack of face validity) and, consequently, not motivating the participants adequately. The generalisability of the results to real clinical settings is then questioned.

3. Selection bias is a potential threat to the validity of both types of studies of clinical reasoning. Senior clinicians in any clinical domain can decline to participate in research far more easily than can medical students or house officers in the same domain. Therefore, the more experienced participants in a study are usually volunteers. Attention should be paid to issues of selection bias and response rate as potential limitations; thought should be given to their possible effects on the validity and generalisability of the results of the study.

4. Behavioural decision research conducted to date has been concerned primarily with demonstrating that a particular phenomenon exists, for example demonstrating biases in probability estimation, such as availability and representativeness. Statistical tests of significance are used to demonstrate the phenomena. From an educational standpoint, we ought to be more interested in identifying how prevalent these biases are and which are most likely to affect treatment and management. Thus, more research is needed to assess the prevalence of these errors and to determine how often treatment choices are affected by diagnostic errors caused by these biases. If these facts were known, a more rational, systematic curriculum could be developed.

Conclusion

This chapter has selectively reviewed 30 years of psychological research on clinical diagnostic reasoning, focusing on problem solving and decision making as the dominant paradigms of the field. This research demonstrates the limitations of human judgement, although the research designs employed make it difficult to estimate their prevalence. Problem based learning and evidence-based medicine are both justified by the psychological research about judgement limitations, violations of bayesian principles in everyday clinical reasoning, and the finding of limited transfer across clinical situations, although we do not believe that these innovations were initially directed by an awareness of cognitive limitations. Within graduate medical education (residency training), the introduction of practice guidelines based on evidence has been controversial because guidelines may be perceived as efforts to restrict the authority of clinicians and to ration care. The psychological research helps to explain why formal statistical decision supports are both needed and likely to evoke controversy.

Preparation of this review was supported in part by grant RO1 LM5630 from the National Library of Medicine.

References

1 Newell A, Simon HA. *Human problem solving*. Englewood Cliffs (NJ): Prentice-Hall, 1972.
2 Elstein AS, Shulman LS, Sprafka SA. *Medical problem solving: An analysis of clinical reasoning*. Cambridge MA: Harvard University Press, 1978.
3 Bordage G, Lemieux M. Semantic structures and diagnostic thinking of experts and novices. *Acad Med* 1991;**66**(9 Suppl):S70–S72.
4 Bordage G, Zacks R. The structure of medical knowledge in the memories of medical students and general practitioners: categories and prototypes. *Med Educ* 1984;**18**:406–16.
5 Schmidt HG, Norman GR, Boshuizen HPA. A cognitive perspective on medical expertise: theory and implications. *Acad Med* 1990;**65**:611–21.
6 Friedman MH, Connell KJ, Olthoff AJ, Sinacore J, Bordage G. Medical student errors in making a diagnosis. *Acad Med* 1998;**73**(10 Suppl):S19–S21.
7 Kahneman D, Slovic P, Tversky A (eds.) *Judgment under uncertainty: Heuristics and biases*. New York: Cambridge University Press, 1982.
8 Baron J. *Thinking and deciding*. New York: Cambridge University Press, 1988.
9 Mellers BA, Schwartz A, Cooke ADJ. Judgment and decision making. *Annu Rev Psychol* 1998;**49**:447–77.
10 Weinstein MC, Fineberg HV, Elstein AS, *et al. Clinical decision analysis*. Philadelphia: WB Saunders, 1980.
11 Sox HC Jr, Blatt MA, Higgins MC, Marton KI. *Medical decision making*. Stoneham (MA): Butterworths, 1988.
12 Pauker SG. Clinical decision making: handling and analyzing clinical data. In: Bennett JC, Plum F, eds. *Cecil's Textbook of Medicine*, 20th edn. Philadelphia: WB Saunders, 1996;78–83.
13 Panzer RJ, Black ER, Griner PF. *Diagnostic strategies for common medical problems*. Philadelphia: American College of Physicians, 1991.
14 Sackett DL, Richardson WS, Rosenberg W, Haynes RB. *Evidence-based medicine: how to practice and teach EBM*. New York: Churchill Livingstone, 1997.
15 Chapman GB, Bergus GR, Elstein AS. Order of information affects clinical judgment. *J Behav Decision Making* 1996;**9**:201–11.
16 Moskowitz AJ, Kuipers BJ, Kassirer JP. Dealing with uncertainty, risks, and tradeoffs in clinical decisions: a cognitive science approach. *Ann Intern Med* 1988;**108**:435–49.
17 Kassirer JP, Kopelman RI. *Learning clinical reasoning*. Baltimore: Williams & Wilkins, 1991.
18 Joseph GM, Patel VL. Domain knowledge and hypothesis generation in diagnostic reasoning. *Med Decision Making* 1990;**10**:31–46.
19 Patel VL, Groen G. Knowledge-based solution strategies in medical reasoning. *Cogn Sci* 1986;**10**:91–116.
20 Wigton RS, Hoellerich VL, Patil KD. How physicians use clinical information in diagnosing pulmonary embolism: an application of conjoint analysis. *Med Decision Making* 1986;**6**:2–11.

21 Groen GJ, Patel VL. Medical problem-solving: some questionable assumptions. *Med Educ* 1985;**19**:95–100.

22 Brooks LR, Norman GR, Allen SW. Role of specific similarity in a medical diagnostic task. *J Exp Psych: Gen* 1991;**120**:278–87.

23 Eva KW, Neville AJ, Norman GR. Exploring the etiology of content specificity: factors influencing analogic transfer and problem solving. *Acad Med* 1998;**73**(10 Suppl):S1–S5.

24 Elstein AS, Kleinmuntz B, Rabinowitz M, *et al.* Diagnostic reasoning of high- and low-domain knowledge clinicians: a re-analysis. *Med Decision Making* 1993;**13**:21–9.

25 Davidoff F. *Who has seen a blood sugar? Reflections on medical education.* Philadelphia: American College of Physicians, 1998.

26 Medin DL, Schaffer MM. A context theory of classification learning. *Psychol Rev* 1978;**85**:207–38.

27 Norman GR, Coblentz CL, Brooks LR, Babcock CJ. Expertise in visual diagnosis: a review of the literature. *Acad Med* 1992;**66**:S78–S83.

28 Rosch E, Mervis CB. Family resemblances: studies in the internal structure of categories. *Cogn Psychol* 1975;**7**:573–605.

29 Lemieux M, Bordage G. Propositional versus structural semantic analyses of medical diagnostic thinking. *Cogn Sci* 1992;**16**:185–204.

30 Elstein AS. What goes around comes around: the return of the hypothetico-deductive strategy. *Teach Learn Med* 1994;**6**:121–3.

31 Bordage G. Why did I miss the diagnosis? Some cognitive explanations and educational implications. *Acad Med* 1999;**74**:S138–S142.

32 Janis IL, Mann L. *Decision-making.* New York: Free Press, 1977.

33 Anderson RC, Pichert JW. Recall of previously unrecallable information following a shift in perspective. *J Verb Learning Verb Behav* 1978;**17**:1–12.

34 Bartlett FC. *Remembering: a study in experimental and social psychology.* New York: Macmillan, 1932.

35 Sackett DL, Haynes RB, Guyatt GH, Tugwell P. *Clinical epidemiology: A basic science for clinical medicine,* 2nd edn. Boston: Little, Brown and Company; 1991.

36 Knottnerus JA. Application of logistic regression to the analysis of diagnostic data. *Med Decision Making* 1992;**12**:93–108.

37 Ebell MH. Using decision rules in primary care practice. *Prim Care* 1995;**22**:319–40.

38 Meehl PE. *Clinical versus statistical prediction: A theoretical analysis and review of the evidence.* Minneapolis: University of Minnesota Press, 1954.

39 James PA, Cowan TM, Graham RP, Majeroni BA. Family physicians' attitudes about and use of clinical practice guidelines. *J Fam Pract* 1997;**45**:341–7.

40 Hayward R, Wilson MC, Tunis SR, Bass EB, Guyatt GH, for the Evidence-Based Medicine Working Group. Users' guides to the medical literature. VIII: how to use clinical practice guidelines, A: are the recommendations valid? *JAMA* 1995;**274**:70–4.

41 Wilson MC, Hayward R, Tunis SR, Bass EB, Guyatt GH, for the Evidence-Based Medicine Working Group. Users' guides to the medical literature. VIII: how to use clinical practice guidelines, B: what are the recommendations and will they help me in caring for my patient? *JAMA* 1995;**274**:1630–2.

42 Col NF, Eckman MH, Karas RH, *et al.* Patient-specific decisions about hormone replacement therapy in postmenopausal women. *JAMA* 1997;**277**:1140–7.

43 Tversky A, Kahneman D. Judgment under uncertainty: heuristics and biases. *Science* 1974;**185**:1124–31.

44 Elstein AS. Heuristics and biases: selected errors in clinical reasoning. *Acad Med* 1999;**74**:791–4.

45 Eddy DM. Probabilistic reasoning in clinical medicine: problems and opportunities. In: Kahneman D, Slovic P, Tversky A, eds. *Judgment under uncertainty: Heuristics and biases.* New York: Cambridge University Press; 1982;249–67.

46 Dawes, RM. *Rational choice in an uncertain world.* New York: Harcourt Brace Jovanovich, 1988.

47 Tversky A, Kahneman D. The framing of decisions and the psychology of choice. *Science* 1982;**211**:453–8.

48 Tversky A, Kahneman D. Advances in prospect theory: cumulative representation of uncertainty. *J Risk Uncertain* 1992;**5**:297–323.

49 Fischhoff B, Bostrom A, Quadrell MJ. Risk perception and communication. *Annu Rev Pub Health* 1993;**14**:183–203.

50 Einhorn HJ, Hogarth RM. Decision making under ambiguity. *J Business* 1986; **59**(Suppl):S225–S250.

51 Tversky A, Koehler DJ. Support theory: a nonextensional representation of subjective probability. *Psychol Rev* 1994;**101**:547–67.

52 Rottenstreich Y, Tversky A. Unpacking, repacking, and anchoring: advances in support theory. *Psychol Rev* 1997;**104**:406–15.

53 Redelmeier DA, Koehler DJ, Liberman V, Tversky A. Probability judgment in medicine: discounting unspecified probabilities. *Med Decision Making* 1995;**15**:227–30.

54 Wolf FM, Gruppen LD, Billi JE. Differential diagnosis and the competing hypotheses heuristic: A practical approach to judgment under uncertainty and Bayesian probability. *JAMA* 1985;**253**:2858–62.

55 Gruppen LD, Wolf FM, Billi JE. Information gathering and integration as sources of error in diagnostic decision making. *Med Decision Making* 1991;**11**:233–9.

56 Edwards W. Conservatism in human information processing. In: Kleinmuntz B, ed. *Formal representation of human judgment.* New York, Wiley, 1969. pp. 17–52.

57 Wallsten TS. Physician and medical student bias in evaluating information. *Med Decision Making* 1981;**1**:145–64.

58 Poses RM, Cebul RD, Collins M, Fager SS. The accuracy of experienced physicians' probability estimates for patients with sore throats. *JAMA* 1985;**254**:925–9.

59 Kern L, Doherty ME. "Pseudodiagnosticity" in an idealized medical problem-solving environment. *J Med Educ* 1982;**57**:100–4.

60 Hatala R, Norman GR, Brooks LR. Influence of a single example on subsequent electrocardiogram interpretation. *Teach Learn Med* 1999;**11**:110–17.

61 Wason PC, Johnson-Laird PN. *Psychology of reasoning: Structure and content.* Cambridge (MA): Harvard University Press, 1972.

62 Bergus GR, Chapman GB, Gjerde C, Elstein AS. Clinical reasoning about new symptoms in the face of pre-existing disease: sources of error and order effects. *Fam Med* 1995; **27**:314–20.

63 Barrows HS. Problem-based, self-directed learning. *JAMA* 1983;**250**:3077–80.

64 Barrows HS. A taxonomy of problem-based learning methods. *Med Educ* 1986;**20**:481–6.

65 Schmidt HG. Problem-based learning: rationale and description. *Med Educ* 1983; **17**:11–16.

66 Norman GR. Problem-solving skills, solving problems and problem-based learning. *Med Educ* 1988;**22**:279–86.

67 Gruppen LD. Implications of cognitive research for ambulatory care education. *Acad Med* 1997;**72**:117–20.

68 Bordage G. The curriculum: overloaded and too general? *Med Educ* 1987;**21**:183–8.

69 Ludmerer KM. *Time to heal: American medical education from the turn of the century to the era of managed care.* New York: Oxford University Press, 1999.

70 Fagan TJ. Nomogram for Bayes' theorem. *N Engl J Med* [Letter] 1975;**293**:257.

71 Schwartz A. Nomogram for Bayes' theorem. Available at http://araw.mede.uic.edu/ cgi-bin/testcalc.pl.

11 Improving test ordering and diagnostic cost effectiveness in clinical practice – bridging the gap between clinical research and routine health care

RON AG WINKENS, GEERT-JAN DINANT

Summary box

- In recent decades the number of diagnostic tests ordered by doctors has increased enormously, despite the often absent or disappointing results from studies into their accuracy.
- Contradictions between scientific evidence and daily practice can be obstacles to improving test ordering behaviour.
- Evidence-based clinical guidelines are needed to formalise optimal diagnostic performance, but will not work unless implemented properly.
- There is no "one and only ideal implementation strategy". Often, a combination of supportive interventions is the best approach.
- Interventions should provide both knowledge on what to do and insight into one's own performance. Such interventions are audit, individual feedback, peer review, and computer reminders.
- From a viewpoint of cost effectiveness, computer interventions look promising.

- More attention must be paid to the perpetuation of interventions once they have been started, and to the measurement and scientific evaluation of their effects over time.
- Although the randomised controlled trial remains the "gold standard" for evaluation studies, inherent methodological challenges, such as the required randomisation of doctors, need special attention.
- More research into the ways to improve test ordering is urgently needed, in particular for patients suffering from recurrent non-specific or unexplained complaints.

Introduction

An important part of making a proper diagnosis is using diagnostic tests, such as blood and radiographic investigations. In recent decades the total number of diagnostic tests ordered by doctors has increased substantially, despite the often disappointing results from studies into their diagnostic accuracy. Apparently, arguments other than scientific ones for test ordering are relevant. Furthermore, it might be questioned to what extent current knowledge, insights into the correct use of diagnostic tests, and results from research have been properly and adequately implemented in daily practice. This chapter will discuss how to bridge the gap between evidence from clinical research and routine health care.

The need to change

For several reasons there is a need to improve test ordering behaviour. The use of medical resources in western countries is growing annually and consistently. In the Netherlands, for example, there is a relatively stable growth in nationwide expenditures for health care of approximately 7% per year. The growth in expenditure for diagnostic tests is similar. However, whereas expenditure increases, health status does not seem to improve accordingly. This at least suggests that there is a widespread and general overuse of diagnostic tests.

The following factors may be responsible for the increasing use of diagnostic tests. First, the mere availability and technological imperative of more test facilities is an important determinant. In view of the interaction between supply and demand in health care, the simple fact that tests can be ordered will lead to their actual ordering. This applies especially to new tests, which are sometimes used primarily out of curiosity. Another factor is the increasing demand for care, caused partly by the ageing of the population and an increasing number of chronically ill people. Also, new insights from scientific evidence and guidelines often provide recommendations for additional diagnostic testing.

Doctors might wish to perform additional testing once an abnormal test result is found, even in the absence of clinical suspicion, while ignoring that a test result outside reference ranges may generally be found in 50% of a healthy population. A cascade of testing may then be the result.

Furthermore, over the years, higher standards of care (adopted by the public, patients, and healthcare professionals) and defensive behaviours from doctors have contributed to the increased use of healthcare services, one of them being diagnostic testing.

In summary, despite the introduction of guidelines focusing on rational use of diagnostic tests, in daily practice reasons for ignoring evidence-based recommendations (such as fear of patients, and the doctor's wish to gain time) are numerous and hard to grasp.

Altogether, the ensuing problem is threefold. First, there are reasons to believe that some of the tests requested are non-rational. Second, contradictions between scientific evidence and daily practice can be ultimate obstacles to changing test ordering behaviour. And third, there is an increasing tension between volume growth and financial constraints. With this in mind, it is clear that there is a need to achieve a more efficient use of diagnostic tests. If interventions meant to put a stop to the unbridled growth in the number of tests ordered were to focus especially on situations where their use is clearly inappropriate, healthcare expenditure might be reduced and the quality of care might even improve.

Can we make the change?

In terms of quality improvement and cost containment there are sufficient arguments for attempting to change test ordering behaviour. To do so, it is recommended that certain steps be taken, from orientation to perpetuation. The individual steps are described in the implementation cycle[1] (Figure 11.1).

Following the implementation cycle, several things need to be done. First, insight into the problem is needed. The problem needs to be well defined and must be made clear to those whose performance we wish to change. Next, the optimal – "gold standard" – situation should be determined, and communicated as such. Usually this means the development and dissemination of guidelines. Also, an assessment of actual performance (the level of actual care) is needed. Then, the desired changes need to be determined and an implementation strategy set up to achieve the actual change. After this, the results should be monitored. The outcome of this monitoring can be used as new input for further improvement and for defining new goals for quality assurance, thereby re-entering the implementation cycle. It should be noted that these general rules apply

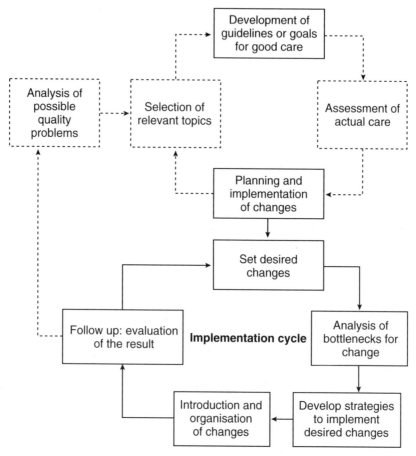

Figure 11.1 The implementation cycle.[1]

not only to test ordering behaviour, but also to other actions (such as prescribing drugs and referring to hospital care). The following highlights a number of steps in the implementation cycle.

If we are to change the test ordering behaviour of clinicians the first move is to assess and establish what the desired optimal situation would be and how the actual performance should look. Guidelines, protocols and standards are needed to formalise this optimal situation. In the past there have been various moves toward guideline development. By and large, these guidelines are problem oriented and address clinical problems as a whole, such as taking care of diabetes patients, or diagnosing and managing dyspepsia. The diagnostic work up of a clinical problem and the resulting recommendations for specific tests – if necessary – are then important aspects to be dealt with. A good example of a comprehensive set of guidelines is the development of standards for Dutch GPs by the Dutch College of General Practitioners.[2] Starting in 1989, the College has set up almost 70 guidelines on a variety of common clinical problems. In the meantime, many of these standards have been revised in line with new evidence from scientific research. One of the guidelines specifically addresses the principles of rational ordering of blood tests.[3]

The development of guidelines does not automatically lead to the desired behavioural change, especially when their dissemination is limited to the distribution of written material. In other words, simply publishing and mailing the guidelines does not make clinicians act accordingly. Implementation strategies are needed to bring about actual change. Implementation actually includes a whole range of activities to stimulate the use of guidelines. Such activities may include communication and information, giving insight into the problem and the need to change, and specific activities to achieve the actual change in behaviour.

One of the oldest and most frequently used interventions is postgraduate continuous medical education (CME), varying from lectures to comprehensive courses and training sessions. Nowadays, CME is increasingly connected to (re)certification. Another intervention that can be considered an implementation strategy is written material through books, papers in the literature, and protocol manuals. Although part of the written material is intended as a way to distribute research findings and to increase the level of up to date scientific knowledge, among clinicians it is often also focused as improving clinical performance. There is a range of interventions that combine the provision of knowledge with giving more specific insight into one's own performance. Such interventions include audit, individual feedback, peer review, and computer reminders.

Audit represents a monitoring system on specific aspects of care. It is often a rather formal system, set up and organised by colleges and regional or national committees.[4] The subject of an audit system may vary strongly, and the same applies for the intensity of the related interventions. Feedback resembles audit in many ways, although it tends to be less formal and its development is often dependent on local or even personal initiatives. In peer review, actual performance is reviewed by expert colleagues. Peer review is used not only to improve aspects of clinical care, but also to improve organisational aspects such as practice management. An intervention that needs special attention is the provision of computer reminders. Having the same background and intentions as audit and feedback, these do not generally involve the monitoring of the performance of specific groups or individual doctors. Here the computer may take over, but the intention is still to provide knowledge and give insight into one's own performance. From the viewpoint of the observed clinician, "anonymised" computer reminder systems may appear less threatening:

there are no peers directly involved who must review the actions of those whose behaviour is monitored.

Organisational interventions are focused on facilitating or reducing certain (diagnostic) actions. Examples are changing test ordering forms by restricting the number of tests that can be ordered, and introducing specific prerequisites or criteria that must be met before a test is ordered. There are two structural implementation strategies that can be used to change test ordering. Regulations include interventions where financial incentives or penalties can be easily introduced. Reimbursement systems by health insurance companies or the government may act as a stimulus to urge clinicians to move in the desired direction. Combinations of regulatory steps and financial changes are also conceivable. In several western countries the healthcare system includes payment for tests ordered by doctors, even if the tests are performed by another professional or institution. Adaptation of the healthcare regulations could change this payment system, which might reduce the ordering of too many tests, thereby directly increasing clinicians' income. Even negative incentives for non-rational test ordering can be built in, acting more or less as a financial penalty.

For obvious reasons we should seek and apply methods that both improve the rationality of test ordering and can stop the increase in the use of tests. Ideally, such instruments combine a more rational test ordering behaviour with a reduction in requests. To determine these, a closer look at the performance of the specific implementation strategies is needed. However, not all of these instruments have been used on a regular basis. Some have been regularly applied on a variety of topics (such as changing test ordering), whereas others have been used only incidentally. Most implementation strategies try to change clinicians' behaviour. Although evidence showing relevant effects is required to justify their implementation in practice, because of the nature of the intervention it is not always possible to perform a proper effect evaluation. Especially in large-scale interventions, such as changes in the law or healthcare regulations (nationwide), it is virtually impossible to obtain a concurrent control group. Nevertheless, a number of (randomised) trials have been performed, albeit predominantly on relatively small-scale implementation strategies. The next section gives an overview of the experience so far with most of the aforementioned instruments.

Is a change feasible?

Implementation strategies

As shown above, a variety of implementation strategies is available. However, not all of them are successful: some strategies have proved to be effective, but others have been disappointing. This section gives a review of the literature to assess which implementation strategies are potentially successful and which are not. There have been a number of published reviews focusing on the effectiveness of implementation strategies. Although their conclusions vary, some general consensus can be observed: there are some implementation strategies that on the whole seem to fail and some that are at least promising.

One of the reasons for the increasing use of tests is the simple fact that tests are both available and accessible. Consequently, a simple strategy would be to reduce the availability of tests on forms, or to request an explicit justification for the test(s) ordered. Such interventions have by and large proved to be effective, with a low input of additional costs and effort: Zaat and Smithuis[5,6] found reductions of 20–50%. A drawback of these interventions, however, is that they risk a possible underuse of tests when the test order form is reduced too extensively and unselectively. Therefore, the changes to the form should be selected and designed very carefully.

Among the implementation strategies that have been used and studied regularly in the past are audit and feedback. To that end, tests ordered are reviewed and discussed by (expert) peers or audit panels. Within this group of interventions there is a huge variation in what is reviewed and discussed, in how often and to whom it is directed, and in the way the review is presented. It may not be surprising that the evaluation of various types of peer review does not allow a uniform conclusion. An intervention with substantial effects, also proven in a randomised trial, was feedback given to individual general practitioners, focusing on the rationality of tests ordered.[7] After 9 years there was a clear and constant reduction in test use, mainly due to a decrease in non-rational requests. Not all interventions are so successful. In studies by Wones[8] and Everett,[9] feedback was restricted to information about the costs of tests ordered; it did not show any effect. Nevertheless, there is evidence suggesting that feedback under specific conditions is an effective method to bring about change. Feedback is more effective when the information provided can be used directly in daily practice, when the doctor is individually addressed, and when the expert peer is generally respected and accepted.

An increasingly popular implementation strategy is the use of computer reminders. This is stimulated by the explosive growth in the use of computer technology in health care, especially in the last decade. The results of computer reminders are promising. It appears to be a potentially effective method requiring relatively little effort. Reminders have significant but variable effects in reducing unnecessary tests, and seem to improve adherence to guidelines.[10] To date, there are relatively few studies on computer reminders. It may be expected, however, that in the near future more interventions on the basis of computer reminders will be performed as a direct spin-off of the growing use of computer-supported communication facilities in health care.

For one implementation strategy in regular use it is clear that the effects on test ordering behaviour are only marginal, if not absent. For many years much effort has been put into postgraduate education courses and in writing papers for clinical journals. The goal of both is to improve the clinical competence of a large target group. Nowadays there is evidence that the direct effects of these methods are disappointing. In a recently published systematic Cochrane Review, Davis et al.[11] concluded that "didactic sessions do not appear to be effective in changing physician performance". In another Cochrane Review by van der Weijden et al.,[12] it was found that the effects of written material on test ordering was small.

Perpetuation and continuation

One aspect that needs more attention in the future is the perpetuation of interventions once they have been started. It is by no means assured that effects, when achieved, will continue when the intervention itself is stopped. In most studies, the effects after stopping the intervention are not monitored. As one of the exceptions, Tierney[13] performed a follow up after ending his intervention through computer reminders on test ordering. The effects of the intervention disappeared 6 months after it was stopped. On the other hand, Winkens[7] found that feedback was still effective after being continued over a 9-year period. This argues in favour of a continuation of an implementation strategy once it is started.

Evaluating the effects

There is a growing awareness that the effects of interventions are by no means guaranteed. Consequently, to discriminate between interventions that are successful and those that are not, we need evidence from scientific evaluations. However, after a series of decades where many scientific evaluations of implementation strategies have been performed and a number of reviews have been published, many questions remain and final conclusions cannot yet be drawn. In a dynamic environment such as the (para)medical profession, it is almost inevitable that the effects of interventions are dynamic and variable over time too. Hence there will always be a need for scientific evaluation.

As is the case with all scientific evaluations, there are quality criteria that studies should meet.[14] Regarding these criteria, evaluation studies on implementation strategies do not essentially differ from other evaluations. The randomised controlled trial still remains the "gold standard". However, there are some circumstances that need special attention.[15] A striking one is the following. In most studies on improving test ordering behaviour, the doctor is the one whose decisions are to be influenced. This automatically means that the unit of randomisation, and hence the unit of analysis, is the individual doctor. As the number of doctors participating in a study is often limited, this may have a considerably negative effect on the power of the study. A potential solution to this problem may be found in multilevel analyses.[16]

Cost effectiveness of implementation

As far as the cost effectiveness of intervention strategies is concerned, those that combine good effects with the least effort and lowest costs are to be preferred. On the other hand, we may question whether strategies that so far have not proved to be effective should be continued. Should we continue to put much effort into CME, especially in single training courses or lectures? Who should we try to reach through scientific and didactic papers: the clinicians in daily practice, or only the scientist and policy maker with special interest? Should we have to choose the most effective intervention method, regardless of the effort that is needed? If we start an intervention to change test ordering, does this mean it has to be continued for years? There is no general answer to these questions, although the various reviews that have been published argue in favour of combined, tailormade interventions. How such a combination is composed depends on the specific situation (such as local needs and healthcare routines, and the availability of experts and facilities). Generalisable recommendations for specific combinations are therefore not possible or useful. However, if we look at costs in the long term, computer interventions look quite promising.

From scientific evidence to daily practice

An important objective in influencing test ordering behaviour is the change in the rationality and volume of orders, thereby reducing costs or achieving a better (so-called) cost–benefit ratio. However, the ultimate goal is to improve the quality of care for the individual patient. It might be asked to what extent patients are willing to pay for expensive diagnostic activities, weighing the possibility of achieving better health through doing (and paying) the diagnostics, versus the risk of not diagnosing the disease and staying ill (or getting worse) because of not doing so. In other words, how is the cost–utility ratio of diagnostic testing assessed by the patient? In this context the specific positive or negative (side) effects of (not) testing on the health status of the individual patient are difficult to assess independently of other influences. On the other hand, a reduced use in unnecessary, non-rational tests is not likely to cause adverse effects for the individual.

Despite the increasing research evidence showing the need for changes in test ordering behaviour, doctors will always decide on more than merely scientific evidence when the question whether or not to order a test for a certain patient is at stake.[17] Low diagnostic accuracy or high costs of testing may conflict with a patient's explicit wish to have tests ordered, or with the doctor's wish to gain time, the fear of missing an important diagnosis, his or her feeling insecure, and the wish of both patient and doctor to be reassured. These dilemmas are influenced by a variety of doctor and patient related aspects. Regarding the doctor, one could think of the way in which they were trained, how long they have been active in patient care, the number of patients on their list, their relationship with their patients, and their personal experience with "missing" relevant diseases in the past. The patient might suffer from a chronic disease, or from recurrent vague or unexplained complaints, making them question the skills of the doctor. For this latter category of patients in particular, doctors might order more tests than are strictly necessary. Research into the ways of improving test ordering in these situations is urgently needed.

References

1 Grol RPTM, van Everdingen JJE, Casparie AF. *Invoering van richtlijnen en veranderingen.* Utrecht, De Tijdstroom:1994.
2 (a) Geijer RMM, Burgers JS, van der Laan JR, *et al. NHG-Standaarden voor de huisarts I*, 2nd edn. Utrecht, Bunge:1999.(b) Thomas S, Geijer RMM, van der Laan JR, *et al. NHG-Standaarden voor de huisarts II.* Utrecht, Bunge:1996.
3 Dinant GJ, van Wijk MAM, Janssens HJEM, *et al.* NHG-Standaard Bloedonderzoek. *Huisarts Wet* 1994;**37**:202–11.
4 Smith R. *Audit in action.* London, BMJ Publishers:1992.
5 Zaat JO, van Eijk JT, Bonte HA. Laboratory test form design influences test ordering by general practitioners in the Netherlands. *Med Care* 1992;**30**:189–98.
6 Smithuis LOMJ, van Geldrop WJ, Lucassen PLBJ. Beperking van het laboratorium-onderzoek door een probleemgeorienteerd aanvraagformulier [abstract in English]. *Huisarts Wet* 1994;**37**:464–6.
7 Winkens RAG, Pop P, Grol RPTM, *et al.* Effects of routine individual feedback over nine years on general practitioners' requests for tests. *BMJ* 1996;**312**:490.
8 Wones RG. Failure of low-cost audits with feedback to reduce laboratory test utilization. *Med Care* 1987;**25**:78–82.
9 Everett GD, de Blois CS, Chang PF, Holets T. Effects of cost education, cost audits, and faculty chart review on the use of laboratory services. *Arch Intern Med* 1983;**143**:942–4.
10 Buntinx F, Winkens RAG, Grol RPTM, Knottnerus JA. Influencing diagnostic and preventive performance in ambulatory care by feedback and reminders. A review. *Fam Pract* 1993;**10**:219–28.
11 Davis D, O'Brien MA, Freemantle N, *et al.* Impact of formal continuing medical education: do conferences, workshops, rounds, and other traditional continuing education activities change physician behavior or health care outcomes? *JAMA* 1999;**282**:867–74.
12 van der Weijden T, Wensing M, Grol RPTM, *et al.* Interventions aimed at influencing the use of diagnostic test. The Cochrane Library, Bunge 2001 (accepted for publication).
13 Tierney WM, Miller ME, McDonald CJ. The effect on test ordering of informing physicians of the charges for outpatient diagnostic tests. *N Engl J Med* 1990;**322**: 1499–504.

14 Pocock SJ. *Clinical trials: a practical approach*. Chichester, John Wiley & Sons: 1991.
15 Winkens RAG, Knottnerus JA, Kester ADM, Grol RPTM, Pop P. Fitting a routine health-care activity into a randomized trial: an experiment possible without informed consent? *J Clin Epidemiol*. 1997;**50**:435–9.
16 Campbell MK, Mollison J, Steen N, Grimshaw JM, Eccles M. Analysis of cluster randomized trials in primary care: a practical approach. *Fam Pract* 2000; **17**: 192–6.
17 Knottnerus JA, Dinant GJ. Medicine-based evidence, a prerequisite for evidence-based medicine. *BMJ* 1997;**315**:1109–10.

12 Epilogue: overview of evaluation strategy and challenges

J ANDRÉ KNOTTNERUS

Summary box

- The first phase in the evaluation of diagnostic procedures consists of (1), specifying the clinical problem, the diagnostic procedures(s), and the research question; (2), a systematic search and review of the literature, to decide whether the question can already be answered or whether a new clinical study is necessary.
- In preparing a new clinical study, the investigator must decide about the need for (1), evaluation of test accuracy in circumstances of maximum contrast or, as a further step, in the "indicated" clinical population; (2), evaluation of the impact of the test on clinical decision making or prognosis. The answers to these questions are decisive for the study design.
- Systematic reviews and meta-analysis, clinical decision analysis, cost effectiveness analysis, and expert panels can help to construct and update clinical guidelines.
- Implementation of guidelines should be professionally supported and evaluated, in view of what is known about how clinicians approach diagnostic problems.
- Further developments in three fields are especially important: innovation of (bio)medical knowledge relevant for diagnostic testing; the development of information and communication technology in relation to clinical research and practice; and, further exploration of methodological challenges in research on diagnostic problems.

Introduction

The chapters in this book speak for themselves and there is no need to repeat them or summarise their contents. However, a compact overview of important steps in the evaluation of diagnostic procedures may be useful. In addition, challenges for future work are outlined.

Important steps

The most important steps are represented in a flow diagram of the evaluation strategy (Figure 12.1), with reference to chapters in the book.

The first step is to specify the clinical problem and the diagnostic procedure(s) to be evaluated, and the aim of the study. Are we looking for the (added) diagnostic value of the procedure, the impact of the procedure on clinical management or on the patient's prognosis, or its cost effectiveness? After having formulated the research question accordingly, we should search and systematically review the literature and decide whether sufficient research data are already available. If not, a new clinical study should be considered.

In preparing a clinical study, to choose the appropriate design the following questions need to be answered: (1) is evaluation of accuracy of the test procedure in ideal circumstances of maximum contrast (still) necessary? (2) has this already been successfully achieved, and should accuracy still be established in the "indicated" clinical population? (3) is the impact of the diagnostic procedure on clinical decision making or prognosis yet unknown? The answers to these questions are decisive for the study design, as shown in Figure 12.1. It is sometimes possible to include more than one type of design in one study. For example, test accuracy can sometimes be determined in the context of a randomised trial or a before–after study.

In preparing and reporting the results of a clinical study, the generalisability or external (clinical) validity should be carefully considered. If the study is unique with regard to clinical applicability, the results represent an important evidence base themselves. More often they contribute to a broader knowledge base and can be included in a systematic review or meta-analysis. Clinical decision analysis, cost effectiveness analysis, and expert panels are helpful in constructing or updating clinical guidelines. The implementation of guidelines in clinical practice should be professionally supported and evaluated, in view of the acquired insights into the way clinicians approach diagnostic problems.

Challenges

Throughout this book a comprehensive range ("architecture") of methodological options have been described. At the same time, it has become clear that there are important challenges for future work.

210

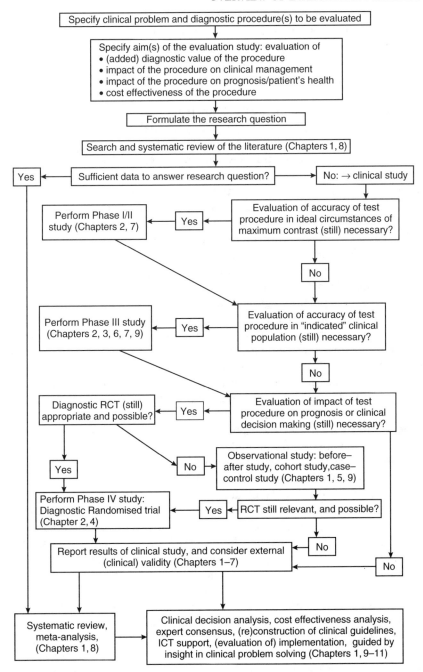

Figure 12.1 Important steps in the evaluation of diagnostic procedures.

Developments in three fields are especially important. First, (bio)medical knowledge will continue to be innovated, cumulated and refined. Second, information and communication technology will further develop and its use in daily practice will be more and more facilitated. Third, in research on diagnostic problems, methodological requirements and limitations are to be increasingly explored.

Innovation of biomedical knowledge and understanding of pathophysiological processes are the principal requirements for the development and evaluation of better diagnostic tests. A clear example is the current work to develop DNA tests in various clinical fields. In future these will not only be supportive of genetic counselling and prenatal screening, but also for clinical diagnostic and prognostic purposes. In addition, the ambition is to use DNA testing to improve the targeting and dosing of therapeutic and preventive interventions ("diagnostic effect modification"). Much work in this field is being done, for example, in cardiovascular medicine,[1] oncology,[2,3] and psychiatry.[4] However, it will be quite some time before these promises will really have an impact on daily patient care. Considerable efforts are still needed, both in the laboratory and in clinical epidemiological research. It was recently shown that the clinical epidemiological quality of many molecular genetic studies was poor: of 40 evaluated research papers, 35 failed to comply with one or more of seven essential methodologic criteria.[5] Furthermore, long-term follow up to clinically validate diagnostic and prognostic predictions needs more attention. In view of the ambition to develop a more tailormade, perhaps even individualised, diagnostic process, population oriented validations will be increasingly unsatisfactory. Also, ethical issues regarding the privacy of genetic information and the right to (not) know have to be dealt with. Doctors and patients, traditionally struggling to reduce diagnostic and prognostic uncertainty, must now learn to cope with approaching certainty.

Although until now computer decision support systems seem to have had more impact on the quality of drug dosing and preventive care than on diagnosis,[6] the growing body and complexity of knowledge enhances the need for (online) diagnostic support systems. The development and evaluation of such systems will therefore remain an important challenge. The same applies to the provision of appropriate input, that is, valid diagnostic and prognostic knowledge. However, performing individual studies in large study populations is very expensive and will always cover only a limited part of diagnostic management. Moreover, such studies may produce results with rather limited generalisability in place and time. Consequently, ways are sought to more efficiently and permanently harvest clinical knowledge and experience. It is therefore worth considering whether and under what conditions accuracy studies, RCTs, quasi-experimental studies, and before–after studies can be more embedded in routine health care.[7] In view of continuity, up to date results, and (external)

212

clinical validity, much is expected from standardised clinical databases, with international connections, to be used as sampling frames for research. As these databases will be closely related to or even integrated into routine health care, additional efforts are required to meet basic quality and methodological standards and to avoid biases, as discussed in Chapter 10.[8] In the context of such an integrated approach, the implementation of new findings can be studied and monitored in real practice.[9–11]

Diagnostic research should be refined with respect to strategy, spectrum and selection effects, prognostic reference standards,[12] and the assessment of the clinical impact of testing. Data analysis needs progress with regard to "diagnostic effect modification", multiple test and disease outcome categories, and estimation of sample size for multivariate problems. In addition, more flexible modelling is needed to identify alternative but clinically and pathophysiologically equivalent models, appropriate to classify subgroups with varying sets of clinical characteristics with a maximum of predictive power.[13,14] Better methods to improve and evaluate external clinical validity are also required. Furthermore, one must neither forget nor underestimate the diagnostic power of "real life doctors": at least, the performance of proposed diagnostic innovations should be compared with the achievements of experienced clinicians, before they are recommended as bringing new possibilities. We also need more understanding of the "doctor's black box" of diagnostic decision making, using cognitive psychological methods. This can help in more efficient diagnostic reasoning, and in the development of custom-made support systems.[15] Efficiency and speed in the evaluation of the impact of diagnostic procedures can be gained if new data on a specific aspect (for example a diagnostic test) can be inserted into the mosaic of available evidence on a clinical problem, rather than studying the whole problem again whenever one element has changed. For this purpose, flexible scenario models of current clinical knowledge are needed.

Systematic review and meta-analysis of diagnostic studies[16,17] must become a permanent routine activity of professional organisations producing and updating clinical guidelines. Meta-analysis should not only be performed on already reported data, but increasingly also on original and even prospectively developing databases. Such databases can originate from specific (collaborative) research projects, but sometimes also from health care (for example clinics where systematic work ups for patients with similar clinical presentations are routine, and where the population denominator is well defined). Accordingly, meta-analysis, evaluation research, and health care can become more integrated.

The role of the patient in diagnostic management is becoming more active. People want to be involved in the decision as to what diagnostics are performed, and want to know what the outcome means to them. Patient decision support facilities, at the doctor's office and at home, using e-mail

213

or internet services, are receiving increasing attention. Clinicians have to think about their possible future role in sifting, explaining, and integrating information via these facilities. The question as to which level of certainty is worth which diagnostic procedures, is not always similarly answered by patients and doctors. Patients' perceptions, preferences, and responsibilities should be respected and supported, not excluded, in diagnostic research and guidelines.[18] Sometimes, however, these features are not easily measurable and show substantial inter- and intrasubject variability. A good patient–doctor dialogue therefore remains the core instrument of individual decision making.[19]

Last but not least, formal standards for the evaluation of diagnostics are needed to control acceptance, maintenance, and substitution in the healthcare market. This also requires high quality and transparency of evaluation reports. The initiative to reach international agreement on Standards for Reporting Diagnostic Accuracy (STARD) therefore deserves full support from the scientific and healthcare community.[20]

References

1 Aitkins GP, Christopher PD, Kesteven PJL, et al. Association of polymorphisms in the cytochrome P450 CYP2C9 with warfarin dose requirement and risk of bleeding complications. Lancet 1999;**353**:717–19.
2 McLeod HL, Murray GI. Tumour markers of prognosis in colorectal cancer. Br J Cancer 1999;**79**:191–203.
3 Midley R, Kerr D. Towards post-genomic investigation of colorectal cancer. Lancet 2000; **355**:669–70.
4 Joober R, Benkelfat C, Brisebois K, et al. T102C polymorphism in the 5HTA gene and schizophrenia: relation to phenotype and drug response variability. J Psychiatry Neurosci 1999;**24**:141–6.
5 Bogardus ST Jr, Concato J, Feinstein AR. Clinical epidemiological quality in molecular genetic research. The need for methodological standards. JAMA 1999;**281**:1919–26.
6 Hunt DL, Haynes RB, Hanna SE, Smith K. Effects of computer-based clinical decision support systems on physician performance and patient outcomes: a systematic review. JAMA 1998;**280**:1339–46.
7 van Wijk MA, van Der Lei J, Mosseveld M, Bohnen AM, van Bemmel JH. Assessment of decision support for blood test ordering in primary care. A randomized trial. Ann Intern Med 2001;**134**:274–81.
8 Knottnerus JA. The role of electronic patient records in the development of general practice in the Netherlands. Meth Info Med 1999;**38**:350–5.
9 Haines A, Rogers S. Integrating research evidence into practice. In: Silagy C, Haines A, eds. Evidence based practice in primary care. London: BMJ Books, 1998;pp.144–59.
10 Baker R, Grol R. Evaluating the application of evidence. In: Silagy C, Haines A, eds. Evidence based practice in primary care. London: BMJ Books, 1998;pp.75–88.
11 Kidd M, Purves I. Role of information technology. In: Silagy C, Haines A, eds. Evidence based practice in primary care. London: BMJ Books, 1998;pp.123–8.
12 Lijmer JG. Evaluation of diagnostic tests: from accuracy to outcome. Thesis. Amsterdam: University of Amsterdam, 2001.
13 Heckerling PS, Conant RC, Tape TG, Wigton RS. Reproducibility of predictor variables from a validated clinical rule. Med Decision Making 1992;**12**:280–5.
14 Knottnerus JA. Diagnostic prediction rules: principles, requirements and pitfalls. Primary Care 1995;**22**:341–63.

15 Friedman CP, Elstein AS, Wolf FM, *et al.* Enhancement of clinicians' diagnostic reasoning by computer-based consultation: a multisite study of 2 systems. *JAMA* 1999;**282**:1851–6.

16 Irwig L, Tosteson AN, Gatsonis C, *et al.* Guidelines for meta-analyses evaluating diagnostic tests. *Ann Intern Med* 1994;**120**:667–76.

17 Kester AD, Buntinx F. Meta-analysis of ROC curves. *Med Decision Making* 2000; **20**:430–39.

18 Nease RF, Owens DK. A method for estimating the cost-effectiveness of incorporating patient preferences into practice guidelines. *Med Decision Making* 1994;**14**:382–92.

19 Sackett DL. Evidence-based medicine. *Semin Perinatol* 1997;**21**:3–5.

20 STARD Steering Committee. The STARD project. Standards for Reporting Diagnostic Accuracy. Amsterdam: Department of Clinical Epidemiology, Academic Medical Center Amsterdam, 16–17 December 2000.

Index

Page numbers in **bold** type refer to figures; those in *italic* refer to tables or boxed material

abnormal test results, randomising 66, **67**
abstractions, construction of 183, 190
accuracy 39–59, 117, 145–166
additional testing 46, 199
  see also before-after studies
adjustment, diagnostic opinions 188
adverse effects 3, 55, 62
aetiologic data analysis 7, 56, 57
allocation concealment *62*, 77
ambispective approach 45
analysis of variance 156
anchoring, diagnostic opinions 89, 188
angiography, as "gold" standard 7–8
appendicitis
  abdominal rigidity *35*
  reference standard for tests 101
  right lower quadrant tenderness 33–4
  study profile flow diagram **110**
  ultrasonography/clinical assessment RCT 77–8
architecture, diagnostic research 19–37
  "normal" and "normal range" 21–4
  research question 24–37
    Phase I studies 25–6
    Phase II studies 26–8
    Phase III studies 28–33
    Phase IV studies 36–7
  summary *19–20*
area under ROC curve 5, *99*, 109, *117*, 128, **129**
  pooling 160
artefactual variation *95*, 96, 100
asthma, long-acting β agonists study 174–5
asymptomatic disease, population screening
  breast cancer 13
  Phase IV questions 36
  study population 53

audit 201, 203
automatic mental processes 191–2
availability bias 192

background information 154
bayesian approach, data interpretation and diagnosis 181–2, 190–1
bayesian properties, diagnostic tests 36
Bayes' theorem 47, 97, 98, *117*, 130–2, *179*, 180, 181, 184–6, 189
before-after studies 11, *12*, 13, 81–93
  limitations 92
  research question 83–6
  summary *81–2*
  working out study 86–92
    diagnostic testing 87–8
    modified approaches 91–2
    post-test outcome 88–9
    pretest baseline 86–7
    sample size and analysis 91
    study subjects, selection 90–1
    time factor 89–90
behavioural decision research 180, 181, 187, 192
best evidence synthesis 154
between-population variability 112
between-site variability 112, 113
bias 135
  availability 192
  "confirmation" 189
  incorporation 49, 51
  observer 9
  in phase III studies 32
  publication 148
  selection 8, 150, 192
  spectrum 8
  "test review" and "diagnosis review" 48–9
  verification 152
bivariate analysis *40*, 56

blinding 9, 31, 48, 51
  before-after studies *81*, 89
  delayed-type cross-sectional studies
    50
  randomised controlled trials *62*, 77
blood pressure, therapeutic definition
  of "normal" 23
blood tests, routine 10
breast cancer screening 13
B-type natriuretic peptide (BNP), LVD
  diagnosis 20–1
  "normal" and "normal" range
    21–4
  research question 24–5
    Phase I 25–6
    Phase II 26–8
    Phase III 28–31

CAGE questionnaire, data extraction
  difficulties 153
calibration, diagnostic tests 97–8, *99*,
  107, 109
CARE consortium 35–6
carotid stenosis, duplex
  ultrasonography, prognostic
  value 63–4, 65, 66, 67
case-control study 11, *12*, 13
case-referent study 11, *12*, 44
  sample size estimation 55
case specificity 182, 190
categories
  case diagnosis 183
  test results 107
  thresholds between 98
central randomisation procedure 77
chance-adjusted agreement, systematic
  reviews *146*, 150
citation tracking 148–9
clinical decision analysis 14, 185,
  186
clinical prediction rules 7, 111, 185
clinical problem
  defining 42–3, 210
  see also target condition
clinical signs, appendicitis diagnosis
  33–5, 77–8
clinical spectrum see spectrum
clinicians
  blinding to allocation 77
  doctor as unit of randomisation
    204–5

Cochrane Methods Group on
  Screening and Diagnostic Tests
  150
coded data, medical records 174
cognitive research literature review
  179–93
  diagnosis as opinion revision 184–6
  educational implications 189–91
  hypothesis generation and
    restructuring, errors in 184
  hypothesis selection 181–2
  methodological guideline 191–2
  pattern recognition 182–3
  probability estimation, errors in 186–8
  probability revision, errors in 188–9
  summary *179–80*
cohort studies 11, *12*, 13
colorectal cancer screening, systematic
  review 36–7
combined predictive power 56
comorbidity 54, 85
complications of test see adverse effects
confidence intervals 56, *117*, 121–3
  tables 136–43
  theory of calculation 123
"confirmation bias" 189
confounding by indication 50, 174–5
confounding probability 188
confounding variables 47, 56, 85, 91
"conjunction fallacy" 186
consensus methods 11, 14
conservatism 188
context
  and long-term memory activation
    184
  reducing dependence on 190
continuous medical education (CME)
  201, 205
continuous tests 107
  dichotomisation and
    trichotomisation 126–30
  weighted linear regression 160
contrast evaluation, defining research
  question *39*, 41
cost effectiveness 5, 11, 14
  changing test ordering 205
costs
  changes in 11
  diagnostic tests 6
  randomised controlled trial designs
    76

cost-utility ratio, diagnostic testing 205
covariables 56, 87
critiquing systems 172
cross-sectional studies 1, 11, 12,
    39–57
  adverse effects 55
  delayed type 7, 50–1
  design outline 43–5
  external validation 57
  operationalising determinants and
      outcome 45–52
  research question 41–3
  statistical aspects 55–7
  study population, specifiying 53–4
  summary *39–40*
    of steps to take 41
"culturally desirable" definition of
    normal 22–3
cumulative prospect theory (CPT) 187
cut point for test *5*, 98, *117, 128*, **129**
  decision analytical approach 132–3
  searching for in meta-analysis 155–6
  selection of 33
  SROC curve 157, **158**, 159
    formula 165

data analysis 7, 41, 56–7, 117–43, 213
  Bayes' theorem 130–2
  before-after studies 91
  clinical example 118–20
  confidence intervals 121–3
    tables 136–43
  cut-off value, decision analytical
      approach 132–3
  dichotomisation and
      trichotomisation, continuous
      tests 126–30
  error rate 124–5
  likelihood ratio 125–6
    see also likelihood ratio (LR)
  logistic regression 133–5
  odds ratio 126
    see also odds ratio (OR)
  pre- and post-test probability 123–4,
      130–2
    see also post-test probability;
        pretest probability
  sensitivity analysis 133
  sensitivity and specificity,
      dichotomous test 120–1
    see also sensitivity; specificity
  software 135, 136

summary *117–18*
systematic reviews 153–61
  see also subgroup analysis
databases 171, 213
  observational 172–5, 176
  searching electronic 147–9, 162
data collection 41
  direction of 44–5
  selective 181
  thoroughness of 182
data extraction, systematic reviews
    152–3
data interpretation in problem solving
    181–2
data presentation, systematic reviews
    161–2
decision analysis approach 14, 185,
    186
decision making *179*, 213
  behavioural decision research 180,
      181, 187, 192
  calibration, test results 107
  diagnosis as opinion revision
      184–6
  process 3, 5, 6
  randomisation at time of decision
      71, 72, 79
decision support 167–76
  observational databases 172–5
  summary *167–8*
  systems 171–2, 212
delayed type cross-sectional studies 7,
    50–1
dependent variables 45, 46, 56
design 1, 11–15, 210
  before-after studies *see* before-after
      studies
  cross-sectional studies 11, 12, *39*, 41,
      43–5
  randomised controlled trials (RCT)
      12–13, *61*
    alternative 68–9
    choice of 74, 75–6
    comparing test strategies
        69–74
    practical issues 76–8
    single test 64–7
  determinants, operationalising *39*, 41,
      45–7
developmental screening in childhood
    trial 37
"diagnosis review bias" 49

diagnostic accuracy studies *see* cross-sectional studies
diagnostic certainty, increasing 3
diagnostic classification 40
diagnostic definition of normal 23
diagnostic odds ratio (DOR) *see* odds ratio (OR)
diagnostic prediction model 56
dichotomous tests 126–9
  comparing prognostic value 69–71
  data analysis 56
  meta-analysis 152–3
  sample size estimation 55
  sensitivity and specificity 120–1
disclosure, test results, random 37, 71, *73*
discordance rate calculations 78, 79
discordant test results, randomising 71, *72*, 79
discrimination of test 107
  measures of 3, *4*, 12, 97, *99*, 109
    see also likelihood ratio (LR); odds ratio (OR); predictive value; sensitivity; specificity
  and usefulness of test 9–10
  for various target disorders *5*
disease
  definitions of 98
  monitoring course 3
  ratio to non-disease 98
  spectrum of 98, 102–3
  see also target condition
distribution, test results, transferability 98, **99**
DNA testing 52, 212
Doppler ultrasonography, umbilical artery RCT 68–9
duplex ultrasonography
  patient selection, anticoagulation in acute stroke 65, *66*
  prognostic value 63–4, 65, 66, 67
Dutch College of General Practitioners 201

echocardiography study, LVD patients 28, *29*
ectopic pregnancy, serum hCG test 106
educational implications, cognitive instructional theory 189–91
effect modifying variables 46, 47, 56, 85, 87, 91

electronic literature databases, searching 147–9, 162
electronic medical records *167–8*, 169, 170–1, 176
  observational databases 172–5
Elias medical record system 170–1
EMBASE, searching 147
endoscopy
  FEESST trial 72, *73*
  therapeutic impact study 10
error rate 124–5, 132, 133
  see also standard error, calculating
erythrocyte sedimentation rate (ESR) studies
  accuracy and reproducibility 47
  pre- and post-test assessment 83–4
evidence-based clinical guidelines *197*
evidence-based medicine (EBM) 185, 186, 189, 190–1
exclusion criteria 13, 41, 53–4
exemplar based recognition 183
exercise ECG in primary care 51–2
expected utility theory 187
expert panel 50, 51
experts
  clinical reasoning 180, 182, 183
  consulting to identify studies 148
explanatory studies, diagnostic tests and treatments *27*, 28
external (clinical) validation *40*, 54, 57, 210, 212–13
external validity criteria 150
  urine dipsticks in UTI reviews *151*

faecal occult blood testing, systematic review 36–7
feedback 190, 201, 203
financial incentives/penalties, test ordering 202
findings, synthesising with clinical expertise 13–14
Fisher's exact test 154
fixed effect model, statistical pooling 157, 159
flexible endoscopic evaluation of swallowing with sensory testing (FEESST) trial 72, *73*
flow diagram, research question formulation **110**
forms
  changing test ordering 202, 203
  data extraction 153

forward reasoning 183
free text in medical records 173
funding, diagnostic evaluation studies 2

Galbraith plot 156, **157**
gaussian definition of normal 21
general models, need for 11
generic search strategy 147
genetic tests, breast cancer 74
    see also DNA testing
global measures, test accuracy
        97, 109
"gold" standard *see* reference standard
guidelines
    clinical *197*, 210
    methodological 191–2
    systematic reviews 145–63
        data analysis 153–61
        data extraction 152–3
        data presentation 161–2
        how to search literature 147–9
        inclusion criteria 149–52
        summary *145–6*
    test ordering 199, 200, 201

Hawthorne effect 45
healthcare expenditure 198
healthcare setting 42
    accuracy of test 103, *104*
    effect of 33–6, *95*, 96
    systematic reviews 149
    transferability between settings
        112–14
health status, baseline 85, 87
Helicobacter pylori serology study,
        evaluating preaddition 74, **75**
heterogeneity 114
    in meta-analysis
        dealing with 156–7, **158**
        dipstick example 152, 157, **158**
        searching for 154, **155**
        statistical pooling 158–9
    predictors of in diagnostic accuracy
        112, *113*
history data 3, 45
homogenous studies, statistical pooling
        158
human chorionic gonadotrophin
        (hCG) test, ectopic pregnancy
        106
hypothesis generation *179*, 181, 183
    errors in 184

hypothetico-deductive method 181–2
    experienced clinicians 182

implementation cycle 199, **200**
implementation research 12, 15
inclusion criteria 13, *40*, 41, 53, 54
    systematic reviews 149–52, 154
        comments 149–50
        methodological quality 150–2
incorporation bias 49, 51
incremental value, test 105–6, 107,
        111, 112
independent expert panel 50, 51
independent variables 45, 46, 56
"indication area" for test 10
information and communication
        technology (ICT) *12*, 15, *167*,
        168, 169
information, integrating in clinical
        practice 14–15
instance based recognition 183
interassessment period, before-after
        study 89–90
internal validity criteria 150
    urine dipsticks in UTI reviews *151*
international cooperation 15
interobserver variability 49
interpretation 155–6
    and diagnostic hypothesis 181–2
    incorrect 189
intraobserver variability 49
intrauterine growth retardation
        (IUGR) RCT 68–9
invasive tests 3, 14
    reference standard 49
IPCI database 174

"kit" form tests 107

language, published studies 149
latent class analysis 109
left ventricular dysfunction (LVD) *see*
        B-type natriuretic peptide (BNP),
        LVD diagnosis
lesions, localisation 40
likelihood ratio (LR) *4*, *26*, 97, *99*, 107,
        109, *117*, 125–6, 127, **129**, 185, 190
    answering Phase III question with
        29, **30**, 32
    pooling in meta-analysis 159–60
    statistical formula 165
    various target disorders *5*

literature search 147–9
liver tests
  discrimination of 7
  function tests 3
logarithmic transformed DOR
    (lnDOR) 156, **157**
logistic regression 46, 56, 133–5, 185
  formula 134
  see also multiple logistic regression
long-acting β agonists (LBA) cohort
    study 174–5

medical informatics 168–9
  clinical decision support systems
    171–2
  observational databases 172–5
medical knowledge, clinical decision
    support systems 171–2
MEDION database 147–8
MEDLINE
  research on diagnostic tests 2
  search strategy 147, *148*
memory
  long-term, activating stored
    knowledge 184
  working 181
meta-analysis *1*, 11, *12*, 14, *40*, 136,
    146, 153, 213
  cut-off point effect, searching for
    155–6
  discussion 162–3
  heterogeneity
    dealing with 156–7
    searching for 154, **155**
  individual study results, describing
    154
  statistical pooling 159–61
    deciding on model 157, 158–9
methodological challenges *1*, 6–11
  changes over time 10–11
  complex relations 6–7
  discrimination and influence on
    management 9–10
  "gold" standard problem 7–8
  indication area and prior probability
    10
  observer variability and bias 9
  "soft" measures 9
  spectrum and selection bias 8
methodological guidelines, decision
    making 191–2

methodological quality, systematic
    reviews 150–2, 162
misclassification 88
  of reference standard 101, *102*,
    109, 113
modified barium swallow test (MBS)
    dysphagia trial 72, *73*
monitoring disease course 3
"mosaic" of evidence 10–11, 15
MRI scans 10
  nerve root compression,
    intraobserver variability 49
multiple logistic regression 56, *118*,
    135
multiple tests, evaluating 46, 56
  how to compare strategies
    69–74
multivariable statistical techniques 7
multivariate analysis *40*, 56, 57, 91

natural prognostic value 65, 67
negative predictive value (NPV) 123,
    124
new tests
  evaluation 6, 42, 73–4, 106–7
  ordering of 198
nomogram
  pretest to post-test likelihoods
    conversion **30**
  use of 191
non-disease
  diagnosis of 21
    "upper-limit syndrome of" 22
  variation in test specificity 103
non-English publications 149
non-invasive tests 3, 14
normal
  definitions of *19*, 21–4
  selection of "upper limit" 33
  see also non-disease

objectives, diagnostic testing *1*,
    2–6
observational databases 172–5,
    176
  confounding by indication 174–5
observer variability
  and bias 9
  reducing 47
  see also intraobserver variability
"occurrence" relation 45–6

odds ratio (OR) *4*, 97, *99*, 107, 109, *117*, 126
  duplex ultrasonography trial 65, *66*
  meta-analysis 154
    logarithmic transformed DOR (lnDOR) 156, **157**
    pooled OR 161
  and prevalence of target condition 101, 102
  various target disorders *5*
operator variability 111
order effects 189
ordering of tests, changing 197–206
  feasibility of change 202–5
    cost effectiveness 205
    evaluating effects 204–5
    implementation strategies 202–4
    perpetuation and continuation 204
  making the change 199–202
  need to change 198–9
  summary *197–8*
outcome
  before-after study 88–9, 90
  effect of test on 87
  health 36
  operationalising 41, 47–52
    principles 47–9
outcome data, systematic reviews 149
outcome measurement
  blinding 77
  systematic reviews 154
outliers 156
overview, evaluation strategy 209–14
  challenges 210, 212–14
  important steps 210, **211**
  summary *209*

patient registers, sampling from 54
patients
  blinding to allocation 77
  characteristics 46
  impact of test on 62
  role in diagnostic management 213–14
  selection of 53
  see also study population
  self-testing 85
patient-specific advice, decision support systems 172
pattern recognition *179*, 182–3
peer review 201, 203
percentile definiton of normal 21–2
performance, diagnostic test

assumptions for transfering test characteristics *99*
measures of 97–8
variation in *95*, 96
Phase I studies *19*, 25–6, 43, 44
Phase II studies *19*, 26–8, 44
Phase III studies *19–20*, 28–36, 44–5
Phase IV studies *20*, 36–7
physical fitness measurement 3
pilot searches 148
pilot studies 47
placebos 12
  placebo effect 62
point estimates 56
pooling results 159–61, 163
  deciding on model 157, *158–9*
  formulae 165
positive predictive value (PPV) 123, 124
postaddition 73, 74
post-test outcome, before-after study 88–9, 90
post-test probability *4*, 29, **30**, 47, 123–4, 130–2, 185
  Bayes' theorem formula 131
  confusing with sensitivity 186
pragmatic studies, diagnostic tests and treatments 27
preaddition 73
  designs to evaluate 74, **75**
prediction model 56
prediction rules 7, 111, 185
predictive value *4*, 97, *99*, *117*, 123–4
  see also post-test probability; pretest probability
prejudice towards method 9
pretest baseline, before-after study 85, 86–7
pretest probability *4*, 29, **30**, 36, 47, 123–4, 130, 184, 185
prevalence, target condition 101, 102, 113
primary care settings 33, 103
  accuracy of tests *104*
  appendicitis, accuracy of diagnosis 34, 35
probability
  estimation, errors in 186–8
    distortions 187
    support theory 187–8
  prior 10
  revision, errors in 188–9

probability – *Continued*
  see also post-test probability; pretest
    probability
problem based learning *180*, 189–90
problem solving *179*, 180
  diagnosis as hypothesis selection
    181–2
  pattern recognition 182–3
  see also decision making
prognosis, assessing 3, 13, *61*
  comparing multiple test strategies
    69–74
  how to measure prognostic impact
    63–4
  need to assess prognostic impact
    62–3
prognostic criterion *40*, 52
proportions, pooling of 159
  statistical formulae 165
prospective data collection 44, 45
prospect theory (PT) 187
prototypes, construction of 183, 190
"pseudodiagnosticity" 189
psychiatric illness, diagnostic research
    51
publication bias 148
PubMed (MEDLINE), search strategy
    147, *148*

qualitative approach and decision
    making 5, 6
qualitative models, decision support
    systems 172
quality, medical record data 170
quantitative approach and decision
    making 5, 6, 14
quantitative models, decision support
    systems 172
quasi experimental comparison 92
questions, diagnostic research *see*
    research question

random disclosure, test results 37, 71,
    73
random effect model, statistical pooling
    158
random error 57
randomised controlled trials (RCT)
    1, 61–79, 82
  colorectal cancer screening 36–7
  and decision support systems
    176

prognostic impact
  how to assess 63–4
  need to assess 62–3
randomised designs 11, 12–13
  alternative 68–9
  choice of design 74, 75–6
  how to compare test strategies
    69–74
  practical issues 76–8
  for single test 64–7
  summary *61–2*
rank-dependent utility theories 187
rare conditions, overemphasising 186
ratio, disease to non-disease, constancy
    98
reader variability 111
recruitment procedure *40*, 41, 54
redundant evidence, acquiring 189
reference standard 7–8, 20, 31, 32,
    39–40, 46, 47–52
  adverse effects 55
  choosing 108
  clinical follow up 50–1
  differences in 98
  error in 109
  independent expert panel 50
  misclassification 101, *102*, 109, 113
  pragmatic criteria 49–50
  prognostic criterion 52
  standard shift as result of new insight
    52
  systematic reviews 149, 152
  tailormade standard protocol 51–2
referral filter 103–5, 111
reflection 190
reimbursement systems, changing test
    ordering 202
reliability, clinical data 170
reminder systems 172, 176, 201–2, 203
renal artery stenosis (RAS) 118–19
  diagnostic questions and concepts
    119–20
  dichotomous and trichotomous tests
    126–30
  error rate of test 124–5
  likelihood ratio 126
  prediction of 120–1, *122*
    likelihood ratio 125
    pre- and post-test probability 123–4
replacement tests 106–7, 111
reports, diagnostic research 148
reproducibility, test 47

research question *19–20*, 24–5, 210
  before-after studies 83–6
  cross-sectional studies 41–3
  formulating, flow diagram **110**
  Phase I studies *19*, 25–6, 43, 44
  Phase II studies *19*, 26–8
  Phase III studies *19–20*, 28–31
    limits to applicability of studies
      33–6
    threats to validity of studies
      31–3
  Phase IV studies *20*, 36–7
retrospective data 13, 45, 91
risk factor definition of normal 22
ROC curve 5, 26, 97, 107, 109, 128,
  129, 156
  pooling 160–1
  SROC curve 157, **158**, 159, 165

sample size 10, 37
  before-after studies 91
  cross-sectional studies 55–6
  Phase III studies 45
  randomised controlled trials (RCT)
    62, 77–8
sampling
  cross-sectional studies 44
  variability 121–3
Science Citation Index 149
search strategy, systematic reviews
  145, 147
secondary care settings 33
selection bias 8, 150, 192
selection of patients 53, 109–10
  see also study population
self-testing, patient 85
sensitivity *4*, 97, *99*
  confusing with post-test probability
    186
  for dichotomous test 120–1
  homogenous 159
    statistical formulae 165
  variation in
    biased inflation of 32
    healthcare setting 33, 103, *104*
    prevalence of target condition
      101, 102
    spectrum of disease 102–3
  various target disorders *5*
sensitivity analysis *117*, 133
sequential information and clinical
  reasoning 182

serum creatinine concentration, RAS
  diagnosis
  dichotomised values *128*
  ROC curve **129**
  trichotomised values *130*
setting *see* healthcare setting
severity indicators, absence of 175
single tests, evaluation 46
  data analysis 56
  randomised designs 64–7
  see also dichotomous tests
"soft" measures 9
software, statistical 135, 136
Spearman correlation coefficient 156
specificity *4*, 10, 97, *99*, 111
  for dichotomous test 120–1
  homogeneous 159
    statistical formulae 165
  variation in
    biased inflation of 32
    healthcare setting 33, 34, 35, 103,
      104
    prevalence of target condition 101,
      102
    spectrum of non-disease 103
  various target disorders *5*
spectrum 33, 42, 54
  bias 8
  characteristics, measuring 47
  of disease/non-disease 98, 102–3,
    111
split-half analysis 57
SROC curve 157, **158**, 159
  formula 165
standard error, calculating 123
standardised data extraction forms 153
standardised (simulated) patients
  91–2
Standards for Reporting Diagnostic
  Accuracy (STARD) initiative xi,
  214
statistical pooling 159–61, 163
  deciding on model 157, 158–9
  formulae 165
straight-leg raising test review,
  subgroup analysis **161**, 162
stratified analysis 46
stroke, duplex
  ultrasonography/anticoagulation
  RCT 65–6
study population
  before-after study 90–1

study population – *Continued*
  cross-sectional study 41, 44, 53–4
  heterogeneous *96*
  selecting 53, 109–10
  systematic reviews 149
  and test performance 102–6
subgroup analysis 46, 71, *146*, 149,
    156, 156–7, **158**, 163
  variation in findings, different groups
    111–12
subject characteristics 46
subject specific search strategy 147,
    148
support theory 187–8
surveys 11, 12, 43–4, 54
systematic reviews *1*, 11, *12*, 14, *40*,
    145–63, 213
  colorectal cancer screening trials
    36–7
  discussion 162–3
  guidelines 147–53
    data analysis 153–61
    data extraction 152–3
    data presentation 161–2
    how to search literature 147–9
    inclusion criteria 149–52
  summary *145–6*

target condition
  choosing 108
  defining 42, 100
  prevalence 101, 102, 113
  test specificity and sensitivity
    estimation 101, 102, 103
technological innovations, speed of and
    test evaluation 10–11, 15
telediagnosis 169, 171
tertiary care settings 33, 103
  appendicitis, accuracy of diagnosis
    34, 35
test based enrolment 44
test ordering *see* ordering of tests,
    changing

test result-based sampling 11
"test review bias" 48
therapeutic definition of normal 23
therapy
  and diagnostic test objectives 3
  effective and efficient 2
  treatment protocols 76
transferability, test accuracy 95–114
  questions before designing study
    108–14
  summary *95–6*
  true variability in test accuracy
    97–108
    discrimination and calibration
      97–8
    facilitating transferability
      98–100
    lack of transferability 100–8
Treeage-DATA 136
trichotomisation 130

urine dipstick review
  data extraction 152
  data presentation **162**
  dealing with heterogenity 157,
    158
  poor methodological quality 150
useless testing, examples 6

validation, external (clinical) *40*, 54,
    57, 210, 212–13
validity criteria, diagnostic research
    150, 153, 162–3
  urine dipsticks in UTI reviews
    151
verification bias 152
Visual Bayes 136

weighted linear regression 160
working memory 181
written medical records 170

χ^2 test 154

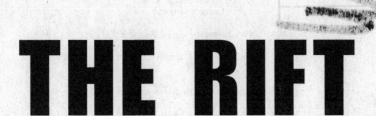

THE RIFT

UPRISING

AMY S. FOSTER

HARPER
Voyager

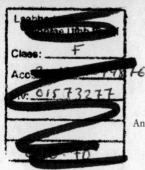

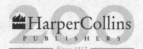

Harper*Voyager*
An imprint of HarperCollins*Publishers*
1 London Bridge Street
London SE1 9GF

www.harpervoyagerbooks.co.uk

This Paperback Original 2017
1

Copyright © Amy S. Foster 2016

First published in Great Britain by
Harper*Voyager* 2016

Cover layout design © HarperCollinsPublishers Ltd 2016

Amy S. Foster asserts the moral right to
be identified as the author of this work

A catalogue record for this book is
available from the British Library

ISBN: 978-0-00-817926-7

Printed and bound in Great Britain by Clays Ltd, St Ives plc

This novel is entirely a work of fiction.
The names, characters and incidents portrayed in it are
the work of the author's imagination. Any resemblance to
actual persons, living or dead, events or localities is
entirely coincidental.

All rights reserved. No part of this publication may be
reproduced, stored in a retrieval system, or transmitted,
in any form or by any means, electronic, mechanical,
photocopying, recording or otherwise, without the prior
permission of the publishers.

MIX
Paper from
responsible sources
FSC
www.fsc.org   FSC C007454

FSC™ is a non-profit international organisation established to promote
the responsible management of the world's forests. Products carrying the
FSC label are independently certified to assure consumers that they come
from forests that are managed to meet the social, economic and
ecological needs of present and future generations,
and other controlled sources.

Find out more about HarperCollins and the environment at
www.harpercollins.co.uk/green

For my daughter Mikeala,
who taught Ryn how to be brave

'məltē͵vərs/

noun

an infinite realm of being or potential being of which
the universe is regarded as a part or instance.

2005 A highly classified experiment in Livermore, California, attempting to understand the properties of dark matter results in a doorway to the Multiverse that scientists name The Rift. Within hours, thirteen more Rifts open, each one getting sequentially smaller as they move east around the world in Battle Ground, Washington; Brazil; France; Algeria; Zimbabwe; Poland; Saudi Arabia; Russia; Siberia; Myanmar; China; Australia; and New Zealand. The Rifts are portals not to other planets, but to an infinite number of other Earths.

2005 Out of fear that the Rifts would cause mass hysteria, a global effort is launched to keep them a secret. World leaders meet and form ARC: the Allied Rift Coalition.

2005 ARC is tested almost immediately when all manner of dangerous creatures spill out of the Rifts. These creatures are a panacea of evolutionary biology, as humanity learns that *Homo sapiens* are only one of many sentient beings that could have evolved on Earth.

2005 One month after the Rifts open, seventy-three Roones enter Earth. The Roones are a highly evolved humanoid species that promises to help ARC deal with the Rifts.

2006 With technology developed by the Roones, human trials begin with military troops. Soldiers are implanted with a chip intended to make them exponentially stronger, smarter, faster, and more agile. The test subjects are unable to handle the metamorphosis the brain must undergo to allow for these new "super" abilities. Each subject dies.

2006 ARC theorizes that by changing the microprocessor in the implant and delaying the time the chip takes to activate by seven years, a child's young biology can better accept and adapt to the massive changes their bodies would undergo. ARC agrees to let the Roones implant children with the chip.

2006 Seven-year-olds within a two-hundred-mile radius of each Rift site are tested in school. ARC chooses one hundred with the most average test scores. They do not want to take a potentially bright future away from a gifted child and they want their "super" soldiers to appear as unremarkable as possible.

2006 Without these children's parents' consent, the first crop of one hundred children is implanted with the chip.

2007 The first Village is created outside the Battle Ground Rift. This is where ARC takes all Immigrants (anyone or anything that Rifts to this Earth from another) to be held in captivity, away from the general population.

2007 A second crop of children is implanted.

2008 Militaries from around the world continue to deal with the hostile Immigrants exiting the Rifts; there are numerous casualties on both sides.

2008 Construction begins on six more global Village sites.

2008 A third crop of children is implanted with the chip.

2009 Levi Branach and a fourth crop of children are implanted with the chip.

2010 Henry Gibbon, Violet Henshaw, Boone Castor, and Ryn Whittaker are all implanted and join a fifth crop of children.

2011 A sixth crop is implanted.

2012 A seventh crop is implanted.

2012 ARC creates an elaborate subterfuge to relocate the families of the implanted children. ARC tells the parents of these children that its acronym stands for Accelerated Rate Curriculum. It is staged as the most prestigious program in the world for gifted students. It guarantees a bright and successful future. Parents believe their kids will attend a highly competitive high school program when in reality they will be policing The Rift.

2013 The first crop of implanted children is activated. ARC calls these new soldiers Citadels.

2013 The Karekins immigrate to this Earth. They are a deadly and highly advanced humanoid race. Their attacks become increasingly brutal and frequent.

2013 An eighth crop of children is implanted.

2014 A ninth crop of children is implanted.

2015 A tenth crop of children is implanted.

2016 An eleventh crop of children is implanted.

2016 Levi Branach is activated and becomes a Citadel.

2017 A twelfth crop of children is implanted.

2017 Henry, Violet, Boone, and Ryn become active Citadels.

2018 A thirteenth crop of children is implanted.

2019 A fourteenth crop of children is implanted.

2020 Present day.

2020 Ryn's parents believe she is a junior in high school and a fifteenth crop of children has just been implanted . . .

CHAPTER 1

"Command Center, this is Gamma Team in Nest four. There is no visual. Over." The voice crackles in my earpiece. I tap the small device without thinking. It's not a hardware issue, not with the kind of equipment we use. More than likely it's interference. We are the closest team to The Rift. I wait for the other teams to check in, but it's protocol at this point. They aren't going to see anything before we do. We hear from Lambda, Phi, Rho, and Omega. The reserves are farther back, in the denser part of the forest, waiting in case something really bad comes through, like a column of Karekins. Karekins are the most dangerous enemy we face in The Rift game. They are humanoid but proportionally much, much bigger—at least eight feet tall. Whenever I see one, I think of the Titans from Greek mythology. Maybe the big shots at ARC thought the same thing when they divided us all into groups using the Greek alphabet.

The scientists at The Allied Rift Coalition created sophisticated machines that spike and beep whenever The Rift is about to dump something out.

We don't need them.

Citadels are in tune with the opening. I don't even think it's our heightened senses. We just spend so much time around the damn thing that we've grown accustomed to its habits. I am Beta Team's leader. I was surprised at first when I got the rank. I am not the fastest or strongest among us. When we first deployed, it didn't take long to see that I think quickly on my feet. I'm a natural tactician and I don't make sentimental decisions. In the beginning of all this, I would never have volunteered for a command. After so much time on active duty, however, it's clear the rank is a good fit. The fact that ARC figured out my strengths before I did still pisses me off. It's like swallowing one of those huge horse vitamins without water. The truth that they somehow know me better than I know myself will always burn right in my center.

I try not to think about how or why anymore. It's pointless and distracting, and I need to focus. I'm here and in charge, responsible for my team. We are holding our positions. The four of us are crouched behind a large rock that sits just off to the left of The Rift. The rock was strategically placed here so that we can see what's coming out, but they can't see us.

No, we can't actually see through solid rock or anything . . . though that *would* be cool. Instead, the rock has a couple holes bored through, covered and camouflaged on The Rift side with paint and sieved metal. It's kind of like a two-way mirror. No one would notice the holes unless they got right up and put their face up to them, and by that point, well, more than likely they would have already been neutralized.

I study my three teammates for a moment. They look so

badass they could be on the cover of a comic book. Three years ago, Christopher Seelye—the head of ARC—told us we had all been chosen because of our incredible "averageness." He got that one wrong by a mile. Maybe it was bad math, or maybe it's the chip they implanted us with to give us all these crazy superpowers. Either way, we are far from average. Citadels are striking. People look at us and can't look away. We are sleek and dangerously fascinating, like any other large predator, which makes it impossible for any of us to fly under the radar. Am I pretty? No, not conventionally. But we all have a strange and complicated beauty that's undeniable. We have become used to being watched and stared at. I wonder what our parents think sometimes. Do they notice, or are they just used to us? I wouldn't dare ask them, and because of the role I am forced to play at home, they wouldn't expect me to.

I am snapped back into the moment when Boone checks in on the mic, trying to sound all official. "Command, this is Brony Team. We still don't have a visual." He smirks beside me. I roll my eyes. Always the comedian.

"Repeat," Command demands through our earpieces.

"This is Team Rainbow Sparkle and we have a negative on a visual."

Violet gives Boone a smack, and per usual Henry says nothing at all. Henry has no sense of humor. He's as immovable as the rock we are crouched behind.

Colonel Applebaum's voice cuts through the static. "Cut the shit, Boone. After we're done here today you can go home and play with all your little action figurines, but since we know something is about to come through, maybe you'd like to focus so that we can save some lives."

It's an inside joke, years old, that Boone never gets tired of. When we first met Applebaum we were so intimidated that it was difficult for most of us to even speak, let alone answer one of the dozens of questions he would scream in our faces during basic training. It was Boone who came up with the idea that his last name sounded like a My Little Pony character. Boone can be a smart-ass, but he can always defuse a tense situation. After we started associating Applebaum with a children's cartoon, the colonel seemed far less terrifying.

"Ryn?" he asks.

"I'm on it, sir." I shoot Boone a look. A look that says everything without me having to use any actual words. And then I feel the hair on my arms begin to stand up. I know that I am the first one to sense that The Rift is about to open. I always am. I think that's another reason I was made team leader: I have a hypersensitivity to it. I hold my hand up and make a fist. It's a gesture that means business, and my team knows me well enough to stop the nonsense and follow my lead. I keep my head down and close my eyes. I can feel the tug of The Rift's giant mouth in my belly. I know we won't be sucked in, because all the mathematicians have calculated the exact safe distance from The Rift. It's one of the few things ARC has told us that I believe absolutely, because we haven't yet lost a Citadel that way.

But it doesn't mean the pull doesn't bother me every time.

My heart begins to beat a little faster, the adrenaline starts to course through my veins. The Rift's rippling intensifies.

"Command, this is Beta Team leader. We have a visual. Stage one. Repeat: We have a visual. Stage one." Through the rock I can see the shimmering air undulate like a hummingbird's wings and then, from The Rift's center, a purple dot begins to bleed out toward the edges. "That's Stage two, Command. Copy," I say swiftly.

"We copy, Team Leader. Hold your position."

I grit my teeth. They don't need to tell me what to do. I know exactly what needs to happen next. I'm about to put my life on the line and they are safely sitting on their asses a mile away, watching this all on a bunch of camera feeds. I take a breath. Irritation won't help me if things turn ugly. I have to empty myself of every emotion. I have to become a thing instead of a person if I want to survive the next ten minutes. It's why we're called Citadels and not soldiers. Solid, immovable objects, not malleable beings.

Ready to withstand anything.

The purple in The Rift begins to darken until it is pure black. It's not a normal black but the darkest color my eyes can register. It is the inky night of the universe. I look at my team. They are ready. Focused. Intense.

"Stage three, Command. Stand by." We all wait for the sound. The Rift always opens with a muffled sonic boom. It's not ear piercing. It's not even all that unpleasant. In fact it comes as sort of a relief. No more waiting. No more guessing. It's time.

The boom happens.

It is an echo of a thing started a million or a billion Earths away from our own Earth. The ground shakes ever so slightly.

"That's it. Stage four. Weapons ready," I say calmly. I peer through the rock. The view isn't perfect through the tiny holes perforated in the metal on the other side, but it's enough. The Rift opens completely and a person comes tumbling out. Just as quickly, The Rift closes and turns back into the neon green tower of energy that it is. It always closes with far less ceremony than it opens—like a guest who's overstayed his welcome and hustles to get out of there before things get awkward.

"It looks like we have a solo passenger, Command. I repeat: a lone individual, a man or possibly . . ." I peer through the grate in the rock. It's ten A.M., so he's pretty easy to see from my clumsy vantage point, even though there are fifty feet between us. He's tall but a bit wiry, a swimmer's build. He looks pretty young, maybe my age or a bit older. "A youth. Not a child, though," I add hastily.

"Roger that, Team Leader. Let's give him The Five," Applebaum says cautiously.

"Yes, sir, going silent," I say softly. The Five is what we give every Immigrant—human or otherwise—who comes through The Rift. There are a few species we simply attack, like the Karekins, because we know they are a threat and have shown no desire throughout the years to negotiate.

For the rest of what or whoever ends up here, we have a pretty decent method of threat assessment: We watch them for five minutes. It becomes clear almost right away what we are dealing with. They are all afraid. How that fear manifests itself is the key. Some get panicked and desperate. Some cry. Some wail. Some simply sit down and look at The Rift, staring into its sickly green abyss, clearly in shock over what has just happened to them. Some get very, very, violent.

I breathe out slowly. There is an unlikely chance things will turn ugly this morning. This young man is wearing a flannel shirt and jeans, and sporting a backpack that makes him look like he's from a version of Earth very similar to our own. Obviously we've seen more benign-looking beings step through and wreak havoc, but my gut says he's not about to go on a rampage. And yet I'm troubled.

He is also standing just a little too close to The Rift.

Regardless of whether their five minutes are up, we can't ever let them go back through. Who knows where they would end up? The chances of making it back to their exact same Earth of origin are almost nonexistent. Anything that has the misfortune of stumbling through becomes our responsibility, and we wouldn't want them jumping back in and ending up God knows where—an Earth without an atmosphere? A Kare-kin Earth? The sharpshooters are ready with a tranq gun up in one of the tree towers, or Nests, just in case.

"He's awfully close," Applebaum says, as if reading my mind, but I know he's just looking at one of the video feeds back at Command Center.

"Just give him a second," I whisper. The young man cups his hands over his eyes and steps back, as if he's trying to get a better view. He's taking it in.

He looks around. All he will be able to see is forest. He looks back at The Rift. "What the hell?" he asks in plain English. He reaches around for his backpack and then stops, bites his lip and slips it over his shoulder once again. "Oh my God." His voice is just barely loud enough for me to hear. My hearing is enhanced, so he must have almost whispered it. The minutes tick by. He scratches his head and begins to pace. He's trying to figure it out. He's trying to analyze. I recognize this approach. I've seen it in others. There is no real logic to what's happened to him, though. Well, there is—in a "PhD in quantum physics" type of way—but this guy doesn't look old enough to have that. Besides, even if he could wrap his mind around how this happened, there is no rhyme or reason for *why* it happened to him. It's moot at this point, though.

The Five are up.

"Command, this is Beta Team leader. I'm going in." My team begins to stand up, and I immediately stop them. "I'm going in alone," I say with finality. I register their looks of annoyance. I don't care. This guy is not a threat and he doesn't need to be scared half to death by a bunch of commandos jumping out from behind a rock.

"Not a good idea, Ryn," I hear Applebaum say with authority. "What if there is a weapon in that backpack of his?"

Applebaum doesn't care about me personally one way or another. What he does care about is losing *any* Citadel—probably because of the expense that goes into training us. It's hard to think of Applebaum caring about an actual *person*.

"I don't think there is," I say. "I'm making the call, but it's sweet that you're worried about me." I put my gun down and stand up. I try to imagine what this guy is going to think when he sees me pop out of nowhere. We wear a uniform, of course. A long-sleeved unitard in forest green. The suit was designed by the Roones—one of the first groups that came through The Rift, and the creators of a lot of the tech we use. In terms of the uniform, our outfits are made of a polymer titanium, and spandex for movement. The titanium is spun so lightly and so deftly that it weighs practically nothing, but it is in effect like chain mail, kind of like wearing a bulletproof vest on your whole body. They must have added another compound to the suits, to compensate for the impact of melee weapons, but the Roones don't like to answer questions about exactly how things work. Since the suit has saved me more than a few times, it seems rude to keep asking.

Attached to the bodysuit are strategically placed lengths of quilted black leather. Our knees, shoulders, elbows, and torsos are covered for added heat and protection in hand-to-hand combat. We wear boots, too, though they aren't standard military issue. They look more like motocross meets Mad Max. I wish I could wear them outside of work, but we aren't allowed to take any of these provisions home. How would we explain them to our parents? Especially the utility and weapons holsters? The guys generally choose to put khakis over the suit. I understand why. Tights are a pretty hard sell to a teenage boy.

The girls have no such qualms. The suit helps us fight better and stay alive. I see no reason to alter it, even though we are all acutely aware that our uniform hugs every curve.

I walk around the rock with my hands up. I have taken my holster off. I have no type of weapon on me at all. Granted, every Citadel is basically a living weapon—and yes, Boone loves to make that joke over and over.

And over.

The guy is looking not at me but down at the ground, shaking his head, muttering something to himself. I walk closer and clear my throat.

"Hi," I say with a smile on my face. He looks up and I really see him for the first time. I catch my breath. He is gorgeous—specifically, *my type* of gorgeous. His skin is one shade darker than olive. His hair is tousled and brown, his eyes are azure blue. They look almost unreal, like he's wearing contacts. I push this thought aside. Even from this distance, he doesn't seem like a guy who would wear lenses to enhance the color of his eyes. Then I push *that* thought aside. *How the hell would I know what kind of guy he is?* Yet even as I think that, my heart begins to race and I clench my fists. ARC is monitoring my vitals through my suit. The last thing I want them to see is my attraction. It's so embarrassing. My cheeks flush. I suck in a deep breath and center myself. I'll be fine as long as this kid doesn't come too close or make any sudden moves to reach for me. He looks at me and narrows his eyes. He seems more wary than scared, which is good. He *should* be wary. But he's not panicking, and that is even better.

I force a grin. "Pretty crazy, right?" *What a stupid thing to say.* He looks at me and then at The Rift.

"Where am I?" he asks slowly.

"Washington. State."

"Well, then, *when* am I?"

The question catches me off guard. He's smart. He knows that whatever has happened to him is huge and mind bending.

I walk closer to him, my arms open, my body language showing vulnerability. "When do you think you are?"

"Please don't come any closer," he says politely. He tries to smile, but it's forced. He is standing stock-still but looks as if he could bolt at any second.

"Do you think you've time traveled or something?" I make it sound like that could never happen in a million years, but in a way it's not that far off from the truth.

"I don't know—have I?" He looks down again and then back at The Rift. His gaze finally falls back to my face, but his eyebrows are raised in a way that says he knows something and there's no point in making small talk.

I tell him what year it is and he nods.

"Same year, then," he says hesitantly.

"What's the last thing you remember?" I ask with genuine concern. How disorienting that trip must be. How terrifying.

"I was working in the lab at school. I heard a kind of drumming noise coming from outside. I walked toward the sound to investigate it and I saw this green light. *That* light," he says, pointing to The Rift. "And then the next thing I knew, I don't know . . . it sucked me inside and I couldn't breathe. It felt like I was being dragged underneath a wave and didn't know which end was up. What is it?" His words are cautious and carefully chosen. Most people are in shock when they end up here. Maybe he is, too, but he's holding on to his rationality pretty well.

Our eyes really lock for the first time and something passes between us. Heat maybe? Or just plain interest?

Or maybe wishful thinking. Get it together, Ryn.

"It's a cosmic anomaly—that's really as much as I know. Can I come a little closer? I promise I'm not going to hurt you."

"Okay," he says. Yet his voice is anything but casual. I walk toward him slowly. We are beside each other now.

I hear Violet's voice in my ear. "Watch yourself, Ryn." She's part of my team, so that's not surprising. But she's also my best friend, and that means she knows exactly what's going on in my brain right now. She's not warning me against any kind of sudden attack by him. She knows he's my type. She's heard us talking. She's worried *for him*.

"I'm not really trained to answer all the questions you must have. There are people here who can, though. I can take you to them," I offer. But I don't really want to take him anywhere. I wish we could just stay here for a while. I wish we were two normal people who met by chance, and who decided that they would like to get to know each other better. It's a selfish thought. We are a thousand light-years away from normal and the answers he wants won't bring him anything but pain.

It hurts *me* to think about that, and I start to wonder when in the past couple minutes I stopped being a Citadel and started acting like a teenage girl.

Never mind the fact that I *am* a teenage girl . . .

He looks me up and down. "What are you trained for, then?" he wonders out loud. Is he flirting with me? I'm so crap at this kind of thing, I have no idea.

"I'm like"—I fish for a word—"a guard."

"You're a girl," he says flatly.

Now it's my turn to narrow my eyes. "A girl can't be a guard?"

"A woman can, sure—a female—but you're a *girl*. How old are you?"

His words sting. He thinks I'm a child. I imagine picking

him up by the collar and holding him in the air. He'd change his mind pretty damn quick about me being a little girl.

Definitely back to being a Citadel again.

"I'm seventeen," I say, trying not to sound defensive or pouty. "How old are you?"

"Eighteen. Technically an adult. And last time I checked, you had to be an adult to be in the military, especially if you're guarding something like that," he says as he points to the huge shimmering green pool in the sky. "So again, where are we?"

"We're in Washington, like I said." I have to move things along now. They aren't going to give me forever to get this guy to trust me.

"Yeah, but where exactly in Washington?" he asks—not in a cocky way, but in a way that says he's not going to be distracted from getting an answer.

"Battle Ground," I say.

He jerks his head up and takes a slight step away from me.

"I mean, this isn't a battle ground—at least, not always . . ." I bite my lip. I've never done anything like this before—gone in alone and made first contact without my team. Boone is better at this kind of thing. Way better. "The name of the *town* we're in is Battle Ground, though actually, technically, we're at Camp Bonneville Military Base."

"And why would a seventeen-year-old girl be in charge of a cosmic anomaly?" He cocks his head, almost daring me to answer.

"I'm not so into the tone you're using when you say the word *girl*—just gonna put that out there," I snap back, and he gives me a half smile.

"Sorry. Why would *someone* so young be guarding something so . . . I don't know, what's a synonym for terrifying, but, like, way, way more?"

Now it's my turn to give a hint of a smile. "Have you ever heard of the Multiverse Theory?" I ask tentatively.

"Ryn!" Applebaum barks in my ear. "Enough. You do your job and let the experts do theirs for the intake. You have sixty seconds," he warns.

"Yes, the Multiverse, heard of it, go on," he says warily.

"Okay, so that thing is a portal to different versions of Earth. Some versions are similar to yours and mine and some are different?" It's weird that I'm framing this as a question. Am I trying to be cute? I am not cute. Applebaum is yelling objections through my earpiece and it's throwing me off. I need to take charge here. "I have a very particular skill set to deal with the ummm . . . more dangerous variations of other Earths." I do not take charge with this statement. I sound ridiculous.

"A particular skill set?" he counters immediately with sarcasm. "Like Liam Neeson?"

"Well, no, but yes, I mean, that's great. You have a movie star Liam Neeson on your version of Earth and so do we. We're getting somewhere!" He frowns. I am screwing this up royally.

"Thirty seconds, Ryn," Applebaum growls at me, "and I am not happy at all."

I sigh and then I disable the audio. I don't need the colonel's disappointment buzzing in my ear. I take a step closer to the guy in front of me. I get so close that my mouth is just an inch away from his ear. He smells like the woods and something else, something spicy. I like it, but I do my best to ignore it.

"Look," I whisper, "I don't have time to walk you through this. I know you have no reason at all to trust me. But, if you just let me and my friends escort you away from here, to someplace safer, there will be a bunch of people who are far better equipped than I am to answer all your questions. Okay?"

He turns toward me. His eyes are like turquoise and they are boring into me, making my knees go a little weak. I make a fist and push my short nails into my palm. "What if I say no?"

"Please don't do that," I plead. There must have been something in the tone of my voice because he nods his head slightly. "All right," I say softly, "my friends are going to come over here from behind that rock. Don't be freaked out. They have guns, but it's just standard procedure. That being said, don't, like, make any crazy sudden moves."

"Given that I can barely feel my arms or my legs right now, I don't think that will be a problem," he says, and stands perfectly still.

"Hey, guys, I think we're ready to go back up to Base. We just need to get a reading." Boone, Henry, and Violet pop up from behind the rock and make their way toward us, much faster than I would have liked them to. I can see him tense up beside me. But Boone, with his open face and his casual body language, immediately changes the energy among us all.

"Hey, man," he says, extending his hand. "I'm Boone and this is Violet, Henry, and of course you've already met Katniss."

Vi stifles a giggle.

"Your name is Katniss? Seriously?"

"No, it's not. That's Boone's idea of a joke. My name is Ryn." I hold my hand out and he shakes it and smiles genuinely.

"Ezra."

"Ezra, great!" Boone says. "Okay, we're all friends now and we're gonna get outta here 'cause, I'm not gonna lie, this particular spot is very not safe. All I need to do before we leave is use this little machine," he says, holding up a small silver box about the size of a phone, "to make sure you aren't radioactive. It's cool, right?"

Ezra gulps, and his eyes widen in alarm. "Why would I be radioactive?" Boone doesn't answer his question, nor does he wait for permission; he just waves the machine up and down over Ezra's body. He looks at me, wondering if Boone is kidding again. I mouth the word *sorry* to him and then crane my neck and look at the interface. It's blue. Ezra is fine, which I pretty much knew, but in our line of work you can't take anything at face value.

Even a face as gorgeous as Ezra's.

I suppose I was distracted by what I had just done, and that being so close to Ezra threw my senses totally out of whack, because I'm a bit surprised when he points at The Rift and says, "Why is it doing that?"

I glance over, and my eyes widen: The Rift has escalated to Stage 3. We all look at each other for a moment. This is how quickly things can go wrong here. This is how stupid mistakes can get people killed. I enable my audio right away, report to Command, and I'm instantly treated to an onslaught of expletives from Applebaum.

"We need to get to cover," Henry says calmly, but I can hear the strain in his voice. He's pissed. I feel a pang of guilt that my rash decision to come out and meet Ezra alone has now put us all at risk. I sweep it away. I can't afford to feel anything right now. I have to let my training take over and go back to being a soldier. The Rift doesn't usually open up again so quickly, but of course, this would be the day it does.

"There's no time, everyone, just hold your positions. It could be a dog for all we know. Just calm down and keep your hand on your weapon. Do not draw, though. Repeat: Do not draw your weapons," I say with authority. "The Nests have eyes on our situation and can provide ample backup if we need it." My team listens to me, and Ezra to his credit is also standing perfectly still. A lot of other people would have run, so his staying says something about him.

Of course, he could be doing the whole deer-trapped-in-headlights routine. That happens sometimes, too.

The Rift turns to deadly black and seven men come tumbling out. They aren't Karekins, so at least there's that. But they are very large. They have fair skin and long beards, and long hair, though some have pulled it back in rows of braids. They are wearing leathers and pelts. They are armed with an assortment of weapons, some axes, some broadswords. Each is holding a wooden shield with enough decoration and symbology to give me a clue. Apparently Ezra has the same idea as I do.

"Are those *Vikings*?" he says incredulously.

"Yes, it seems like . . . yes, those look like, uhh, Vikings." I take a step forward, but I do not reach out my arms. If they are anything like the Vikings we had on our Earth, they will not respect passivity.

I put my hands on my hips and give the newest Immigrants what I can only describe as a Peter Pan stance. *"Legg ned våpnene. Jeg gir deg kun en advarsel. Legg ned våpnene nå!"* Which roughly translates into: *Put down your weapons. I'm not going to give you another warning.*

"You speak Viking?" Ezra asks, noticeably shocked. I would argue that the fact that I speak Norwegian is far less fantastic than the fact that real-life Vikings have just tumbled through a Rift of time and space, but bantering seems inappropriate. The warriors shout and shake their weapons.

"Vi har visst dødd og er kommet til Valhalla. Det er vår rett til å ta våre våpen til Odin selv, for å bevise at vi er krigere. Vike trollkvinne!"

Boone can't stop the laugh that escapes full throttle out of his mouth.

"What did he say?" whispers Ezra.

"They think they've died and have arrived at Valhalla. They need their weapons to prove what hard-asses they are to Odin. They also say I'm a witch or demon." I wonder if Ezra thinks that we'll just shoot them. I know that would probably be my initial thought if murderous warriors just popped out in front of me. As easy as shooting them would be, though, things don't work that way. We don't kill people without prejudice. It was our scientists who created this Rift, and the thirteen others around the world, albeit accidentally. I mean, I think it was an accident. That's what we were told. ARC has never fully explained the experiment, and even though we all have advanced intellects capable of understanding the complexities of the exact cause, we've never been given the full debrief. It's been deemed top secret, above our security clearance. I guess they don't want us Citadels blaming any one scientist specifically. Which is ridiculous. As members of ARC, we collectively shoulder the responsibility for what happens with The Rift. We are way past finger-pointing.

Again, though, how or why this happened doesn't matter. It's our fault these men are here. It's our fault that their communities will be broken and their children will grow up without fathers. You can't point a gun at someone and pull the trigger to solve this kind of problem, especially when they can't even wrap their minds around what a gun is, let alone the circumstances that led them to be here. We could tranquilize them—in fact, that's exactly what we used to do. But then we figured out (through trial and error and the input of many anthropologists) that, in cases like this, these men must be defeated on their own terms. They have to be given a fighting chance so that their surrender will be lasting. I don't love combat, but I am good at it, especially hand to hand. Everyone gets a boost when they do something they are really good at. I'm no exception. And these guys . . . it's pretty clear they like a good throw down. Their body language is defiant, tensed. They are ready to bring it.

So am I.

"Vi, stay here with Ezra. Make sure he's covered."

Violet nods and stands in front of him, her hands on her rifle, but as ordered does not draw it. The three of us who remain walk just a few steps forward, and I see out of the corner of my eye Violet backing up, taking Ezra farther away from where the action is bound to happen. We don't run at the men, because we want them to come to us, away from The Rift. The men are screaming in Norwegian and pounding their swords against their shields. As annoying as it is, it's better than getting an earful from the colonel. Applebaum is blessedly silent. He knows well enough not to try to talk to me with the threat right in front of us, though I know he'll go ballistic on me once we return to the base. Now we just have to make sure we *make* it back to the base.

The Vikings begin to move forward, and I take a deep breath. Good. They are gaining distance from The Rift. When we are about twenty feet apart, one of the men throws his ax and it hurtles toward me. I catch it easily with one hand and for a moment the seven men are silent. I turn around and throw the ax in the opposite direction, much farther than he could have thrown it, right into a tree trunk. The Vikings charge anyway.

I have to give them bravery points for that.

The whole encounter lasts less than two minutes. I leap ten feet into the air and use a tree as leverage to make another jump down onto two of the men. I land squarely on the chest of one and kick out hard into the groin of the other. The one on the ground is unconscious. I have just enough time to turn him over and make sure there is no blood, that he hasn't hit a rock. Nope. Just your basic traumatic head injury. The one I kicked has recovered somewhat and lunges toward me. I see both Henry and Boone a few feet away. Henry actually picks up one of the men by the throat and lifts him high enough to throw a few feet. Boone blocks and parries the weapons easily. We all move so much faster than them, it's hardly a contest.

The Viking who lunges at me flips his shield up, presumably to use as a sort of battering ram to knock the wind out of me. I dance easily away, sidestepping him and ending up at his back. I jump on him from behind and wrap my arms around his neck. He tries to shake me loose, but I am so much stronger than he is. I know this shocks him. He probably thinks that women are feeble. I feel a sense of satisfaction as he begins to go down, but this is quickly replaced with the knowledge that he also thinks I'm some sort of demon guarding the gates to his afterlife. This one act of overpowering him is unlikely to change his views on women, but he'll learn soon enough when he gets to the Village. He passes out in my arms and I let him drop to the ground. When I look up, I see that all the Vikings are similarly disabled. I hear Applebaum through my earpiece calling for two teams in the Nest to assist. Eight soldiers jump from their perches high atop the trees and land softly behind us. We begin to zip-tie the Vikings' hands and pull each of the men to their feet. They are dazed and defeated, all of their bravado washed away. I notice the youngest one, probably close to my age. A single tear falls from his eye. If this was their great test, they have failed. All hope must be lost for them now. As my adrenaline recedes, I feel for this young man. I look over at Ezra and my heart breaks a little more. We haven't killed anyone, but in a way they are all dead. As soon as they entered The Rift they were reborn into a new life. Ezra's won't be as bad off as the poor Norsemen. Still, for the first little while, maybe for a long while, they will all be walking ghosts trapped in a new world that will take them years, if not their lifetimes, to understand.

I walk over to Ezra and Violet. "Come on, I'll take you to transport," I say wearily. I'm usually pumped after this kind of exercise, but looking at these newest arrivals I just feel kind of sad. "Violet, we still have another couple hours on duty. Can you get Boone and Henry and go back to our post? I'll be there in a minute."

"Sure," she says softly with a smile. Vi is a lovely person. It's an old-fashioned word, but that's what she is. Lovely. Not a mean bone in her body. What we do, who we are, is harder for her than anyone. The only thing that keeps her going is the knowledge that she saves way more lives than she is forced to take. She gives me these few moments with Ezra without making any kind of big deal about it, and I love her for that. She squeezes my shoulder and walks back down toward the big rock.

Ezra and I head for a separate transport vehicle. He will not be going back to base in the same car as the Vikings.

"So . . ." he says, drawing out the word, "skill set."

I chuckle. "Yep."

Ezra lifts up both hands and wiggles his fingers. "Thanks for not zip-tying me."

I keep my eyes on the ground. I don't want to look at him. I don't want to face any more questions, but I know they are coming.

Sure enough, he asks, "Where are they taking me? And

when will I be able to go home?" He stops walking and so do I. I take a deep breath and exhale slowly. I finally look him in the face, deep into those gorgeous blue eyes of his.

"Oh, Ezra, I'm . . . sorry," I whisper. I don't need to say anything more. He still doesn't know the specifics, but he knows enough now.

He bites his lip and nods. "It's okay. It's not your fault. Thanks for being nice." And then, out of nowhere, he pulls me toward him. He is hugging me. It's not a sexual embrace, but it's not exactly brotherly, either. It's a good thing that I had been feeling so sad; it takes a while for my body to get the signal from my brain that our skin has made contact and my face is now in the crook of his neck, and to notice that smell of his, a spicy earthiness mixed with his fear and wonder and the purity of The Rift. I have just enough time to pat him lightly and step back. We walk a couple more minutes in silence until we are just a few feet from the jeep.

"Just promise me that this won't be the last time I see you?" It's a statement, not really a question. Ezra's intake coordinator, Kendrick, is standing right behind us. I look over at him, and he raises his eyebrows. I stop for a minute and wonder why Ezra would ask me this. Does he like me? Does he think we can hang out later or something? He just saw what I did to those two Vikings. Didn't that freak him out? Or maybe it's because I was just the first person he saw when he got here and I *was* nice.

"Yeah. Okay," I say, and Kendrick gives me a stone-faced look. "Ezra—sorry, what's your last name?"

"Massad."

"Is that Arabic?" I ask, because it would explain his remarkable coloring.

"Well, yeah, my dad is Moroccan and my mom is American."

"Cool. Well, this is Kendrick. Kendrick, this is Ezra. Kendrick is going to be your main guy here for a while and answer all those questions you must have." Kendrick is one of the better intake coordinators. He has a calming vibe about him and is pretty much a straight shooter.

"*As-Salaam-Alaikum,*" Kendrick says, putting his hand out.

Ezra shakes his hand. "*Wa-Alaikum-Salaam.* But I'm not really a practicing Muslim. And after today . . . well, I might have to table the whole religion thing."

Kendrick laughs genuinely and opens the rear passenger door of the car. "I hear ya, man."

Ezra and I look at each other. There is too much to say.

There is nothing to say.

"Bye." I give him the warmest smile I can.

"Bye," he says, also smiling, but his eyes are not happy. "Thanks again." Not sure how to take that thanks, though. Everything above his mouth is a mixed bag of terror and crushing sadness. I watch the car drive off down the path and stare after it. I know Kendrick didn't say anything at the time because he thought it would be easier for me to lie. *Yeah, sure, I'll come and see you. No problem, Ezra.* The thing is, Citadels my age don't go to the Village. You don't have to be an adult to kill here at Battle Ground, but for some reason you need to be one to get posted to the Village. I have always known this, but now, suddenly, it strikes me as extremely worrisome. However, little does Kendrick know that I *was* being honest. Whatever it takes, I'm going to get into the Village.

I have decided that Ezra is going to be the only person in the world I will never lie to.

CHAPTER 2

It always feels surreal to walk away from The Rift, from combat, from hours of intensive training—and then straight into Safeway. But it's my turn to cook, and that means it's my turn to shop. Have to keep up the pretense and all that.

I push my cart up and down the aisles. I notice the cans stacked neatly one on top of the next, the endless rows of cereal boxes and the bright reds and oranges of the fresh peppers in the produce department. Shoppers pull items off the shelves and fill up their carts, totally unaware of what's going on just a few miles away. They might notice me, they might pick up that there is something different about me, but they would never be able to guess that I just put the smackdown on a bunch of actual Vikings.

When I get home, I have about thirty minutes until I have to make dinner. So I decide to just sit on our living room sofa.

It is a couch we rarely use in a room we use even less. We are not a "Game night!" family. We are more of a "Great having dinner with you all, I'm going to my room now" family. I wonder if I caused this. I wonder if the thing in my head programmed me this way and my parents and brother just followed my lead. Or maybe, in a rare stroke of good luck, I was born into a naturally solitary family.

It's not that I don't love them. I just don't *know* them . . . and they certainly don't know me.

The walls in here are like most of the walls in our house—covered with artwork. A lot of the paintings and photographs I just don't get at all. For the most part, those are the ones that were done by my dad's art school friends. Some of the artists are famous now and their stuff is worth a lot of money. My dad never got his big break, even though I think his work is ten times better. He paints portraits mostly. I slide my backpack to the floor and stare at one of my favorite paintings by him. In it, a woman in bed, surrounded by letters, looks out a window. I feel her pain through the canvas. I feel like I know her even though she lives in New York and we have never met. Dad says it was more than twenty years ago and he can't remember the exact circumstances that led her to sit for him, though he knows her name is Patricia and that they both lived in the same dumpy building. Did she ever get over whatever broke her heart so badly? The letters are yellowed and old and she isn't exactly young. I used to think it was a love affair, but as I get older I feel like it's something different; her grief seems deeper. Lately I've begun to wonder if she is even alive anymore. It scares me a little, that I feel so connected to an old woman whose sadness is so unbearable. I look away. Patricia is too much for me to deal with right now.

My father, Dan, is in his office, over our garage. He became a freelance graphic designer once I was born so he could bring in steady money. I'm not the only one in this house who's had to make sacrifices for the greater good, and this connects me to my father in a way that I cannot connect to my mother. I try not to let this favoritism show. I feel guilty enough as it is. I lean back in the sofa and close my eyes. My dad always goes on about how he wants me to sit for him. I will never let this happen. If he stares at and studies me for hours, I am sure his brushes and mixed-up colors will reveal all my secrets. My parents will figure out that I am hiding something and I know that this will hurt them. My dad's talent far outweighs my gift for lying, and that's saying something, because I'm a pretty amazing liar.

My mom's name is Vega, which means "star" in Swedish. I get my blond hair and fair skin from her. My green eyes come from Dad, and I got his dimples, too. When I first became a Citadel I hated my dimples because they made me look cute. "So adorable!" everyone would say whenever I smiled. How was I supposed to be a tough guy? A soldier? *So adorable* might as well be code for *soft*, and a Citadel needs to be anything but. Now that I've been in the field for three years, I am grateful for my dimples. I see death all the time. The hardness comes close to consuming me. My father won't live forever, but I will always see his smile in my reflection, and it's a great reminder that I'm the result of two loving people, and not what ARC has made me.

My mother moved to America from Stockholm for college and met my dad in New York City. My mom is a designer. She had big dreams, too, of being the next Diane von Furstenberg or Miuccia Prada. By the time she graduated from college, I think she let that dream go. Her classmates were risk takers, avant-garde designers who made crazy clothes out of recycled beer cans and raven feathers. She just wanted to make women look good. A school friend helped her get an interview at Nike. Since my dad grew up in Portland and his family was here, it seemed like the right move. They thought that only rich people could raise kids in Manhattan. They wanted children and so they relocated. We are, each of us, a product of decisions that other people made, one long chain of choices that stretch back to the beginning of humanity. Working so closely with The Rift, I have seen this firsthand. People arrive who have never heard of a world war, or who have never seen electricity, or who don't understand how it's possible that we are able to move freely from one country to another. History can be entirely rewritten based on one person's choice. Somewhere out there, through The Rift, is a version of Ryn Whittaker who lives in an apartment building in New York City. She is just a normal seventeen-year-old. I wonder who that girl is and what she'll become when she grows up.

I think a lot about her as I sit on the couch, with its hard cushions and unworn feel. I wonder if she'll ever meet Ezra Massad. Probably not. Then again, I have no idea where he's from. Rifts on the other Earths open and close randomly. They don't stay active like ours but flicker off and on, possibly opening once and never again. Scientists theorize that the Earths closest to ours have more frequent Rift activity, as the dark matter in the universe is drawn to these invisible fissures made by our experiment and strike like lightning. But they don't really know. They can't know anything for sure because no one goes back through The Rift. Ezra will never go back. The Roones are stuck here, too. The one exception is that Karekins keep coming, though no one can figure out how or why. It's such bullshit—all of it. I am so drained from today that I just want to sit here and try to think about nothing for a while.

But I pull myself up from the couch and make my way into the kitchen. We rotate cooking duties in the house. Nike is pretty far from Battle Ground. Sometimes my mom is in the car for two hours a day. Since it's my fault we're even in Battle Ground to begin with, I don't mind picking up some of the slack. My brother, Abel, is three years younger than me and has just started high school. He is useless in the kitchen, so he's exempt. Cooking is one of the few things he can't do. He's one of those people who seem to excel at everything they try. He's a natural athlete, he's artistic like my dad, he gets straight As—but I rarely see him doing much work. He's already over six feet tall and very handsome. He looks Scandinavian, but dark haired, like my dad. Actually, the first time I went to Stockholm to see my grandparents, I saw that most people have brown hair, which surprised me at first. That and the fact that they are insanely good-looking. Like, every random person just walking down the street could be a model. It's weird. I would be jealous of Abel, but honestly, if he had been average, like me, he might have been chosen to be a Citadel. I am so glad that he's not one; I can get past the fact that he is so friggin' good at everything.

I begin to cook sausage in an old Le Creuset pot that my mom has had since before she and my dad were married. I start boiling water for the pasta. I cut up the smooth-skinned peppers with an efficiency that belies my skill with knives. Even as I do these mundane things, I think, *I am a killer.* Not really a murderer, because it's all in the name of defense, of my life and the lives of those in Battle Ground and beyond. But a killer just the same. Sure, the way ARC says it, everything sounds quite reasonable. Heroic, even.

Then why don't I feel like a hero?

Each life I take takes a little something from me. I feel impossibly old for my seventeen years. I am not an innocent. I think about Ezra's hands when he waved them in front of me, thanking me for not restraining him. Where do you even go from there? Is that any kind of beginning to a romance? I roll my eyes. I can't have a romance with Ezra and there are so many reasons why that come tumbling into my thought process, they are beyond counting. I put the peppers into the pot and add some garlic as my mom walks through the front door. I hear her kick off her shoes and the thump of her bag on the formal dining room table.

"That smells good," my mom says. "Pasta?"

"Uh-huh," I reply. I look at her and smile quickly. Her pale blond hair falls loose to her shoulders. She is wearing jeans, a cotton button-down blouse, and sneakers. Since she works at Nike, her clothes are sporty and comfortable, but somehow she always manages to look chic. She layers necklaces, winds scarves brilliantly around her neck, stacks leather and gold bracelets on her wrists, has big chunky belts, and even the cut of her jeans—slouchy but fitted—is elegant. I can attribute this only to her being European. A cultural thing—not genetic—because no one would accuse me of being stylish. I rarely think about what I wear. More often than not it's yoga pants and boxy T-shirts with Converse sneakers in the summer and boots in the winter. In a way, my sartorial choices are great, because the rules are clear: We are not to draw any unnecessary attention to ourselves. I think I've worn makeup maybe twice in my life. I'm sure this must be somewhat disappointing to my fashion-conscious mother, but to her credit she never says anything. She takes a look at me and opens her mouth to say something but closes it. How could she not want a normal daughter who rambles on about boys and clothes and teachers at school? Instead she got me: a kid who talks as little as possible and keeps her mother at arm's length.

I am a good girl. She says that a lot. "Ryn, you're such a good girl . . ." She tries to be validating, because that's what I am. That is all I can offer my parents. I am good. I do not sneak out at night, I don't water down their liquor, I don't come home smelling like weed, I don't break my curfew, I don't date. For a while there, my parents thought I was gay. They sat me down and quite sweetly said they would love me no matter what and that if I liked girls, I should just tell them, get everything out in the open. "I'm not gay," I said softly. "I'm shy."

The thing is, I am not shy. I'm quiet only because I hate that every other word out of my mouth is an untruth. I probably should have just said I was asexual . . . which is pretty much what my job requires of me anyway. Besides, that's a thing now. It would have given them something to research and they would stop smirking at each other every time Boone or Henry comes over . . . and then frown when it's clear nothing is happening between me and either of them.

It's almost like my parents would welcome me having sex. I think they'd breathe a sigh of relief even as they grounded me. And it hurts sometimes that I can't even give them *that*.

"Dinner in fifteen," I say, and go back to stirring the peppers. I am always hyperaware of my body language. I know how to close myself off, how to disinvite a conversation with a slight turn of my chin, a shuffle backward, a drawing in of my shoulder blades as if they were wings that needed hiding. I try not to be dismissive, but I know that's what she sees. We both hear Abel come in, and my mom—with some relief— walks to the door to greet him. He's been at football practice. I pretend I don't know his schedule, like I couldn't give a shit. The truth is I know where Abel is almost every minute of the day. I know where everyone in my family is, because if trouble that can't be contained comes through The Rift, I might need to get to them quickly.

I put the pasta bowls on the kitchen table and neatly set a folded paper towel and a fork beside each one. I fill up a carafe with ice water and lay out four glasses. My family arrives from their separate corners of the house and everyone sits in their chairs. The conversation bounces lightly between them . . . and mostly off of me.

"We just got a prototype of a running jacket that I designed and I'm really excited about it," Mom gushes. "I know you don't run, Ryn, but it's supercute. It would look great on you. You could use it as a light coat when the weather gets cooler." I run, on average, about twenty miles a day—not that my family would know. When I tell my parents I hate working out, this is not exactly a lie. I don't love exercising, but I don't exactly have much choice, either. "I'll order you one when it goes to market—*if* it goes to market. But I'm sure it will; everyone seems really positive about it at work."

"That's great, V," my dad says, and gives her a broad smile.

"Thanks, Mom," I say politely.

"So," my dad begins, "how's varsity looking?"

Abel's mouth is full of food. I have never seen anyone eat as much as Abel does, not even Henry and he's way bigger than my brother. Abel begins to nod his head as he swallows. "It's good. I think it's there if I want, only I'll probably be benched most of the season. Greg Casiano is a great QB, and I'm just a freshman. I don't think I'll get much field time. Maybe I should just do JV so I can really play." Abel takes another mouthful.

"I don't know . . ." Dad ponders, lifting his thumb and index finger to his chin as if to stroke an imaginary beard.

"Playing varsity all four years of high school looks great on a college application."

Abel shrugs. He's fourteen. He's not thinking about college. He just wants to get out there and have some fun. I get it, and I think my mom does, too, but she doesn't say anything. I know she will bring this up to my dad later, when they are alone. I also know what's coming next.

"Speaking of college," my dad says, turning his eyes to me. I groan inwardly but keep my face passive. "I hope you're giving some serious thought about where you want to apply. Now's the time, Ryn, and you have got to do some extracurricular activities. I know you're in ARC, but it might not be enough. It's not just about grades."

My parents believe that ARC stands for Accelerated Rate Curriculum. They think I'm in a highly advanced scholastic program, but it's a cover for the real acronym—Allied Rift Coalition. They moved to Battle Ground from Portland just so that I could be a part of the program. Even though I start my days off at Battle Ground High, I don't even go to school. I don't need to. When I was fourteen and my chip was activated, I had a secondary and post-secondary education downloaded straight into my brain. I still haven't decided if this is the best or worst part of being a Citadel. ARC robbed me of the opportunity to learn like a normal person. I will never have to sit through a boring lecture or do homework or worry about getting to class. I don't know if I got super lucky or completely cheated.

"She does all that volunteer work at the old military base," Abel says brightly, and looks at me. God, my brother is a nice guy. He has so many reasons to be an asshole, but he's just not wired that way. The taller Abel gets, the more protective of me he feels. It's cute. I smile genuinely back at him.

"I just want you to find the right place, Ryn, where you can really open up and find out who you are, you know? A place that will help you come into your own. Nothing would make me happier."

That would make me happy, too. And the fact is, I *will* leave Battle Ground in a couple years. My parents believe I am a junior in high school and think I will be off to college soon. In reality, though, I will be working another Rift site. I feel the dull throb of a headache emerging. I reach back with my hand and rub at an invisible scar at the base of my skull.

"I know, Dad," I respond, but I don't say anything else. There are a couple of seconds of silence before Abel tells me how much he likes the pasta, effectively switching the subject.

"Thanks," I say gratefully. The talk resumes until dinner is over. I have said six words throughout the entire meal. My parents do not know me. They truly have no idea who I am. I hate that The Rift has denied them the opportunity. I excuse myself and walk upstairs to my room, grabbing my knapsack on the way. I close my door, turn some music on, and unzip my bag. I take out a binder, open it, and put it faceup on my bed. It is filled with fake assignments and handouts from non-existent teachers. The ARC program (that is, the Accelerated Rate Curriculum) has us use an iPad instead of textbooks, and it is where all of our papers, written by God knows who, show up in the appropriate folders. I flip the iPad so the attached keyboard sits propped up beneath the screen, so if one of my parents happens to walk in, it'll look like I'm working.

I take out a book, one of my own from the library, and lie down on the bed. I love reading, and every time I finish a book I feel both indulgent and defiant; I process information faster than a regular person. I could, in theory, read the book in my hands in about half an hour, but, through much trial and error, I have learned to slow this process down when I want. Reading should be savored. Each word should be enjoyed. I'm sure our bosses at ARC would prefer we read technical manuals, something practical on bomb making or physics. Actually, they would probably prefer that we spend our downtime doing crunches and pull-ups, which is never, ever going to happen. The reading is mine. It's the one thing I won't let them have.

I love the look on Applebaum's face when I show up at work holding a romance novel.

And yet I can't seem to enjoy reading tonight. I open the book and stare at the words. Each sentence seems to end and then double back on itself. If I truly focused I could let them settle, but I know there is no point. I keep the book cracked and bring it down over my face. Inhaling the ink and paper, I feel my tension slide just a little. This smell—of the library, of stories and childhood and oak shelves—is comforting.

I allow myself the luxury of thinking about Ezra.

I see him in the clearing near The Rift, so brave, so handsome, and so *totally* fucked. I throw the book across the room. It hits the wall with a thud. How can I get to him? Even if I do, what can I do? Be his friend? How can I be around him without wanting to kiss that beautiful mouth of his? I can't. It's impossible and then I'll hurt him—literally. He's been hurt enough. If I was a decent person I would just let it go, let *him* go. I am not a decent person, though. I am a liar and a killer. And I can't stop thinking about him, of him being debriefed and tested back at the base. After that he'll be sent to the Village. No one breaks out of there.

But, just maybe, someone can break in.

CHAPTER 3

The next morning, I throw on some clothes and stuff my things back into my bag. It's early. I know I am the first one awake. Since I need so little sleep, I am up at dawn or even earlier sometimes. I make a pot of tea and turn on the TV. I don't really watch it, but the quiet always seems different first thing in the morning, more depressing somehow. The night feels like it's full of possibilities, full of dreams and escape plans. Mornings are empty. I don't know exactly what my day will bring, but I know that there is zero chance that I can stay home sick or skip, like I could if I was actually in school. I am needed at my post. People always say, "Oh, I have to get my hair done," or "I have to pick up my dry cleaning." In reality there are only a few things you absolutely have to do: eat, sleep, go to the bathroom, and, in my case, show up for my shift at work in front of an interdimensional Rift in time and space.

You know—the usual stuff.

I drink my tea and eat some toast, zoning out. My mom comes downstairs, takes her coffee with her and zooms out the door with a wave good-bye. She's always in a hurry to get to work on time. I probably won't see my dad this morning. He's more of a night owl and doesn't get out of bed till nine or ten. He's his own boss. Must be nice.

It's my job to get Abel out of bed. This is a Herculean effort that generally takes at least three separate wake-up calls and has involved, to a much more minor degree, some of the torture techniques I've been taught as a Citadel. Oddly enough, blaring death metal doesn't work nearly as well on a teenage boy as one might think.

Eventually, after twenty highly annoying minutes (for both of us), Abel comes down dressed and ready for breakfast. He grumbles a simple "hey" in my direction as if the last half hour didn't just happen and pours himself some juice. He then eats two bowls of cereal in under ten minutes. It's impressive. We take turns brushing our teeth and then head out the door to my car.

Every summer I work full-time at The Rift. My parents think I'm a camp counselor. I do actually get paid pretty decently. I mean, I'm not a millionaire, but I will never have to worry about money. Once I turn eighteen and leave home I will get paid even more. In the meantime, as a minor, the majority of my money is held in trust. Isn't that a bitch? At the end of the day, I probably have about as much money in the bank as an average teenager who only works during the summer. I was able to buy a car, though. I needed something fast because, once again, if shit goes sideways at The Rift, I might need to get everyone to safety in a hurry. A Ferrari was out of the question obviously, so I opted for a Dodge Challenger. It's not the most comfortable ride in the world, but it's fast, and big enough to fit my whole family. The choice absolutely baffled my parents. But since I rarely, if ever, ask them for anything, they agreed to sign the loan, especially since I put a large chunk of money down and make the payments myself.

Abel, on the other hand, thinks the car is cool, and that alone makes me happy about my choice. He slides into the passenger seat and I fire up the ignition. The engine purrs into life and I turn up the music, deliberately selecting a song I know my brother likes. I do these little things for him and I hope he's getting old enough now to figure out that it's my way of showing him how much I love him. Abel isn't weak or helpless. But of course I worry about him. I might just love my brother more than anyone in the world, but I can't get too close. The lying is always going to be a wedge, of course. But there's more than that. As a soldier, my brain often goes to worst-case scenarios. Who knows what could happen? What if the Karekins invade and succeed? What if they round up everyone I love and hurt them just to try to get some leverage on me? Because of those thoughts, I must keep everyone at arm's length. Close, just not enough to kill me if I lose them somehow.

The drive to Battle Ground High is uneventful. I park in the lot and my brother and I walk to the entrance.

"Later," Abel says as he goes off in the direction of his locker. I turn right and follow the hallway to a solid metal door. I notice the other students staring at me. I feel their eyes scanning me with a mixture of fear and awe. They know I'm different, though they can't quite figure out why, other than I'm part of the ARC. Whatever. I look forward and ignore them all. I don't have the time or the energy to think about how these kids perceive me. I'm too focused on trying to save their lives.

I walk down a flight of stairs into what is, in theory, the ARC section of school. This section is guarded by what looks like just a normal security guard but who is, in fact, a private in the army. For all intents and purposes the entrance looks like a metal detector, but it's all for show, like the rest of this area. This need for enhanced security was built around a lie that one of the ARC kids pulled a gun and tried to shoot a bunch of students when the first Citadels started working. They said we were under more pressure than the other kids. That the workload was so demanding and the schedule so brutal that extra precautions were necessary. This also handily sets up another lie: that the intensity of the program could be mollified by increased physical activity. As such, they tell our parents we take daily martial arts instruction to reduce stress and anxiety in a productive way. It helps explain if we happen to do something extraordinary ("Oh—we learned that today. It's Krav Maga."), and it's an excellent cover for all the injuries we come home with. The key is our parents will never know it's not true, because no one gets through here without proper ID. I walk through the metal detector and down a long hallway with empty classrooms on either side. Although there are other Citadels here waiting to go through the last bit of security, this is a lonely stretch of linoleum. The classrooms, fully kitted out and ready to hold students, are just another lie. If things were different, I would be right here every day—learning and probably hating it a lot—but all of this seems oddly cruel, like a reminder of what we can't have. ARC has to keep up appearances, though, for open house nights and fake teacher conferences.

I wait for the few people ahead of me to have their retinas scanned, then put my eye up to the device. "Confirmed," a soothing voice says. "Citadel Ryn Whittaker, designation 473. Proceed to transport." Now this . . . this is where it gets interesting. ARC built a train beneath the school, linking it straight to Camp Bonneville. Think of it as a high-speed subway that takes us the few miles to base in just under ten minutes. I hate this thing. If the Karekins ever got through our line and found the entrance at the base, Command Center can remotely blow the whole tunnel so that it collapses and prevents the Karekins from getting into town—and they'll blow it up regardless of whether there are Citadels in the tunnel at the same time or not. You take your chances every time you step in here. It's a death trap. I practically hold my breath during each ride.

When the train slows to a stop, I hightail it out of there and take the stairs up just one level to our locker rooms. I shimmy into my uniform quickly and as I do, I feel the change come over me as well. Once again I'm not a kid anymore. I'm a soldier. I'm ready for action. Today might be the day I die.

God, I'm morbid.

As I pull my hair up into a ponytail, Violet races in. It's clear she has just come from dance practice. Her hair is in a perfect bun. She is wearing tights and leg warmers over a long-sleeved leotard. The irony is so glaringly obvious I don't even need to say anything.

"Oh, good," she says a little frantically as she begins to open her locker. "I thought I was going to be late. I'm actually a little early for a change."

I give her a warm smile. "You're fine." A regular soldier walks in and stands a little nervously in front of me. We have a complicated relationship with the military here. Special Ops used to run the show at The Rift, but they did a pretty piss-poor job of it. There were many casualties on both sides, and so they were taken off the job once the first crop of Citadels was activated. It's only natural that a Navy Seal or a Ranger would resent a fourteen-year-old kid who can not only pull rank but kick your ass in every fight. I never saw it happen, but we've all heard stories of the early years. It created a very us-versus-them mentality. Tensions have only eased as the older, professional soldiers have been transferred out and replaced with younger, greener troops. These newer troops are still resentful, but they are mostly just intimidated. We all kind of respectfully leave one another alone.

"Citadel Ryn?" the soldier says. "Colonel Applebaum wants to see you."

Violet and I exchange glances. I figured that he would have stopped me yesterday before I went home. When he didn't, I assumed I was in the clear.

Apparently not.

"Okay," I say brusquely, and grab the rest of my gear. There are weapons caches all over the bunker. Normally we grab ours from an armory room beside the transport bay right before we go on duty at The Rift site. I'm sure Applebaum wouldn't want to meet any of us for disciplinary action with rifles in our hands. I follow the private out the door, up another flight of stairs to Command. There is nothing much to see at the base from the outside. A few buildings here and there, defunct shooting ranges. But beneath all of that is a bunker, a vast network of offices, control rooms, training facilities, and dorms in case we need to put everyone on lockdown for safety.

The soldier leads us through a maze of corridors until we reach Applebaum's office. I knock once and wait for him to tell me to enter.

When he does, I walk through the door and stand at attention in the middle of the small room. He is seated behind a large wooden desk. It seems out of place in this room; it's more presidential than military, though the office is actually decorated quite nicely, with bookshelves, framed photos on the walls, and an ornate desk lamp that looks like an antique. Fancy. My eyes hover on a picture of Applebaum and Christopher Seelye in the Oval Office. I involuntarily shudder. Applebaum is a prick, but Seelye is something else. If anyone is the villain in this story it could easily be him, the president of ARC. Then again, he could also be the hero. I know he certainly thinks he's the hero, and maybe I would think he is, too, if I didn't feel like taking a shower every time I had to deal with him. His face is happy and light, but his eyes tell a different story. He isn't afraid of us Citadels. Sometimes Applebaum accidentally slips and lets his guard down. The horror of what we do, the carnage we leave behind—it frightens him. Seelye is proud. He makes me feel like a shiny gun or an expensive sports car, like something he *owns*.

"At ease, Ryn." I move my legs apart and put my arms behind my back. We stare at each other in uncomfortable silence for a few seconds.

"Ryn," he begins, "you're a good soldier. A natural leader with superb combat skills. I depend on you."

I keep my gaze fixed above his head, on a photograph of him with the president and first lady. "Thank you, sir," I respond.

"But that stunt yesterday was not only a breach of protocol— it was stupid. You saw a kid your age, you assumed he was an MTI, but that guess endangered you and your team. You could have gotten hurt or worse." Applebaum's voice is level but strained. He pauses. Maybe he thinks I agree with him, but I don't. He closes his eyes for a moment and sighs. "You know why we call them MTIs? Minimal Threat Immigrants? Because there is no such thing as a *Zero* Threat Immigrant. These people, or whatever they happen to be, that come through The Rift are never *not* going to be a threat. It's our fault that they are snatched from their homes and loved ones. It's our fault that they can never return. They have every right in the world to be pissed off about that. We can never let our guard down around them. Do you understand?"

"I understand that you believe that, sir, but I'm not sure I can completely agree," I state calmly.

He looks at me and narrows his eyes. Then he pounds his fist hard on the table. I do not flinch. "No, Ryn, that is unacceptable. You, more than anyone, should know that we can't trust what comes out of that green hellhole." Applebaum's voice is rising with every word and still I do not move, nor do I change the look of indifference on my face. "This isn't Portland. The Rift isn't an organic farm. On a good day it's a hot zone. On a bad day it's a war zone. You can't act like a social worker out here. That's not your job."

"So having empathy and compassion makes me a social worker? I mean, call me crazy, but shouldn't having those things be kind of a prerequisite if you're going to be pointing a gun at someone?" I know I'm speaking out of turn, but I'm getting fed up. He's not the one fighting. He sits on his ass all day while I put mine on the line. Besides, *look what they did to us*. What a hypocrite. I might not have lost my home, but I lost any chance at a normal life when I was seven years old. Don't they get that? That we could be just as dangerous, if not more so, than any Immigrant, for practically the same reason?

"Possibly. The only thing I know for sure is that we can never, *ever* trust them. Period," Applebaum says flatly.

"We trust the Roones," I snap back.

"They're different. I don't even think they are capable of feeling hate, or actually anything for that matter. And they saved us," he says quickly.

I finally look at him. "So says the guy without a chip in his skull."

Applebaum smiles smugly and leans back in his chair,

holding his arms out in front of him and gripping his desk. "You're young. I always forget that about you kids. You fight so well—and don't get me wrong; you all do an excellent job— but it's always a bit like *playing* soldiers, isn't it? What's that thing the nerds do? Larp? Larping? It's like that. No real discipline." He shakes his head and closes his eyes. For a brief moment I imagine punching a hole right through his chest. I imagine taking one of his hands and pulling it all the way back, breaking the bone so that it sticks out from his wrist. The fact that I don't disproves his theory of discipline. Even so, I will not give him the satisfaction of seeing how his truly offensive words have stung me. I will not let him dismiss me as a sulky teenager.

"Will that be all, sir?" I ask in a passive voice.

"Don't let it happen again, Ryn. You're the team leader for a reason. Boone's a clown, Violet is a ballerina, and Henry is coiled so tight I think he might be one mission away from going postal. You're the only one with any sense. Or at least that's what I thought until yesterday. Don't disappoint me again."

I refuse to say anything. I know he's pushing me, though I can't imagine what reason he has for doing so. My own family can't get a reaction out of me—and I *want* to be around them. This guy is getting nothing from me.

After another couple of seconds, he sighs and tells me to go.

I meet the rest of the team at transport to The Rift site. The site is about a mile away, down a graveled road through the forest. We say very little in the car because there are just normal troops accompanying us and we prefer to keep our distance from them. We understand that the things we say get reported back to Command and then to ARC. We're on the same team, but at the same time, we're not. No one trusts anyone here, and either way, I'm happy for the silence.

Today we are working up in one of the seven Nests above ground, in the tree line. The Nests surround The Rift and serve as both lookouts and vantage points for sharpshooting, if it comes to that. The four of us easily scale the rope ladder that leads up to a wood platform suspended in a huge sequoia tree. There are provisions here—water and emergency rations—but no bathrooms. The boys will often piss in empty bottles. The girls have gotten good at holding it until the shift is over in four hours.

Nothing like a little institutional sexism to remind us we're in the military.

Omega Team is at the rock on lookout. We really just have to check in and make sure Command knows we're here if needed. I ask the team to make sure their earpieces are functioning and then we disable the mics so we can talk without being overheard.

"So, did Applebaum cut you a new one this morning?" Boone asks, wasting no time. Before I can even answer he goes off again. "He's an ass. You didn't do anything wrong, Ryn," Boone assures me.

"You really didn't," Vi adds.

I lean back against a wooden slat in the platform. "I shouldn't have gone in alone. Without a weapon. It wasn't the smartest move," I confess.

"It wasn't," Henry says through clenched teeth.

Violet places a hand on my arm. "Oh, please. He was young and cute. It's bad enough that he ended up here. He didn't need a bunch of us ambushing him."

I have to smile at her optimism.

Henry pulls a few pine needles off a close branch and throws them down from the Nest. "He could have been dangerous. You gambled. It worked out okay, but it might not have."

"Stop being such a hard-ass all the time, Henry," Boone says. "It's boring. I think I might have a coronary if you ever cracked a joke." Of course, Boone's sarcasm does not play well with Henry. Henry *is* wound tight. Applebaum hadn't gotten that wrong. At six four, he is the biggest of us. His mom is Korean and his dad is Native American. He'd probably be the total package if you didn't have to go on such a search-and-rescue mission for his personality. The thing about Henry, other than the fact that he's a superb soldier, is that he is loyal as anything. He's taken a bullet for me more than once, multiple punches, and even a knife wound. Whether we are at work or hanging out, he is always just there. I love him. I love his quiet strength and the little things he does to show he cares about us—things that Boone is too clueless to pick up on.

"Knock it off, Boone. It was fine with Applebaum, but to be honest I really don't want to talk about it."

"Fine." Vi tries to negotiate. "We'll leave Applebaum out of it if you tell us why you went out there alone. I meant to ask yesterday, but you went home so fast."

"Whoa, what's with all the questions?" I snap. "It seemed like the right thing to do. That's it. No agenda. I just said I didn't want to talk about it. *God*." My teammates look at each other with raised eyebrows.

"It's okay to think someone is cute," Violet says softly. "It's okay to be attracted to someone, to have feelings for someone even if they come through The Rift."

At that, I have to laugh. I look at her, my eyes widening. "Are you crazy? It's *not* okay to be attracted to anyone. Because obviously, thanks to ARC, we're mature enough to save the world but not mature enough to keep our hormones in check." Without thinking, I pick up my arms and start doing a weird version of jazz hands while talking in an absurdly low voice. "Hey, I'm ARC," I blurt out sarcastically. "We're going to make you superstrong and superfast and supersmart but not smart enough!" I'm off on a tangent now. I see Henry sigh. "You might check for a text from your boyfriend while you're fighting for your life, so we're just going to put this little glitch in your implant that turns you into a maniac if you touch anyone you might be remotely attracted to. Not so much as a little, teeny-tiny, even-Catholics-would-approve-of-it hug. Nope, sorry! No sex for you! Ever!"

"You didn't need to go straight to the Blood Lust, Ryn," Violet says with an undeniable hint of sadness. "It's a long way from liking the way someone looks, and maybe even crushing on them a bit, to activating that part of the chip's programming. It's not like we have no control."

I look up to the sky and shake my head. "Oh, well, *I know that*," I spit back meanly. "Look at you and Boone. You guys have been in love with each other since we were fourteen and you two haven't killed each other." This is common knowledge, but we never speak it. The fact that we are all *just* the best of friends, like family—that is another lie. "It's easy, right? As long as you guys don't touch each other or even brush up against one another. Unless you're fighting. We can always fight. They made damn sure of that."

"Shut up, Ryn," Boone shoots back, clearly wounded.

"And what about poor Henry?" I continue even as Henry shoots me a death stare. "He's gay. I mean, seriously, he's like every gay guy's wet dream. He could get more ass than all of us put together and he can't even jerk off without destroying his bedroom, maybe even his whole house. So yeah, I'm a little skittish. I'm a little fucking sensitive about being attracted to anyone, because I can't even stick my hand down my pants and make this teeth-grinding ache go away." The silence in the Nest becomes a living thing, awkward and full of ugliness. I put my head down on my knees. Shit.

"I'm sorry," I say finally. "That was mean. I don't know what's wrong with me. And so help me God, Boone, if you say 'PMS' I will punch you in the face." Boone puts his hands up in surrender. "Can we please just drop it? I don't know why I went out there or why this Ezra guy should be any different from anyone else. He probably isn't. I'm just . . . I don't know . . ." I rummage around in my head trying to come up with the words to explain how I feel. When I can't, I just apologize again.

Vi reaches over and gives me a hug. "It's okay. We're all just doing the best we can. Some days are better than others," she says, and I nod my head, embarrassed. I hate hurting my friends. And for the most part, Violet was right. The Blood Lust is one of the crueler by-products of the chip, but it's not like we want to kill every person we find attractive. It's always there, though, simmering beneath the surface like a sleeping junkyard dog. As long as we are careful, as long as we don't linger on romantic thoughts or touch someone that we might have—in another life—hooked up with, the dog remains asleep. I understand that the idea behind this wiring was to make us more efficient, but honestly it takes a lot of energy to suppress these urges. ARC must know this, but they continue on with it anyhow. Maybe it's just too late; they can't have some Citadels who can get it on and some who can't without a mutiny. Or maybe it's just another cruel way to control us. I don't know, but if you combine the Blood Lust with our constant lying and living a double life, we can burn out in this job. When that happens, they send the Citadel away for a couple months to recuperate. Sounds great, but it's not something we push for. Our teams depend on us. What if something bad happens while we're gone? Something we might have stopped?

I take hold of her hand. "Thanks, Vi." I watch Boone look at us. We are comforting each other the way best friends do. He turns sharply away, uncomfortable, knowing it's something he'll never be able to safely do with her—yes, even something as benign as holding her hand. There's a lot of pain on this platform, and it's relieved only when I suddenly hear Omega Team in my earpiece. The Rift is opening. I enable my mic, as do the rest of us.

We stand and look out at The Rift. That was quick. We have been on duty for only a matter of minutes. I check in with Command, confirming that we have eyes on the situation and can see The Rift opening. The center of The Rift turns black as tar and then we hear an earsplitting sound.

An explosive detonated by a hand-held rocket launcher deploys as soon as the Karekins enter this Earth. They don't mess around. The rocket destroys a tree about seventy-five feet away from us. Karekins are streaming out of The Rift. I use my enhanced eyesight to count as they come through. A dozen. Two dozen, fifty, one hundred, one hundred fifty, two hundred. That's a significant number. There are about a hundred of us Citadels, so I don't love the odds. The five other teams that have been hiding in trenches will emerge. The reinforcements will come forward. Each Nest team will jump down, leaving the best marksman behind to shoot whomever they can safely. In our case it's Violet. Boone, Henry, and I give each other a nod and do a swan dive off the platform, flipping at the last second so that we land on our feet. I immediately get shot in the shoulder. Karekins use laser technology. I wince in pain and take sharp breaths until I can steady myself. The suit has absorbed most of the impact. I'll have a bruise, but that's about it.

I take about two seconds to calm down. I must not be angry. I must feel nothing. I must run forward when every instinct I have still says, even after all this time, to get the fuck out of there. I take out my gun and shoot one Karekin in the middle of the forehead. I swing around and shoot another in the same place. Karekins, like us, evolved from apes. I think in their case it was more of a King Kong thing. They are eight or nine feet tall, and hairy. Their eyes are small and slit-like. They use sound and smell mostly to fight. Sounds like a big disadvantage, but the research people at ARC think it might be an advanced form of echolocation that allows them to compensate for their poor eyesight. They aren't savage, though. They wear sleek black uniforms and have advanced weaponry—lasers, remember? Most important, they keep coming through, and they seem more prepared each time to deal with us. It's almost as if they are getting to know our weaknesses and adapting, which should be technically impos-sible. Because that would mean that they are reporting back through The Rift, and they should not be able to do that. Yet here they are. Shooting into the trees, into the Nests.

How else would they know to do that?

I feel one of the Karekins pick me up from behind and fling me at least twenty feet to the side. My shoulder takes the brunt of the impact. I know it's been dislocated. I flip up before I can get attacked again. I try to pull my shoulder back into its socket. I can't get the right angle. Bracing myself, I smash it into a tree so that it pops back into place. I hear a Karekin behind me. I kick out, pushing off from the tree trunk. I turn around and he staggers a bit. I leap up, using his shoulders as leverage, and land with my legs around his neck. I squeeze, and we both fall to the ground with a thud. I reach down and pull my bowie knife from my boot and stab him squarely in the throat. I push my body out from underneath him. Just for good measure I slice his throat back and forward. Blood spurts all over me.

Gross.

I almost laugh at that thought—surrounded as I am by all this gore and death—but another Karekin is already racing toward me on the ground. I have just enough time to whip my knife out of the other one's throat and throw it into the approaching Karekin's right eye. Their suits are just as protective as ours, so there is no point in aiming anywhere else. Boone runs up beside the one who is now down on his knees with my knife planted firmly in his eye. Boone shoots him in the forehead and kicks him down to the ground.

There are screams and shouts, and the sound of gunshots and the smell of blood are thick in the morning air. I cannot afford to take the time to really live in the middle of all this. And yet, just for a split second I wonder how I got here. Who put my name down on the list for this? Who guessed that I would make such a good killer? Who would even look at a seven-year-old and be able to imagine such a thing?

"Ryn!" Henry screams at me. He leaps ten feet in the air. I turn just in time to hear a laser pulse whiz past my ear. I can't believe how stupid that was. I lost focus for just a couple seconds and I almost died. Henry is now just a few feet away, but before I can turn and face the enemy to fight, I feel a massive Karekin hand on the back of my neck. He's going to try to snap it and now I have to break free. Henry lunges at him. The Karekin has just enough time to remove his hands and hit me with something large and heavy on the head. When I fall, the sky shifts sideways. It's like it happens in slow motion. One minute I'm up and the next I am floating to the ground. Henry has killed my attacker. From this angle it all looks so different. Like a dance. I can almost hear music in the rifle shots.

"Ryn, are you okay?" Henry screams, but his voice seems far away, like he's on the other side of the forest and not right beside me. I open my mouth to answer, but all my words are gone. I want to say that yes, I am fine, but I am not fine. I am always almost dying and so is he and Violet and Boone. I am not fine, because I will most likely die a virgin. I will never have another profession. I am a liar. I'm not even sure I am capable of telling an absolute truth. My head will heal, but I am not okay. I want to say this, but I can't say anything. Nothing is working on my face. Henry stands guard over me, taking out two or three Karekins as I lie helpless on the ground. The world tilts again and everything goes black.

CHAPTER 4

I awake to the steady electronic beeping of my heart. I am back at the base in the medical facility. I am hooked up to an IV. As my eyes flutter open, I see the plastic tube first, running from the back of my hand to a bag beside me. I try to blink away the fuzzy outline of everything in the room. In short order, the room snaps into focus. I am not lying down but reclined on the gurney. I try to sit completely up, but I feel a small hand gently push me back to the bed.

"Easy, Citadel Ryn. You are safe," the voice purrs. I know immediately that it is a Roone. Their voices are distinctly non-human. They rasp and whirr; it's difficult for the muscles in their throats to push out the words in our language. I recognize the kind blue eyes that are looking back at me with concern. She is smiling, and her skin, like polished onyx, reflects off the fluorescent lights. The Roones are tiny, all of them under five feet. Their bodies are made up of a higher mineral count, so their skin looks like lacquered stone. They vary in color, as rocks and people do. They have no hair and their faces are mostly eyes.

I smile weakly. "Edo, I told you, please just call me Ryn."

"It is a form of respect, Citadel. Like the great castles and fortresses on your Earth, you do so much to keep us safe. Citadels are our greatest defense and it is my job to make sure that you do not become a ruin." Edo checks the electronic pad in her hands and looks at my IV bag. "Though I must say, there are times when you make that increasingly difficult."

I look at the clock on the wall. It's almost one. I have been out for hours. Not good. "Then why don't I call you Doctor Edo, or Nurse Edo, or . . . What are you, again?"

"Because there is no name for what I am in your language," she answers kindly. "But if it makes you more comfortable I will simply call you Ryn." Edo squeezes my shoulders lightly. I feel the pressure of her cold, hard hands, but it is not unpleasant.

"You always say that, but then you forget." She gives me a look that says in a million years she would not forget anything, and I sigh. "How bad is it?"

"Not bad at all. A little concussion. We've given you medicine and the swelling is gone. Your brain is back to normal. We put you to sleep so that you could heal." Edo once again looks at the silver pad in her hands. She could be checking my vitals, but because she is a Roone and the implants were designed by them, I am almost positive she is checking to make sure the chip is functioning at full capacity. I reach back and feel a small metal disk the size of quarter, which is magnetized to attach to my implant. "If I keep getting these little concussions I'm going to turn into one of those football players who goes off the deep end one day."

"I have no idea what you are talking about. But we have repaired all the damage done to the tissue around the concussed area. It's as if it never happened, and your implant . . ." Edo smiles, but the smile is weird, *off* somehow.

"What about my implant?" I ask, immediately sitting up.

"It's fine. I promise." Edo's smile is genuine this time. I can't say why, but I know she is not being totally honest with me. I am an expert in detecting even the barest hint of a lie, and my experiences at The Rift have meant my expertise is not limited to humans. I would push, but I know that I would never get a straight answer. Most Roones remind me of robots. Since they are responsible for the chip that created the Citadels, I am naturally resentful of them. Edo, though, is unlike others of her kind. She is warm and even funny. Still, she is not different enough to confide in me. Instead, I take that one moment when she let me see something in her face that I shouldn't have, and file it away for later.

I pull the magnetized disk off my neck and hold it in my hands. It just looks like a shiny, round piece of metal to me. I examine it for a second or two before handing it back to Edo. She takes the disk and attaches it to her pad.

"My team?" I ask, stretching my back.

"Training. But you are not going with them today. I have put you on twelve hours of bed rest. You can do that here or at home. Your choice."

"Oh my God. Home for sure. No offense." I grin.

Edo looks at me warmly. "You did well today, Citadel Ryn. You killed at least three Karekins. No one from our side was seriously injured. A victory." Edo does not sound victorious.

"Today, yes," I concede. "But what about tomorrow? What about when five hundred come through—or five thousand? What then? And why? Why haven't we been able to get any intel on their agenda? Why isn't everyone more freaked out about what's happening with them?" I try to sound logical—Roones don't deal well with too much emotion—but I'm sure there's a ton of frustration in my voice.

"I don't have an answer to those questions, though they are good ones," Edo says carefully.

"*Come on*," I say, sitting up straighter and giving her a level stare. "The Karekins must have a way of navigating The Rift, of passing information through it. If that's the case, then why isn't every single person on this base—and every other base, for that matter—working their asses off to figure that out? If they did, wouldn't that mean you could go home?"

Edo takes a step away from me and hugs the pad closer to her chest. "I do not think about home anymore. It is pointless and painful. Words, explanations, reasons—none of those things help when tragedy strikes. We just do what we can to continue. To survive." Edo sighs and it sounds like a rush of wings. She steps closer to me. "I am sorry, Citadel Ryn. For the pain that you feel today and every day. I truly am. Why don't you get some rest for a little while longer and then you can leave with your team?" Without waiting for me to say anything in return, Edo walks out the door.

AS VI IS DRIVING ME and Abel home in my car, I feel almost 100 percent, apart from a slight headache that could have nothing to do with the fighting. The conversation I had with Edo is still with me. There was something about it that wasn't right, but since it is only my intuition guiding that feeling, I don't feel confident in sharing my thoughts with Violet or anyone else on the team. I don't even know what I would say to them because I'm not sure if Edo was lying or if she was, in fact, trying to hint at something else—though what that could be, I can't imagine. Something about my implant? We get to our house and Abel gives Violet a funny look. "Aren't we going to drop you off first?" he asks. Man, he's observant for a teenage boy.

"Nah. I'm going to walk home. I know Ryn has a bunch of work she needs to do by tomorrow. I think she wants to get a jump on it." I roll my eyes. Violet is mothering me. She wants me to get to bed after the day I've had, but I feel fine. It's also a terrible lie—I cringe at how lame it sounds. But Abel just shrugs, says good-bye, and runs into the house.

Violet lives less than half a mile away from us. If she runs, she'll be home in less than two minutes. I feel antsy. I don't want to go inside just yet. "I'm going to walk with you."

"Ryn . . ." she starts.

"I need the air. I know I'm supposed to be resting, but as long as you don't mind not running, I think it'll be fine."

"I think you already know I'm fine with not running," Violet says, not bothering to hide the exasperation in her voice.

"Good," I tell her as I head toward the direction of her house. We live in a quiet, leafy part of Battle Ground called Meadow Glade. It's early in the season, so the leaves have not yet turned. Vi is unusually quiet.

"I'm sorry again, about the crack I made about you and Boone. It was shitty."

Violet shrugs. "It *was*. But it was also true. There's a part of me that's glad you said it out loud. Somebody had to." More silence. A couple cars and a kid on a bike pass us. "Do you think you'll ever get it removed?"

I bite my lip, unsure of what to say. I know that I have to say something, just to make my friend feel better, but she wouldn't want my real answer.

"Well, if I make it to thirty, I might," I lie to her. We were told that at thirty, we could have our chips removed and go on and live a normal life. Settle down. Get married. Have kids. It's a wonderful dream to sell us. But I know I will *never* take it out. First of all, I doubt I am going to make it to thirty. Even if I do, I would be so totally messed up from doing this job that I am positive I would be a crap wife and an even worse mom. I would worry all the time about The Rift, but without my enhanced abilities, I would have no way of defending my white-picket-fence life. I am lonely now, but I am useful. Who's to say that I wouldn't be just as lonely without the implant? More than likely I would end up alone anyhow because this life I'm living is taking a toll and I know it. I would be weak and I would never really be normal.

But Vi is not me. We arrive at her house, a quaint and cozy craftsman painted gray with white trim, and I think she might have a chance at this kind of life in the future, even without Boone. Then again, I'm not sure if she wants it. Violet is an only child. Her parents work a lot and she is often alone. This never seems to bother her. She must be lonely, as we all are, but I never see it. She grabs me and pulls me into a long hug.

"I hate it when you get hurt, Ryn. I worry so much about you." We both know that she is not just talking about my injury today. I am the team leader. I carry an extra burden, one that I am happy to accept. Everyone else seems to have some kind of an outlet for their frustration. Violet dances, Boone jokes, and Henry trains pretty much twenty-four hours a day. I strategize—and by that, I mean I overanalyze, running scenarios in which I am able to make sure everyone is safe. My own safety is rarely a priority.

Another person might say I worry.

"I'll be fine. We've got the day off tomorrow, so I'll sleep in and chill," I promise her.

"Yeah, but you are going to Flora's party tomorrow, right?"

I groan inwardly. I do not feel like going to any party. I want as little social interaction as possible over the next twenty-four hours. Vi looks at me expectantly, though, and I know I have to go. I am the buffer between her and Boone. I make it safe for them to be together.

Being team leader doesn't end when you step out of uniform. It's always there. I am never not doing my job. So I finally say, "Of course. She *is* practically my neighbor. It would be kind of rude if I didn't go."

Violet gives me a huffy sort of laugh. "Oh, please, like you give a shit what anyone thinks about you. But thanks. I'll come over a bit early and get ready with you." I nod my head and watch Violet walk into the house. I amble slowly back, trying to block out the swirling thoughts that are beating inside my brain. I just want to not think—about anything. I need a break from my own brooding over Ezra and Edo and the implant and the people I killed today.

It's so hard to fight a war hardly anyone knows about.

When I get home I tell Abel that I don't feel well and that I am going to bed. He's playing a video game. Something with shooting and guns. I practically leap up the stairs to get away from the noise. I skip dinner and my dad comes in eventually to check on me.

"Rynnie?" I see his outline under the door, through the purplish twilight of the day's end.

"Yeah?" I am in bed. My iPad is open beside me. I have been trying to read, but mostly I have been lying here with my eyes closed.

"Can I come in?" I tell him yes, and he walks in and sits gingerly on the edge of my bed. Unlike other teenagers', my room is spotless. Since becoming a Citadel, I have become an obsessive organizer, taking control of the one thing in my life I feel that I can. "What's wrong? Are you coming down with something?" He puts the back of his hand over my cheeks and forehead.

"No, I'm just tired." I don't turn away from him. I like the way his skin feels on my own. Safe. Comforting. I regress to ten years old, when my dad was everything to me. My biggest hero, my greatest champion. I remember what it was like to be so small he could hold me in his arms. My eyes begin to tear, but in the darkness, he won't see. He waits a minute, and then runs a hand over my head.

"I'm sorry if I came on too strong about college. I know you'll make the right choice. I'm your dad, and even though you're such a good kid, I worry about you." A tear spills down my cheek and I turn my head into the pillow to wipe it off. "You used to talk nonstop. You wanted to know how everything worked. 'Why is the sky blue?' 'Do animals have their own heaven?' 'Is gasoline like water for cars?' You had such an imagination, Ryn." My dad laughs, remembering. "We would play the quiet game and you would sit on your hands and stomp your feet, dying to speak. Your face would go red! And now . . ." My dad breaks off. "Well, I suppose it's a teenage thing, or friggin' ARC. I never thought I would miss those millions of questions, but I do, Rynnie. I really do."

"Yeah." I wish I could say more, but I don't trust myself to speak. "Sorry." It's about all I can manage. My dad stands up.

"Don't be sorry. Just, I don't know, reach out once in a while. Let us know what's going on in that magnificent head of yours.

We're here for you. There's nothing you could tell us that would make us love you any less." No, they wouldn't love me any less if they knew the truth, but they would never get over it. They would be furious, worried, half-crazy if they knew.

I roll over on my side, away from him. " 'Kay, 'night."

"Love you, darling girl," he says as he walks toward the door.

"I love you, too," I whisper. My parents are great, truly good people.

I cannot say the same about myself.

CHAPTER 5

Violet has outdone herself with the wardrobe selection. She is wearing super-high-waisted jeans and a skinny belt around her impossibly tiny waist. Her gray silk blouse is unbuttoned low enough to show some cleavage. She is covered from head to toe, but the look is far sexier than the trampy, try-too-hard outfits I know the other girls at the party will be wearing. I tried to get away with a sweatshirt and my yoga pants, and honestly it almost came to blows. After refusing to put on a dress, or a skirt, I finally agreed to short Levi's cutoffs and a cropped black tank. I insisted on my dark brown leather boots with straps, but I did concede to a bunch of jangly bangles. I am wearing my hair long and loose. I almost always wear it back, so even I am a little surprised when I see how long it is—down to the middle of my back. My hair is a Nordic blond with a natural wave. Because I wear it up so often,

I have darker-blond highlights that have been tucked away from the sun. I pull the light strands over my shoulders and twist the ends to make it look smoother. When I realize I am preening at my own reflection, I stop. I'm not used to caring about how I look, but for tonight, I realize how much I want to look pretty. Or at least, I want to know that I can *be* pretty.

I let Vi put makeup on me. Luckily we both agree that, for me, less is more. I only look good wearing makeup if I don't actually look like I have any on. Violet has dark voluminous hair and even darker eyes. Her skin, though, is as fair as mine. She can get away with all kinds of crazy eye shadow colors and, unlike me, not look like a hooker.

We walk to Flora Branach's house and don't bother to knock. We can hear the music blasting, so there's no point. We get more than a few stares when we walk in. I know the boys are imagining all kinds of sexual scenarios when they look at us. What they don't know is that we'd likely crush their windpipes before they would ever find out what we look like without our shirts.

The way some of them are outright leering, the prospect of some broken tracheas appeals to me. I find myself smiling.

The house is jam-packed. I guess we took more time getting ready than I'd thought. Boone comes up behind us and starts dancing right away with Violet. I suppose the fact that they're grooving to a boy-band song from the nineties in a room full of people takes the sex appeal right out of it. Surprisingly, he's actually pretty good. Violet starts doing what I can only assume is the Robot. I laugh, and so does everyone else. People don't, like, *dance* at house parties. But Vi and Boone somehow make it cool. I'm sure that everyone will join them soon enough. Maybe if I drink enough, I will, too. But it takes a *lot* for us Citadels to get drunk.

Flora sees me from the kitchen and starts to shimmy toward me with an extra cup in her hand.

"You came." She looks pleased and also strangely wary. The corners of her mouth are turned up into a smile, but it seems forced.

"I did," I say, smiling back at her. There is an awkward silence for a couple seconds. We both just stand there, grinning like assholes. The thing is, Flora and I used to be absolute best friends. Flora and I had almost every class together in eighth grade and we had an instant connection. We just got each other. We liked all the same things and, with her living so close to me, I think we spent just about every day together. She can be sassy but also really kind. When the headaches came because of the implant, I can vividly remember lying in her lap, her room darkened because the light stung my eyes. She would put a cold washcloth on my forehead and whisper that everything was going to be fine. She talked me through that agony on more than one occasion.

I repaid her by abruptly cutting her out of my life once I became a Citadel.

I was mean about it because I was mad, too. I just couldn't lie to her; she was my best friend. So I avoided her as much as possible. It broke both our hearts. We have gotten over the worst of it by now. We are civil to one another—nice, even. Still, it will never be the same between us. Tonight, though, she seems weird but happy, happier than I have seen her in a long time. Her cheeks are flushed, and I realize part of the reason for her attitude: She is drunk. She passes me a drink and puts a hand on my shoulder.

"I mean . . ." Flora begins, "how can you not even have one ounce of body fat on you? It's, like, not natural." Flora is slurring her words. I take the drink and shrug. What am I supposed to do? Apologize? I look around, suddenly uncomfortable. "I think you . . . something is going on there. I don't know. It's Levi, too. Levi!" she screams over the music, and waves her arm wildly. I catch her older brother's eye. He's on the stairs, behind us. Watching. Slowly he walks down and joins us. Levi and I look at each other, communicating caution without words.

He is tall and muscular but not too beefy—as his sister noted, not an ounce of fat on him, either. His hair is a true auburn, like his sister's, and his eyes are the most remarkable shade of green, far brighter than my own. Another interesting fun fact about Levi is that he tried to work around his implant with his girlfriend, another Citadel, named Ingrid. She ended up in a coma for three weeks, while he got most of his ribs broken. A leg, too.

Oh . . . and he's a jerk.

During one of my first experiences with Karekins at The Rift, I had almost let one get the jump on one of his teammates. When it was over, he just screamed at me. He was the first boy I really crushed on, but after that day any romantic feelings I had for him immediately evaporated. To be fair, he was never really all that nice (hot, yes, but aloof), but after the Ingrid thing he became a downright prick. I generally avoided him as much as I could.

"You two." Flora sways as she says it and points a finger at us both. "What is it with you? You're like aliens. You think I'm stupid? You think I don't know there's some freaky shit going on?" Levi tries to grab the drink from her hand, but she lifts it up and spins away from him. "Fuck off, Levi, you weirdo."

"I think you've had enough to drink," he says sternly, narrowing his eyes.

"Shut up, *Spider-Man*, or whatever the hell you are. I just wanted to tell you both that I don't know exactly what it is, but I know it's something." Flora backs away and walks off into the crowd.

"What was that about?" I take a long swig from the plastic cup in my hands.

"We were in the kitchen last month and she started a grease fire. I put it out very quickly. *Too* quickly, if you know what I mean."

"Ahh."

"And a couple days ago she walked into my room without knocking and I was working out. Doing a handstand. On one hand." I nod my head because I'm not sure what else to say. Finally, though, I can't stand his eyes boring into me.

"You think I should go talk to her or something?" I ask. I really don't want to go talk to her, but I feel like it's the right thing to do, even though I have no idea how a conversation like that would play out.

"Nah, she's too drunk to reason with. You'd probably just make things worse." I roll my eyes. I don't really know Flora anymore, but I'm sure I could say something that might make her feel less paranoid about the vibes she's been feeling. Before I can say anything, though, Levi turns around and leaves. He's about as sensitive as a bag of rocks. I shrug and join Boone and Violet, who are dancing happily in the living room. I don't exactly start to dance, but I tap my boots to the rhythm of the music. Henry has arrived. I see him at the fireplace with his arms crossed, looking like a bouncer. No wonder kids think everyone in ARC is a freak.

I drink some more. I feel myself loosening up. I can't believe it, but I actually think I'm having a good time. After about an hour, though, I get a pang about Flora. I really should go find her and make sure she is okay. I look throughout the house for her and then outside where the party has spilled out around a fire pit. I see Levi talking to another Citadel his age, a year older than me, a supposed senior at Battle Ground High. When I don't see Flora, I ask Levi if he has. He says he hasn't, sighs with annoyance, and together we walk into the house.

I grab a random girl on the stairs and ask her if she's seen our host.

"She went up to her room," the girl says drunkenly. "With two guys," she whispers, and stumbles a bit on the step. I see Levi tense. I can see he's about to leap up the remaining flight of stairs, but I grab the back of his arm and push him up against the wall, pinning him to it. Anyone looking would assume that we're about to hook up. I speak softly in his ear.

"Take it easy, Levi."

He turns his head and looks at me, his eyes burning. His voice goes deathly quiet. "Get off of me, Ryn."

"I will go and deal with this," I assure him. Levi pushes forward and I push him back harder.

"She's *my* sister."

"Yeah, but if you go in there, you'll kill them. Me?" I smile. "I'll just hurt them." Levi rolls his eyes and then nods his head. I race up the stairs, and throw open the door to Flora's room. I see my friend naked on the bed. She is totally passed out. One guy is on top of her, and the other, beside me, has his phone out and shirt off, and is clearly filming the action.

"Hey, girl, you wanna join the party?" the guy next to me says. *Oh my God, did he just say that? The* party? Dumbass must think we are in an actual porno, because that's the only situation where I think a girl would be down with this rapey shit.

I consider how much restraint I actually want to show. My conclusion: very little.

"Oh, yeah, I really do." My voice is a soft purr. I quickly

reach out and grab the guy's phone and throw it hard against the wall so that it smashes into pieces.

"What the hell?" he screams. The guy on the bed turns around. His pants are open, but it doesn't look like he has done anything . . . yet.

Thank God.

"She brought us up here, she wanted to do this and it's a free country, so get naked or get the fuck out," Bed Boy snarls. "Oh, yeah, and you can pay for my buddy's phone, too, you crazy bitch."

Restraint level: virtually zero.

"You think this is cool?" I yell. "She is passed-out drunk. Any alarm bells go off in your head? Even you two morons must know that this is wrong."

The guy closest to me goes to grab me by the arm. I'm not sure what he was thinking, but now the gloves are off. Maybe he was going to try to force me onto the bed, too, or maybe he was just trying to throw me out of the room. Either way, he should not have touched me. I grab his hand and bend it back the wrong way. I sidestep him as he yelps in pain. I easily maneuver my arms around his neck to put him in a choke hold. I squeeze, applying just enough pressure to make him pass out. His body slumps, I push him off of me, and he falls to the ground with a thud.

The guy in the bed scrambles up. He's about six feet tall with sandy-colored hair and brown eyes. He's not exactly ugly, but there is something distinctly ratlike about his nose and mouth. He looks at me with a mix of surprise and anger. "What did you just do? Did you just kill him?"

I walk closer to him and see that he's breathing hard. His chest is puffed out. If his body has gone into fight-or-flight mode, I know he's going to choose the first option. It's a *big* mistake.

"Thought about it, but no. He's sleeping." I can't help but give a little laugh. I am wearing a dangerous smirk. This idiot has no idea who I am or what I can do. I'm grinning because he thinks he has a chance, and I'm happy because there are so many cruel boys like him in the world and so many helpless girls. I don't really believe in Karma. I've seen too many good people die and too many assholes win, but tonight is different. It feels like the universe put me in this room for a reason, and on behalf of so many defenseless women, I'm about to tip the scales in their favor—for once.

"You're disgusting," I tell him as I lose the smile. "All the therapy in the world won't help you. There is something dark and twisted inside of you; I can see it in your eyes. A person like you understands only two things: fear and violence. And since you're clearly not afraid of me . . ."

The boy gets inches in front of my face. The veins in his neck bulge. His eyes widen and shift erratically back and forth. "Shut up!" he screams. "All you ARC brats are the same. You walk around thinking that you're better than us, *smarter* than us—"

"We are," I interrupt, which only pisses him off more.

"There is something not right with you people. I don't even know if *you are* people." Now he's the one to laugh, and he throws his hands up wildly. "You're all fucking robots or aliens or something, but you don't scare me. You think I won't hit someone just because they're a girl?"

I narrow my eyes at him. I know I'm goading him, but I can't help it. He is a truly vile individual.

"I'm *counting* on it."

He lunges at me and I grab his fist and squeeze, breaking every bone in his hand. He whimpers and goes down on his knees. I twist behind him and deliver one swift kick to his kidney, which lands him on the floor, howling in pain. I spin once more and hit him in the face. Then I hit him again. I keep hitting, knowing that I'm inflicting damage, but I'm holding back because I do not want to kill him. Though, frankly, I kind of think the world would be a better place without him. His face is a bloody mess.

I crouch down beside him. He is sputtering blood, coughing, trying to catch his breath. "Pay attention," I say in a soothing tone. "There is a lesson to be learned with every defeat. Like I told you: fear and violence—that's all you understand. You'll think twice now before you try something like this again. Really, you should be thanking me. Maybe you won't end up in prison."

"Screw you," he manages to wheeze out of his swollen lips.

I stand up and look down at him. "No. Clearly that won't be happening. I guess you haven't learned your lesson after all. So I suppose we'll just have to stick to violence. I know who you are and if I ever, *ever* hear that you've been inappropriate with a girl, I will come back and finish you. I *will* kill you, and I will get away with it."

The boy says nothing. I lean down and grab his face with my hand. I rear my other fist back to punch him again. He whimpers and shies away. "No, no, please don't." He is crying now. "I heard you. I won't. Please!" I let his face go. I grab his T-shirt from the floor by the bed and wipe as much blood off my hands as I can manage.

"Now, pick up your friend and get out of this house. And don't even think of telling anyone what happened here." I throw the shirt in his face and he gingerly puts it back on. He picks himself up slowly and then grabs his buddy, who is just coming around. Somehow he manages to pull the other guy to his feet.

"How am I going to explain this?" he asks, pointing to his face. "I'm probably going to have to go to the hospital. I think my jaw is broken—and my *hand* . . ." He really is pathetic, asking me for answers. Such typical behavior in an alpha who has been kicked out of his dominant place. I roll my eyes. He's surrendered all his power. I've seen it too many times to count.

"I dunno, tell them you walked into a door or tripped down the stairs. Women have had to use those lines for years." I turn away from him, toward the bed. He has been dismissed. He will leave and say nothing more, and because he's such an unevolved human being he won't even really understand why. I look down at my knuckles, which are raw and scratched. I saved Flora. I may have saved some other girl from the same fate. I don't feel guilty for what I've done, but I resent the fact that I had to do it. I just wanted to go to a party. I feel like I drag violence along with me everywhere I go, the same way a mother has to drag her screaming toddler around a grocery store. It's just life. Things have to be done. I look down at a bloodstain on the carpet. This is who I am. This is more than just my job, and all the times I just wish for something normal are starting to feel like wallowing.

I walk lightly over to Flora, who hasn't awakened. *Thank God.* I check her vitals. She's fine, just drunk as hell. I go to her chest of drawers and pull out a pair of sweats and a T-shirt. Gently, I dress her. I pull back the covers, put her into the bed, and tuck her in. I walk out the door, turning the light off as I go.

I walk down the hallway and see Levi waiting for me at the top of the stairs, his arms folded, his face like stone.

"I saw them leave," he says through a clenched jaw.

"I told you I would handle it. I did," I offer. There is silence between us. A silence that reaches up and stretches outward beyond whatever explanation I could give.

"Did they hurt her? Did they . . ." Levi can't continue from there. The words seem to stick in his throat and he clears it. I hear pain in that half-strangled cough. He breaks eye contact and looks away. I watch his hands, they twitch and his fingers curl into fists. Without even thinking, I reach out and cover them with my own hands. His skin is hot to the touch.

"They tried, but I stopped them before anything happened. She's so drunk, I doubt she'll even remember bringing them in there. Does she do this a lot? Is this a thing with her now?" I was referring to both the drinking and the guys, but my tone was soft, as tender as I could manage.

Instead of answering, Levi stares down at our hands. He looks back up at me, at first confused and then angry. He jerks himself free. "What are you doing? Don't do that. Don't touch me, Ryn, *ever.*"

"Seriously?" I ask him, thoroughly insulted. I was just trying to be nice. Then it dawns on me why he wouldn't want me touching him. "Oh," I say, looking at my hands and then at him. "I . . . didn't know that you thought of me in that—"

Levi huffs and scowls at me. "Please," he condescends. "You've got tits and I'm a dude. I won't let *any* female touch me."

I fold my arms and consider this typically rude statement, and Levi snaps his game face on. I know this face. I've seen creatures and beasts whimper at this face. His eyes become terrifyingly vacant. His features become still and hard, as though sculpted out of marble. And then something changes in his eyes. He begins to stare intently at me. It's not attraction I'm getting—at least, not the obvious kind. It's something else. If I had to name it, I would say hunger, like he wants to pull me apart and eat me bit by bit. He is *so* screwed up, though; who knows what he's thinking? He probably can't want something without wanting to hurt it, or maybe he just wants to hurt everyone. He's not like the boys who were up in Flora's room. He doesn't have an abusive nature. He's not a bully. I've never seen him be unnecessarily violent . . . but I think there's a part of him that wants everyone to hurt as badly as he does.

It's a feeling that I can totally relate to.

Eventually he looks away and I am only partly relieved. Like I said, my crush on Levi came to an end long ago, but I'm messed up, too. The way he stared at me should have made me uncomfortable, but it didn't. It's strangely hot, to think of him eating me, to imagine him biting into my flesh and tearing off the muscle and bone. Every Citadel is twisted up in some way. I thought my fucked-up-ness came in the form of over-the-top control freak. It scares me to think that it can come in the form of something so much darker.

"I suppose this means I owe you one."

His voice snaps me out of my own brooding. I cock my head suddenly. I did not expect him to say that. Maybe I just imagined whatever it was that passed between us, because his question makes me think that he doesn't really remember me at all. I used to practically live in his house. His sister and I were best friends. He does not owe me anything. I didn't *do* anything for him. But a plan is forming in my mind, just the barest hint of an idea.

"Yeah, you do," I lie. And with that I walk past him, down the stairs, and out the door.

CHAPTER 6

Beta Team is on reserve duty the following Monday. We are staggered throughout the forest with almost seventy troops, about three-quarters of a mile from The Rift. The four of us sit underneath a canopy of tree branches. A weak sun dapples through them and the shapes throw down pockmarked shadows. We are not at attention, but we are not relaxed, either. We are ready to push forward should the need arise at a moment's notice. We hear the other teams check in. The Rift is silent, a closed mouth. No fighting today.

When our rotation is up, we take the transport back to base. My team is unusually quiet.

I wonder if my team is annoyed at me for leaving without saying good-bye, but I don't provide a reason for leaving and they don't ask for one. I wonder, too, if Henry had to step in at some point and make sure Boone and Vi didn't spend too much time alone. That would be reason enough for all three of them to be irritated.

When we arrive back at the base we go to our separate changing rooms and dress for training. Our training uniforms are much like our combat ones, only black and with less padding. The four of us spend an hour doing circuit training, which is kind of like an amped-up version of CrossFit, in the facility's large gym. Then we spend another hour working on agility and hand-to-hand combat skills in a different part of the building that is a huge room with padded floors divided into dozens of small rings. We do a lot of stretching to keep our muscles limber and flexible—Violet has us all beat on this front, but what's always so surprising is how giant Henry can contort his body.

Like I said: every gay guy's fantasy come true, and probably most straight women's, when it comes down to it.

Then we spar in a style that is, for the most part, mixed martial arts but with an emphasis on a particular martial art given our individual strengths. For me, it's Krav Maga.

When that's done, we spend an hour outside with weapons. The base already had a significant target range; our group just enhanced it. We shoot for a while. Then we practice knife throwing—at the same distance we shot. Sometimes we work with explosives. We know how to build bombs and how to detonate much more sophisticated ones. Sometimes we do survival weaponry, which means we learn how to turn a dead branch into a spear, or we make our own arrows from flint and fallen logs. There is an array of bows hidden throughout the forest, just in case things get truly terrible and we run out of ammo. This hour also sometimes incorporates survival training. We hunt game and learn how to skin and cook it. We learn about the medicinal properties of plants and how to make a fire without matches. The boys universally love this hour—some of the girls do, too, but it really feeds into all the boys' *Red Dawn* fantasies. I generally excel when I'm in survival mode, but please, give me a hot shower and a comfortable bed any day.

For the last hour of training we run. As Citadels, we run fast and we run hard. Our speed is inhuman, almost faster than a human eye can track. There is a number that we have maxed out at, miles-per-hour-wise, but I prefer not to know it. They were smart like that, to give us the choice. Some people like Boone and Henry want to know how fast the fastest Citadel can run. Me? I prefer not to know. I don't want to know my limits. I don't want to have to make those calculations in my head if I am fleeing a nightmare. I'd rather go on thinking I have a fighting chance to escape to safety or, at least, to fight another day.

Of course, I don't like running. For one thing, I prefer fighting rather than fleeing, and I'd rather spend my time training at that more. Hell, I think I may even prefer hunting and skinning to running. Sure, it's vital that we keep our stamina up, but I find it so . . . stupid.

Maybe I should clarify: I don't dislike racing through the uneven terrain of the camp because it's exhausting—it takes a lot more than that to tire out a Citadel, even after the three hours of training that went on before—it's just, well, *boring*. Henry, as well as other Citadels, finds the running soothing, like meditation. I wish I could zone out like that. My brain won't stop turning, though. I'm always imagining other things I could be doing, *would rather* be doing, like reading or watching some lame TV show (if I'm being completely honest with myself).

Thankfully, it's not only running we do. Very rarely are we

on clear terrain, so it's crucial that we use the trees and other aspects of the forest to give us an advantage: a kind of bastardized version of parkour. We don't use traditional obstacle courses and obviously we aren't around much cement. But the woods provide more than enough to work with. We spin and leap and flip over rock formations and logs. We use the soft moss covering the firs to swing for momentum and jump down. We use the massive tree trunks by pushing the tread of our boots into the bark for traction to spring up and out in any direction. I prefer this to running. As a woman I can use my flexibility to my advantage and my light weight to scramble up places that are almost impossible for someone like Henry to get to.

More important, this comes naturally to me, and unlike while sprinting along the roads of Camp Bonneville, I *can* let my mind wander. So today I use this hour to strategize even as I leap through and fly over the green and brown at my feet. My focus: I have a way to get into the Village.

The problem is, I have no real idea what the Village is like inside. Citadels who are old enough to work there are not permitted to talk about what goes on with those of us who aren't. As soldiers, we accept the hierarchy of secrets. It has always made sense to me before, but as I look at it now, it seems illogical. Why does the Village even need to be a secret? What is ARC hiding from us there?

And now my imagination is in full overdrive.

They wouldn't make Immigrants live in tents, would they? Always cold, never truly comfortable. Surely they would have built proper barracks. If they imagine Immigrants living out their natural lives in the Village, then even barracks wouldn't cut it. They must have prefab homes, even neighborhoods. Maybe. Or maybe it's built like a prison. Maybe they keep the

Immigrants in cells, behind bars. The idea of that makes me suddenly nauseous.

How can I not know?

And the answer is more than just how well ARC keeps its secrets. The fact is, it's been three years and all I've thought about is The Rift. I have been obsessed with keeping everyone safe: my fellow soldiers, my family. I don't know why that concern has never extended as far as the Village, and I am ashamed. The Immigrants, as part of this Earth now, deserve my protection, too.

I jump ten feet in the air, grab a tree branch, swing myself up onto a thick limb, and squat down, bracing my back up against the trunk. I guess I have chalked up what happens with the Immigrants to bad luck. That's my go-to response— it's like cancer or a hurricane or a car accident.

Like getting chosen to be a Citadel. The bitterness of this thought surprises me.

And like us, they get pulled here terribly, but it's beyond anyone's control. Vi brings it up a lot, and I am forever changing the subject. Don't we have enough to worry about? That's been my excuse. As I've gotten older, the excuse has worn thin. I am getting past my own bad luck. I suppose this is what it means to grow up. You realize that everyone has something dark and hidden that seems colossally unfair. It's not right anymore that I should just dismiss these other stories out of hand because mine feels so much worse. The truth is that, compared to nearly getting raped like Flora, or a lifetime in a wheelchair because of an accident, or losing your mom to breast cancer like Boone did when he was only nine, my story is definitely not worse.

I leap down and start running again. I hear the others swish through the undergrowth not too far away, and I know they're focusing on their own training. I get back to musing.

Once I get into the Village, though, then what? I have to find Ezra, obviously. But, just as obvious, that won't be easy. I will need help with that. And then, once I do find him, what am I supposed to say? We can't go off and talk. We can't go for coffee and compare life stories. I will have to remain with him wherever he is and hope I can get a few minutes of privacy. Given that I know nothing about the Village, this could be a tall order.

When our hour is up, I realize I'm still basically nowhere in terms of a plan.

We run back to the base. Upon arriving down in the facility we are given a massive protein drink that the doctors and scientists must watch us finish before our training is officially over. We expend so many calories a day, and this elixir, invented by the Roones, keeps our nutrition up. As I gulp down the shake, I see Boone is almost finished with his. I need to catch him before he goes into his locker room.

"Boone," I say, grabbing his arm before he can leave.

"Yeah?" Boone has a towel and he's wiping off the sweat and grime of our training.

I take a deep breath. I try to sound casual. "Can you do me a favor and ask Levi to meet me at Old Town Burger before he goes home? I know he just got off duty, so he should be in there changing."

Boone smirks. "Levi, huh?" He crosses his arms and cocks his head. "Well, does Saint Ryn have the hots for someone?" I do not smile—if anything, I do the opposite of smile—and the grin on Boone's face disappears. "Fine, but don't expect me to pass him any notes in math class, okay? I'll ask him, then leave me out of it. That guy is bad news, Ryn."

Boone is sneering and I'm a little shocked. I know what happened with Levi and Ingrid—it's common knowledge that they tried to have sex and failed. It was consensual, something they both wanted, and everyone knows that, too. Is Boone blaming Levi for that? I suppose Boone's own predicament with Violet makes him sensitive to the issue. I don't get any more insights from him and he disappears through his locker room door. I walk to the other side of the hall and go into mine.

I shower quickly and throw my hair up into one giant knot on my head. On go my yoga pants. I pair them with Converse and an old T-shirt of my mom's with some grunge band on it that she used to love. I look at myself in the mirror and, unlike the way I felt on the night of Flora's party, I'm not thrilled with what I see. I don't care about impressing Levi, but I am beginning to think that at some point I should put a little more effort into the way I present myself to the world. Maybe going to the party awoke something in me that had long been dormant. That thought seems way more exhausting than the four hours of training I just put in, though.

I take the train to the school. I don't need to worry about driving Abel because he has football practice and Mom will pick him up on her way home. The burger restaurant is almost exactly across the street from Battle Ground High. When I walk in, there are about a dozen students, and Levi is waiting at one of the only free tables. He must have been on the train before me. I slide into the booth so that we are facing each other.

"That was fast," he says by way of a hello.

"Yeah, well, I just jumped in the shower and got the first train I could." I say this impassively. I don't want Levi thinking that I was racing to *meet him*.

"No, I mean that you want to use your favor pretty quickly. I have to admit I'm curious. Obviously, I can't give you just

anything." He smirks and leans back in the booth, every gesture dripping with aggression. Even his neutral look smolders.
Wait. When he said *anything,* did he mean his *body?* Does he
think because he admitted to me that I was an actual girl,
with boobs, that I want to confess my love to him or something? I don't know a lot about guys, but I know it doesn't take
much to get one sexually attracted to you. Does he actually
believe I'm naive enough to confuse normal teenage lust with
real feelings? Is this his version of flirting?

I'm so out of my element, I wonder if this is *everyone's* version of flirting. But Levi is so singular in his wretchedness, I
have to think it's just him.

"Uhh . . ." I pause, because even though I am itching to tell
him that he is not actually God's gift to the universe and that,
no, I am not interested in him in that way, I need him to agree
to this. If I piss him off, he won't. If I butter him up too much,
though, he won't do it just to spite me.

He's like an enigma wrapped in a mystery wearing a smirk
that makes me want to never stop slapping him.

Instead, I take a deep breath and decide to just take the
plunge. "Well, there is actually one thing you can do . . ." He
raises an eyebrow in question. "I need you to get me into the
Village." I smile brightly, innocently. Levi does not return the
smile. Instead he glowers at me. An awkward silence settles
between us and my smile fades.

Levi's lip curls sufficiently high to almost reach his eyeball.
"What?" he demands. "No, even better: *Why?*"

"I captured an MTI from The Rift. He was very nice, very
confused, obviously. And then I promised him I would come
and see him and make sure he was okay." This is not a lie.
It isn't the whole entire truth, but I am not lying to him. It
feels good.

"Oh," Levi responds coolly. He's clearly unimpressed with my answer. "I get it, you have a crush on a boy. So you want me to help you break into one of the most heavily guarded areas on Earth so you can—what? Ask him to homecoming?" Levi laughs, and there's a cutting cruelty to it that makes my cheeks burn.

"Don't laugh. It's not funny," I protest, my back straightening. "I don't have a crush on him. I don't even know him. I just made a promise. It was a stupid promise, I know, but I did it and after what he's been through I don't want to be an asshole . . . not that you'd know what not being an asshole is like."

"Ooh, you got me!" he says, grabbing at his chest like he's wounded. He really *is* an asshole. He sits up. "Listen, Ryn, he's going to be in there for the rest of his life. Just wait until next year, when you turn eighteen. You'll get assigned a Village rotation. You can see him then." Something about the way Levi says it—with such obvious disdain—it's like it just doesn't compute that there is anyone on Earth who can compare with him, especially an Immigrant, and he thought it was important I know that.

I bite my tongue and count to five in my head. I need him to help me. It's taking a lot of work not to antagonize him. I lean in close so that no one else can overhear. "I don't understand—aren't we both on the same side here? I'm a Citadel, you're a Citadel. I'm not a spy. I don't see what the problem is. In fact, I don't see what the big deal is in general. What is it with the Village that we aren't supposed to see it till we are eighteen?"

"Seriously?" Levi asks through gritted teeth, in a voice just barely above a whisper but stern enough to get my adrenaline going. "It's fucking monsters and demons and crazy shit that we don't even have words for in the English language, it's so out there. It's also normal people like you and me who will basically be in prison, not because they are criminals, but because they were in the wrong place at the wrong time. So yeah, they don't want kids near there."

"I *am not* a kid."

Levi lets out a loud, disrespectful laugh. "A kid calls in a marker to go and meet a boy regardless of consequences. Grown-ups don't do shit like that. You're so immature. I can't believe you're a team leader. I wouldn't let you be in charge of a picnic. I wouldn't let you babysit my cousin, and she's ten."

It hurts, and it hurts more than I thought it would. I couldn't care less if he liked me or not, but to not *respect* me?

"You are so mean, Levi. Honestly, you're the meanest person I know. Why are you acting this way? Why would you even say that? We've fought side by side and I've held my own. I deal with those monsters and demons and whatever all the time! I've saved people and put the safety of my team before my own. You've seen that! So why say such horrible things to me? I am not an adult. You're right. But you're going to sit there like a pompous jerk and tell me grown-ups are smarter? 'Grown-ups,'" I say, using my hands to make quotation marks, "are the reason you and I will never have a normal life. Adults opened The Rift and they made children police it. Adults are the reason you and Ingrid nearly killed each other."

Levi gives me a dead-level stare. He shakes his head. "I can't believe you went there."

"I went there and I'll go further. Either you help me or I tell Flora the real deal about us. I miss your sister. I would love nothing more than to tell her the truth, so please give me a reason to." The fury is building inside of him, I can see it. Levi clenches his fists and releases them.

"You have no idea" is all he says.

I am breathing hard. I'm angry, ready to fight, and so is he. No one pushes my buttons more than Levi. His tone, his arrogance, the fact that, realistically, he's a better Citadel than me, or at least a more lethal one—it all gets to me. But I need to get to the Village. I slow my heart rate down. I take a deep breath. I have to get him on my side. "You're right. I don't have any real idea about the Village or what you've gone through and that is part of the problem. I'm tired of being in the dark. I'm not scared of them. They *need* us." I look at him calmly. He really is beautiful but so, so broken. "The question is, why are you so scared? What are they going to do to you? Make you a Citadel? *Again?*" Levi leans back in the booth, eyeing me. I don't know what he could be thinking. Maybe he wants to slam my head into the table. Maybe he wants to kiss me. Maybe he wants to slam my head into the table because he wants to kiss me. I've just told him I was willing to risk God knows what to see a boy, threatened him, *and* emasculated him all at once. Levi hates to lose—I know, because I'm the same way. I also know he is not going to help me and I'm starting to wonder if he's going to say anything else.

"Fine. I'll find a way in without you." I grab my bag and go to stand up.

"Hey." Levi kicks my leg gently under the table.

"Don't worry. I won't tell Flora. She doesn't need to know anything. I mean, look what happened when she saw you do a handstand. She invited two thugs up to her bedroom for a drunken threesome. Imagine what she would do if she knew the real truth. Our secret is safe."

"Ryn, stop," Levi says firmly, and I turn back in the booth to face him. "I will get you in, okay? Somehow. I've got a shift at the Village coming up this Sunday. What's Prince Charming's name?"

"Ezra Massad," I answer with relief. I'm in shock. I cannot believe he is going to help me.

"You have to promise me you'll be careful. Don't tell anyone on your team and don't get your hopes up. You can't touch him. You can't even think about it, not for one second. Do you think you can manage that?"

I want to tell him to screw off. Of course I can manage that. I'm not a lunatic. I don't hurt people on purpose. He's the sick fuck who tried to get it on with his girlfriend. I would never be so dumb. I can't exactly say that, though, because although I can be sassy, I'm not rude like he is.

"I won't tell anyone and there will be no touching. Promise."

Levi lets out a long sigh. He seems resigned. He isn't angry anymore. He looks so different when he's not mad. Younger. Sadder. Once more I think the word *broken*.

"I will come to your house Saturday afternoon with a plan. Around four?" I don't know if he's asking or telling.

"Just text me with the details. You don't need to come over," I offer.

"Oh, man, you really are a kid." Levi shakes his head and stands up. Then he leans over to whisper in my ear. I can feel the heat of his breath. His lips are so close I have to close my eyes and dig my nails into my palm.

"You think they don't read our texts?"

CHAPTER 7

The following Sunday I'm waiting high up in a tree canopy. Both my feet are planted on a thick branch and I am braced and ready to jump more than twenty feet to the ground below. This is the first part of Levi's plan. I cannot go through the main entrance of the Village without the proper credentials. So I am here in this tree, and in exactly one minute I will avoid the electrified fence by swinging my body over it and landing in The Menagerie.

The Village is a little over ten miles northeast of Camp Bonneville. I parked my car about six miles away off a graveled utility road and hid it as best I could inside the tree line. I ran to this exact spot, which Levi gave me via a set of coordinates that I have managed to find quite easily thanks to our extensive survival-skills training . . . and Google. I still have no real idea of the scope of this place. The Menagerie would not have been my first choice, but Levi has assured me that this particular section I'm jumping into has nothing more than a bunch of flightless birds. I imagine they must be something close to chickens or maybe turkeys. I also imagine that my idea of harmless and Levi's idea might not be the same thing.

When the time is exactly right, I jump down into the pen. I pop back up right away. I don't have a gun. I was able to steal my uniform out of my locker room, but I could not gain access to a rifle. There are several coops around the pen, and sure enough, there are birds on the ground. They do look like large chickens, but their feathers are a scarlet red shot through with a few bright yellow plumes. I walk slowly. I don't like the idea of being pecked by them. I don't even want to touch them. I only like birds when they are plucked, gutted, and part of a meal.

I know—not very forgiving. But birds give me the creeps, and that's that.

The good news is that I won't be staying long, and I soon reach the inner fence. It's electrified, and not as high, maybe ten feet. There is a regular gate that people who work here use to exit, but it requires a swipe card, which I don't have. What I do have are leg muscles that would give the Bionic Woman an inferiority complex.

I crouch down and push up with all my strength to lunge over the fence, using the roof of a coop for extra leverage. I clear the fence, roll, and then jump back onto my feet. Levi has told me to think of The Menagerie as a massive wildlife preserve. It is, after all, where all the animal Immigrants end up. It is many acres deep, and the species that might kill each other are separated by the high-voltage fences. However, the whole thing is accessible via a maintenance path I am currently on. I have only a few minutes now to book it to where

Levi is meeting me at one of the entrances. As I start sprinting, I barely have time to look at the animals around me, but what I do see is extraordinary. Not the species themselves—I have, of course, captured many animals that have come through The Rift, so I'm familiar with many of them—but to see them all now, suddenly laid out before me, is a wonder. It's almost enough for me to lose focus.

Thankfully, ARC has been drilling discipline in me since I was fourteen years old, so I keep to my mission—I have been distracted enough this week. When Levi told me that all of our texts were monitored, it threw me. I couldn't believe it at first, but then the more I thought about it, the more it made sense. I cannot really be trusted. Hell, look what I was doing at this moment. No Citadel—not even the most ardent, gung ho, Kool-Aid-gulping Citadel—is honest. We lie to everyone around us out of necessity. So, yeah, not surprised that a group of trained liars would be led by men and women lying to us in turn. I suppose the powers that be need to track what we are saying and to whom. I get it, strategically, but I don't like it. My thoughts aren't even my own anymore, neither are my opinions. Comparatively, in the big scheme of things, this lack of privacy is just a drop in the bucket. But as those drops start to add up, that bucket is getting heavier to lug around by the day.

Maybe that's why I am doing this now. I want to prove I am not wholly owned by them. I can still make a choice or two of my own. I *need* this. Each clandestine step I take into the Village binds together my sense of self. I run faster. I pass a herd of woolly mammoths. I dodge the cameras I know are out there. Levi drew a map of my course, highlighting the cameras with big black *X*s. Past the prehistoric elephants there is a species of ten or twelve animals I don't recognize. They are as tall as giraffes, with stouter legs, sleek ebony fur, and long horns that remind me of the thin spires on top of a gazelle's head.

More running. I pass something that looks like a bear but with a decidedly feline face. I remember having to capture one of these a few years back—not a fun day.

I have been lucky so far. There aren't any employees out, as a shift is just ending, which is why Levi's timing is perfect. However, I doubt anyone who loves animals would go strictly by the clock, especially when they are animals such as these. I have a basic knowledge of biology, but being here, it strikes me how incredible evolution is. One degree warmer or colder, one less predator, one type of a certain grass can change a species into something unrecognizable.

In order to avoid the dinosaurs, which Levi says I absolutely must, I have to cut across another pen. They have a real-life Jurassic Park at The Menagerie. Dinosaurs are pretty common at The Rift. They come from versions of Earth that are behind our own evolutionary time line, or they come from Earths where there was no meteor, no cataclysmic event that led to their extinction. There must be countless Earths filled with dinosaurs and no people. I am fine with bypassing this section of the preserve. I've seen enough of these things, and some of them, while majestic, are downright terrifying. I leap over another fence, into a large penned meadow, and keep up my steady pace. I stop short at a white horse grazing in the grass.

At first the animal looks normal enough, but when it raises its head I see a horn poking through its forelock.

Yep. It's a unicorn.

It doesn't seem real. I feel like I'm in a scene from a movie, with the unicorn shaking its head and the sun hitting its luminous white hide. I am transfixed. Even I, cynical soldier that I am, cannot help myself. *It's a friggin' unicorn.* I walk slowly toward the extraordinary creature with my hand held out. There are just a few paces between us, and the unicorn does not move. I take this as an encouraging sign and come up right in front of it. I raise my hand and touch the animal's nose. I stroke its mane, which shimmers with pearlescent ivories, pinks, and muted blues. I touch its horn and trace the horn's ochre rings. I look deep into the creature's eyes, which are as black as a moonless midnight, and see my own face reflected back. It seems to see through me, to know me somehow, and I think I might weep. The unicorn puts its head down onto my shoulder and I put my face into its silken mane. Could this truly be a magical being? In this moment it feels like it must be, because it is clearly comforting me, a Citadel. I personally did not capture this animal, but someone who looked like me did. I feel an overwhelming sense of compassion, not from myself, but emanating from the unicorn, which doesn't make sense. Aren't I the enemy? Isn't this beautiful thing a prisoner now? He or she will never run wild again. I do not deserve its kindness. A hot lick of guilt spreads up my neck, reddening my face.

"She's beautiful, isn't she?"

I tense and turn, slowly. About ten feet away from me is a Sissnovar. I chide myself for being so lost in the moment that someone was able to sneak up on me. I dismiss the thought quickly. There is no time for that. I have to think fast.

"She is, yes," I say confidently. Sissnovars are a dominant species from a version of Earth that evolved from reptiles instead of apes. This one seems tame, a male, wearing loose pants and a knitted turtleneck sweater. They don't do well in cold climates and I am surprised he is in this Village and not one in the desert or the Everglades. Maybe he was a vet or something on his Earth. The Menagerie here is the biggest in the world, but he must need layers and layers to stay warm. He is wearing a fisherman's tuque, though I know there is not any hair on his head. He looks like how you would imagine a snake man would look: reptilian skin, small yellow eyes, no nose. Yet he doesn't appear aggressive.

He smiles, revealing a row of small white teeth and two longer incisor fangs. "I get the sense you are not supposed to be here, Citadel."

"No, I'm not," I confess. I don't see the point in lying to him. Like everyone else involved in Rift business, he will not know the whole truth. "Got a lunch break and thought I would spend some time out here. It's . . . peaceful."

"I cannot blame you," he agrees. "I know this particular species is only a legend on your Earth, which is most understandable. She seems so very *aware*, does she not? For a herd animal?" I wonder what else this Sissnovar knows. Has he caught on to the fact that I don't have a gun?

"Do you look after her?" I ask, walking slowly around the unicorn, toward the fence, which is just a normal paddock. I guess they don't need to electrify this section.

"I do, yes, and a few of the other horses and horse-like animals in The Menagerie."

"I'm surprised that they didn't assign you to the . . . you know . . ." I nod toward the area where the dinosaurs and the more dangerous animals are.

"The snakes, you mean? You must know, because you are a Citadel and smart enough, that dinosaurs are more closely related to birds than reptiles."

Whoa . . . he just roasted me.

"I . . . yes, snakes or other reptiles. I apologize if I've offended you. It's just that in my experience, Sissnovars aren't usually, ummm, gentle. Sorry." Time is ticking. I don't know why I am talking to this person, but he is fascinating to me. So unlike the half-crazed and sometimes deadly Sissnovars we capture from The Rift.

"We are, actually," he says with a little laugh. "It's just that, like most animals, humans included, fear often incites violence. The trip through The Rift is terrifying, so I'm not surprised that would be your first impression of us. You must be very new to the Village, though, if you still feel that way about my people." My heart begins to beat just a fraction faster. He obviously does not recognize me. But if I run away, I will definitely be found out. I must be casual now. And quick.

"I am. Just started, and I must say that your English is very good." The Sissnovar looks at me oddly and slowly undulates his neck from side to side in a most snakelike manner.

"Of course, Citadel. I wouldn't speak anything else. I felt the rule from ARC was harsh in the beginning, as everyone does who first comes here, but I have been here many years. I have been granted the luxury of perspective. English is a tool that keeps the Village free from violence. Without a unified means to communicate, it would be chaos."

He sounded more human than I would have thought. There was a purr on the s's in his speech, as you would expect from a snake, but he did mostly sound like, well, a man. I had no idea that the species in the Village weren't allowed to speak anything other than English. I had worried about that—running into someone and not being able to communicate. Now I knew that wasn't a problem.

"Besides," he says, "there is no need to hold on to our culture, since we are not permitted to have children. We get a few from The Rift, but thankfully, they are small in number."

I had not considered children. Well, I had, but I assumed that a lifetime in the Village meant an actual life. But of course, that could not happen. How stupid of me. ARC could not house and feed a rapidly growing population. Forced sterilization, though—it seems so harsh, so *Nazi*-like.

Then again, at least they could have sex. I wonder if I would make such a trade-off, then immediately shake that thought away.

I turn to leave. I have to go. "Right, well—"

"Oftentimes," the man interrupts, "you Citadels are the youngest people here. Whenever I feel sorry for myself I only have to look at one of you to know that The Rift does not discriminate when it comes to doling out suffering."

I turn to face him abruptly. "What do you mean?" I don't know why I'm asking, because I know exactly what he means.

"Only that you didn't choose this any more than I did and we must take our pleasures where they come, like here in this paddock, with this beautiful creature," he says, pointing to the unicorn. I want to demand what he knows exactly about the Citadels, and who had told him, but I don't have the time. It makes me uncomfortable, his empathy for me. If he had come at me at The Rift, I would have killed him easily enough. But here he is, a stranger knowing a secret about me that not even my parents know. Yet he is gracious and kind and for all intents and purposes *a prisoner*. A prisoner who feels sorry for his jailers.

How fucked up is that?

"I have to go" was all I could manage to say.

"Of course. My name is Zaka. And we call the unicorn Merle. She seems to like you very much. You should come and visit when you can." He crosses one clenched fist over his heart and bows twice.

"You don't have to bow to me. I'm not a queen or anything."

Zaka lets out a little laugh that sounds a bit like a hiss, like a tire slowly losing pressure. "No. I realize that. It's a form of respectful greeting and leaving in my culture. I hope that's all right? I'm speaking English, of course, but with gestures, the line is less clear."

Is this a test of some sort? Why shouldn't he be allowed to greet someone respectfully in *any* way? "It's fine. I'm not even supposed to be here, so it's not like I'll make a report or anything, but I think you knew that already." Zaka gives a slight shrug and smiles. "My name is Ryn. It was nice talking to you." A lie. It was not nice. It was unsettling and distracting. Obviously, though, the Citadels here have relationships with the Immigrants. I don't understand what the relationships are like, but given Zaka's relaxed posture and gentle disposition, they can't be entirely hostile. I jump the paddock fence and run full-out to where I am supposed to meet Levi. There is a Citadel posted at the large metal gate. Levi knows her and she has agreed to let me out of The Menagerie. When I arrive, she smiles brightly.

"You must be Ryn. Hi! I'm Audrey. Have fun in there?"

I stop short. This I wasn't expecting. Audrey is nineteen or twenty with a French accent. She looks French, too, because somehow she has managed to make our basic uniform look chic. Maybe it's her hair, glossy brown and worn in a neat knot at the nape of her neck. It couldn't possibly be the bracelet alone, a slim silver braid around her wrist, but she definitely looks different from most Citadels. There is an exoticism about her, with the accent and all, but I think what sets her apart is that she seems, oddly, *happy*. It's weird. She must be here from the French Rift. It is a different country, but all Rift sites are supposed to operate the same. Maybe they don't. Maybe that's just another lie. "I'm sorry I couldn't meet you, but I can't leave my post. It's wonderful in there, though, isn't it?"

"Yeah," I say skeptically. Where am I again? Aren't I supposed to be sneaking into one of the world's most heavily fortified areas? And here is this European chick offering me the entrance like I'm getting on a ride at Disneyland. What in the hell is going on?

"Well, I hope you find who you are looking for. I am on duty for another three hours. When you come back, I will turn the electric fence off and you can get back out into the forest. So don't be any longer, okay? Or else maybe you will have to spend the night with the monster cats. Ha!" I do not know what the monster cats are and I don't really care. I do know that she is joking with me, though, and I am not in a joking mood. I see Levi in a golf cart just behind her, throwing me a nasty look. Because of Zaka I am already about five minutes behind schedule.

Well, if Miss Frenchy Brighty Pants seems unconcerned, then he can chill, too.

"Okay, I won't be any longer. Thanks."

Audrey swipes her card and I hear the click of the metal turnstile, so I can walk through. So far, this is not going at all like I expected. I sit down beside Levi and he begins to drive down a winding path, away from The Menagerie.

CHAPTER 8

"You're late."

"I know, sorry. I ran into an Immigrant and it required a soft touch to get away," I offer as an explanation.

"Oh, that's just great. What was it?"

"You mean *who* was it?" I ask back, annoyed. I get that he is doing me a favor. But so far, me being here doesn't actually seem to be that big of a deal.

"Yeah, sure . . . who. Or what." I can't help but sigh audibly. Does he always have to be such a jerk?

"Sissnovar. His name is Zaka."

Levi relaxes a bit in his seat. "That's fine. When they aren't being pussies, they kiss ass big time. We don't need to worry about him shooting his mouth off."

I bite my lip because I really don't want to fight with him, but, man, is he making it hard. Levi's anger seems to be a living thing. It carries its own weight and casts its own shadow. I understand his anger, I know it. But it's just me. He doesn't have to be so hostile *with me*, right? We're all in the same boat here.

"He seemed nice enough, and not in an ass-kissy way." I'm not sure why I am defending Zaka, but I feel for some reason I must. Not just for Zaka's kindness itself, but for Levi's sake, too. It's not smart, strategically, to underestimate anyone.

"Look, I'm gonna tell you how it goes because obviously you haven't gotten the memo. You don't trust *anyone*. You don't play nice. You can't be sure who is working who or what anyone's agenda is here and that can include—actually, it *especially* includes—ARC. Got it?"

Okay, so he wasn't underestimating Zaka. He's just paranoid. Well, I'm paranoid, too, but that doesn't mean I'm an asshole all the time. I'm done fighting his natural state, though, so I just say, "Sure," and then look out at the road unwinding before us. Ahead, I see buildings come into view.

"The general layout of the Village is like this," he says. "There are a bunch of different habitats—we call them habs. But almost everyone, regardless of species, eventually ends up in gen pop. The number one goal at the Village is humanization. They may have lived on their own Earth in caves or huts or tree houses or whatever, but it's hard to argue with a memory-foam mattress and HBO."

I whip my head around to face him. "Seriously? HBO? They watch TV here?" The thought hadn't occurred to me. I suppose I was expecting everyone to be dressed in gray and living in concrete bunkers. Sure enough, I see large parcels of forest with dwellings up high in the trees connected by a series of rope bridges. There are people walking and jumping around. *People* is the wrong word—they look something like a cross between human-sized monkeys and koalas. Or maybe it is the right word. Maybe what makes someone a person has little to do with being human.

I look at Levi and consider *his* personhood. He doesn't seem to notice.

"Those are the Cajas. They do better in their own habs. They aren't very smart. Small brains. Or, I dunno, maybe they haven't had a chance to evolve into something else on their Earth. We get variants of this species, some a little brighter than others." We drive some more and pass large rock formations with pitch-black holes about twenty feet high.

"ARC made those mountains to look like cave entrances, and inside are actual caves—for the Hailee. You've seen them, right? Come through The Rift?"

I nod my head. The Hailee are batlike humanoids with furry rust-colored faces and bodies. Imagine Ewoks but bigger, with wings, and not as cute. They don't talk as much as screech, but they are smart. I can see why they would prefer to be on their own.

Levi continues. "Okay, so you know that there are fourteen Rifts and only seven Villages worldwide. Two of them are here in the States. For now, we have about a dozen different habs for the species that are unlikely, if ever, to humanize. Those particular species are here, though, because the climate of the Pacific Northwest is the closest to what they lived in on their Earth. Of course, the number of habs could change if we get an influx of another species through a Rift. Most of these species Rifted through from other locations and were shipped here."

I look out at the terrain of habs. It looks like a twisted version of an amusement park with different worlds. We drive by one with a giant crane holding a massive tube about sixty-five feet in length over a forested area. The tube is shooting out steady droplets of water as it swings back and forth. It looks like a giant sprinkler.

"That's for the Grenillys. Have you seen them? They're kind of like toad people. Very big, very slimy, very large gross factor. They can't talk much, either, and when they do it's like . . . remember when you drank soda as a kid and burped the alphabet? They sound like that."

"Lovely," I respond, but I am looking at the Grenillys' hab, trying to suss it out.

"They need lots of rain, so ARC rigged up this system. They also built a bunch of ponds in there. I've only been in once, to deliver some insects." I must have looked at him funny, because he laughed. "Seriously—two dozen crates of crickets and stuff. Had nightmares for a few days after that. They're just so disgusting. I can't imagine they'll be worth a fraction of the effort we put into keeping them so fucking happy." I stare at the crane and the fence surrounding the hab. I doubt very much that they are happy.

"Do you ever actually listen to the words that come out of your mouth?" I ask him while keeping my voice at a steady pitch. It's taking a hell of a lot of willpower not to call him on his—well, I guess it would be *human* supremacist bullshit. "We put the effort in because they are a sentient species and our actions brought them here. The fact that ARC makes sure they are as comfortable as possible is pretty amazing considering it's ARC—not the most moral organization."

Levi lets out that loud, cruel laugh he's perfected. He looks at me and then laughs again. "Seriously? You can't possibly be so dumb. Is that part of your deal? Like, you let people think you're stupid so they'll underestimate you? Is it a strategy thing?"

I stare at him. He's not joking. He's serious. I've been accused of many things, but being dumb has never been one of them. Now I'm pissed. "I don't know, Levi. Let's each of us call our friends and ask them how smart they think we are. Ohhh, right. You can't do that because you don't have any friends. So you tell me. Who's the dumb one? Because in our line of work, it's very, very good to have friends."

"Whatever," Levi snorts, but I can tell my comment stung. "It's just stupid to think that ARC is noble in any way. They keep the Grenillys alive because one day they might figure out that their skin cures cancer or some shit."

The Grenilly paddock is behind us now. Still, Levi seems to be driving pretty slow for someone on a schedule. He's so hard to figure out, which is clearly, based on his statement to me, something he feels gives him an advantage. It's a dangerous way to think when you're part of a team. "Don't you ever get sick of it?" I ask him sincerely. "Being so aloof and guarded . . . the Tim Riggins of it all? Don't you ever just want to relax and not be a dick all the time?"

"I'd rather know my enemy. *All* of my enemies," Levi snaps.

"How exhausting for you."

He gives me a look. A look that might be "Fuck you" or "Thank you for noticing how hard my life is." I can't tell which one it is, so I turn my head away. We sit in silence for a few seconds.

"So what do you know about the Villages?" Levi asks. I suppose that's his idea of an olive branch and, for now, it's one I'll happily take.

"I know the other American Village is in the Everglades, built specifically for species, and people, too, I guess, who prefer hot and humid. The other Villages are in Africa, Australia, Lapland, Canada, and Brazil. Everyone wants a posting in the

American Villages, though, because of how close they are to actual civilization."

We don't really get to choose for those years when we are supposed to be in college. We go where they tell us. But we do get to choose which of the fourteen Rifts we want to settle. Or we can choose a Village. That's what they *say*. They could be lying about all that, too.

Who knows.

"Yeah, well, there aren't as many humans in the other Villages outside this country. The weather is pretty extreme. It just depends. Those Vikings you picked up the other day. They want to go to Lapland. It happens. Though the whole idea of nationalism in an internment camp seems pretty fucking stupid."

I blanch. I have never heard anyone call a Village what it really is. The casualness of it is a little scary.

We get past the habs, and what looks like a small town begins to emerge. This is so not what I thought it was going to be at all. It does actually look like a little village. There are stores and restaurants and all manner of people and species coming and going. It all looks . . . quaint. Eerily so. I mean, if you're the type of person who thinks *Star Trek* can be quaint, which I am.

On the walls of buildings and posted to streetlights are large, graphically illustrated posters depicting different species all dressed like humans and doing very human things, like riding a bike or having a picnic. There are words like *peace* and *solidarity* printed at the bottom in a big, bold font.

"I don't get it," I blurt out. "It's cute."

Levi gives me a snide look and huffs. "This is the commercial area of the Village. As you can see, it functions a lot like a Main Street in any other small town." He slows the golf cart and I watch the collection of picturesque buildings as we glide by. I immediately notice that there isn't one distinct style of architecture. Rather, there's an odd assortment, bound together by a similar color scheme so that it is pleasing to the eye. An adobe apartment sits beside a Tudor building. A modern, modular box (what I pictured, really, when I thought about the Village) seems to fit perfectly with a southern farmhouse, complete with a wraparound porch. The farmhouse is a bookstore, and, bizarrely, I have a hankering to stop and go inside, as if I was a tourist or something.

"There is an industrial and manufacturing area just northwest of here, and beyond that are the farms," Levi explains.

"Industrial? I don't get it. They make things here? Isn't everything just shipped in from somewhere else?" I ask, still not grasping the scope of what I am seeing.

"The people, human or otherwise, that come through The Rift all have skills. Furniture makers, artists, journalists, actors, math teachers. They can't be expected to just sit in their houses all day. That would be bad for morale. ARC gives everyone a job, a place, a function so they can contribute to their society. Otherwise there would be thousands of disgruntled Immigrants itching for a fight." I let that statement sink in. It makes sense. If I had to control a vast population of people who were, in effect, prisoners, the smartest way for me to go about doing it would be to make them forget that they are prisoners at all.

"We are going into the neighborhoods now. Each neighborhood is reflective of a city here on this Earth. There's a Marrakech, Kyoto, the Cotswolds, Siena, Stockholm, Tel Aviv, Shanghai, and two American neighborhoods, New York City and Cape Cod." As Levi is speaking, the Marrakech neighborhood comes into view. It's amazing. There are small winding alleys and streets and large stucco buildings with gorgeous

Moorish tilework and intricately carved wood panels on the doors. I know enough about this part of the world to guess that each of these big buildings must be, in fact, *riads*—large structures containing small apartments or rooms around a single courtyard.

"It's like Epcot, right? I mean, that's what this all reminds me of," I say out loud with a heavy dose of awe in my voice. "Is Ezra here? In Marrakech?

"You think he would be, with a last name like Massad, right? But that is one of the rules—you can decide which neighborhood you want to be in as long as you don't really belong to that culture. It's all about integration, right? Though they are pretty lax when it comes to other versions of Earth's Americans choosing either the U.S. neighborhoods or the U.K. one. Americans get preferential treatment, though they swear they aren't supposed to."

We get past Marrakech and into the quaint adorableness that is the Cotswolds. The cottages look like something out of a fairy tale. Row upon row of the cutest little houses I have ever seen. Most have gardens in front and rustic fences. I decide that if I was in the Village, this is where I would choose to live. "Why not? I mean, we are in the United States. Aren't we paying for all this?"

"Yes. But almost every country in the world contributes to the enormous cost of the Villages. We are here to humanize the Immigrants, not *Westernize* them. We have a synagogue, a mosque, different churches, and temples. All religions are welcome, but fundamentalism of any sort is not allowed. For example, a woman cannot veil in anything more extreme than a hijab. They don't put up with that burka shit, so at least there's that."

I myself find burkas misogynistic, but I don't pretend to

understand all the cultural implications of wearing them. Levi dismissing them so out of hand just rubs me the wrong way. There is no point in getting into this with him, though. We are so naturally combative with each other that I think we would each take opposing sides just so we could argue.

"I suppose it would make you one way or the other, wouldn't it?" I say instead, changing the subject. "Going through The Rift would make you either super religious or an atheist."

"I think just working there does that," Levi says with a little more laid-back tone. We leave the Cotswolds and pass through a bunch of lovely modern houses and apartments with pagoda-like tiles on the roofs. I assume this must be Kyoto.

Then suddenly we are in New York. I do a double take just to make sure. I've been to New York a few times with my parents to visit their old friends, and I swear to God, I feel like I am in a residential street in the West Village. Row upon row of brownstones with tons of character line a wide street. There are stoops and fire hydrants and open windows with curtains fluttering out. It is so bizarre.

"Your boyfriend lives half a block up there. The address is 675 and it's apartment 3B. I can't take you any farther because this is the one place on the street where there is a blind spot for the cameras, but please don't tell him that. When you walk, angle your body so that the video won't pick up on the fact that you don't have a weapon. Technically, I am running errands for a superior officer, but I don't have all day. So be as fast as you can."

"Thanks," I say genuinely, but then have to add, "and *he's not* my boyfriend. Jesus."

I get out of the golf cart and walk around it. Levi grabs my arm as I pass him. His fingers dig into my uniform. So much for the not-touching thing. "Please remember your promise to me, Ryn. I'm trusting you and I don't just do that. For any-one." Now he looks concerned. I want to sigh out loud. It's insulting that he thinks so little of me.

I gently pull my arm back. "I made a promise to one of my own, Levi. That means something to me. I wouldn't screw you over and I wouldn't put this person's safety at risk. I'm not like that. I don't know what else I can do or say to assure you."

Levi gives me a brief, reluctant smile. "Okay. You can't blame me for being paranoid, though."

"You don't have to be. Not with me. Not ever." I start to walk away, and I realize what I just said was true. He can always trust me. But I can't get into Levi's bizarre drama right now. I have to focus. I walk up to Ezra's building. I open the door and take a deep breath. Now that I am here, I half wish I wasn't. I practiced many things that I would say to him, but since I have actually seen the Village with my own eyes, I'm not sure that any of those things apply. If he's looking for fur-ther explanations, about anything concerning this place, I cannot provide him with any.

I whip up the three flights of stairs and find his apartment easily enough. I bite my lip and steel myself. This is so crazy. Why am I doing this again? I shake my head, hoping to clear it, and I hesitate for a moment before knocking on the door. This is a person I'm attracted to, and I'm about to be alone with him. Right now, ARC is not the immediate danger—I am. If I slip up, if I allow myself to get distracted even one time, I will kill this boy. I try to concentrate on the idea that not every encoun-ter where there is chemistry leads to romance. Sometimes the attraction takes a different path and ends up at friendship. That has to be my goal right now. Ezra and I are going to be friends. I repeat this a few times to myself and then I knock on the door. It takes a second or so for someone to answer, and the door swings open. Now Ezra Massad is standing right here in front of me. Good Lord, he looks gorgeous.

Shit, my whole friendship theory just went down the friggin' toilet.

This stupid choice I've made to come here practically hits me in the gut. My body tenses the way it does right before The Rift opens, but instead of fighting, words start to pour out of my mouth in an awkward rapid fire. "Hi! I promised you I would come and see you and here I am!" The smile I have planted on my face has got to look ridiculous. My eyebrows are arched up practically to my hairline and my body is so rigid, I'm not sure I can get my feet to move into his apartment.

"You are, yes," Ezra says, giving me a quizzical look. He does not seem happy to see me. Maybe this is because I am so over-the-top happy for both of us.

"It's Ryn," I offer, wondering if somehow he's forgotten me. Maybe he's blocked that whole Rift day from his mind, which wouldn't be surprising. "Can I come in?" I say eventually, because I'm not sure he is actually going to invite me to do so.

"Sure." Ezra opens the door wide enough for me to slip through and I now find myself in a man's apartment. Alone. I hadn't considered that.

"This is nice," I say, and I mean it. There is exposed brick on one wall and a large flat-screen TV on the other. There is a fairly simple couch and an open-concept kitchen with a couple bar stools at an eat-in counter. The appliances are stainless steel and I notice there are a couple more doors at the other end. A bathroom, presumably, and a bedroom. It would probably cost a million dollars or more if it was actually in New York.

"It came like this, but they tell me that after I get a few months of work in I'll have enough creds to make it my own." Ezra smiles for the first time. It's about as genuine as my weird Cheshire cat grin was at the door. Mine was because of nerves, however. His is sarcastic. There is an awful, awkward silence. He does not offer me a seat or anything to drink. It is pretty clear from his body language that he does not want me here. This stings. I didn't expect he would be happy to see me. But I didn't expect he would resent my showing up, either.

Actually, no, I *did* think he would be happy to see me, because he's the one who asked me to come.

And now I'm just a bit pissed off.

It's not like I didn't just have to ask a favor from someone who drives me crazy, or have to sneak past my own people, and basically risk everything just to say hey.

But I am here, and it seems stupid to have gone through that simply to get into a fight. "I just . . ." I begin, and then stop. I want to choose my words carefully. I scratch my neck and bite my lip again. "I just wanted to make sure you're okay. That you've settled in all right, I guess." This is not a lie. This is the absolute truth. It isn't the whole truth. I didn't mention that I hadn't been able to stop thinking about him, but mentioning that part would only increase the awkward factor to an intolerable level.

"Oh, yeah," Ezra begins with mock enthusiasm. "I love it here. It's awesome. First I was poked and prodded in places that no eighteen-year-old heterosexual guy—and I'm pretty sure most homosexual guys—should be poked and prodded. Then I was interrogated for days like I was at Guantanamo, which was super fun."

"Ezra, stop—" I try to speak, but he's opened the floodgates now and is all riled up.

"Then I was tested like a lab rat and put through a bunch of machines that are still making my head buzz. Then I had to take actual tests like the SAT times a thousand. *So amazing.* And then they bring me to this psycho 'Stepford meets It's a Small World' village and tell me how great it's going to be here—get this—*for the rest of my life.* Oh, yeah, it's so wonderful here that I'll never want to leave, which is really great because if I try to, I will be shot on sight. I'm okay, Ryn. I'm fucking brilliant. How are you? How's your special skill set doing?" Ezra's breath is rapid. He is furious. There really is nothing to say to any of that except one thing.

"I'm so sorry, Ezra, that this happened to you." I hope I sound genuine, because I really mean it.

Ezra folds his arms. Clearly my apology isn't going to cut it. "Not sorry enough to warn me what was coming."

I can't hold back anymore. *Don't you get it!* I want to scream. Instead I say, "And then what would you have done? Run? We would have tracked you down. Fight? You would have gotten your ass handed to you. Jump back through The Rift? You could have ended up on an Earth totally devoid of life. There are no happy endings when it comes to The Rift. There are just best- and worst-case scenarios. You got a best-case scenario. I'm not saying you should be thrilled about it, but you'll adapt. Because you're still alive, and some people that come out of The Rift can't say that."

Ezra shakes his head and the anger ebbs away from him, but it has turned into frustration.

"I don't want to adapt. I don't want to just be alive. I want to *live.* I want to travel and have a family and see my parents again. This place might be pretty, but it's a prison. I am a *prisoner* here." His magnificent blue eyes are so sad. I can feel myself begin to pull apart. All the walls over the years that I have built, brick by brick with lies and loneliness, don't feel nearly as solid as they did before I walked into this room. It's as if I am taking his pain and making it my own. And while this idea terrifies me, I am also grateful that I have the ability to feel anything so real and so deep. I honestly didn't think I was capable. I can't think of anything to do other than sit down for a moment. I place my palms on the back of my neck and press hard. It is a force of habit. When the implant felt like it was burning my skull I used to do the same gesture. Now I find myself doing it whenever I hurt.

"Look," I say, "I know you see me as the person who put you here. Maybe you even see me as the person who ruined your life, I don't know." I wait for Ezra to correct me. He doesn't. Great. "I didn't choose this, either, though. You were swept up in The Rift and so was I. They call us Citadels. Do you know that?"

"They told me," Ezra says levelly.

"We're, like, not normal people. I mean, we aren't robots or anything, but we've been enhanced technologically. So. Like . . . Sentries patrol areas. Sentinels are lookouts, but Citadels are the actual physical things that keep people safe. Each one of us is a small army on a fortress that stands between the enemy and the innocent. I didn't volunteer for this job. My parents don't even know what I am. I was seven years old when they put the thing in my brain that makes me able to do what I do. I had seven pretty normal years after I was implanted with the chip, except for the blinding headaches that were so bad that I literally passed out more than once. *Way* more than once. I was fourteen when ARC activated the chip. That's how old I was the first time I killed someone—*fourteen*. I would trade places with you in a minute. I don't mean to undermine what you are feeling; all I'm trying to say is that I never got a choice, either. That *I* am not the enemy."

Ezra looks at me in disbelief. I can see him scrambling, trying to make sense of what I just told him. He sits beside me on the couch. Instinctively I edge away from him. If he notices, he doesn't say anything.

"You know," he begins after a short while, "I was sucked here by a straw full of messed-up string theory. I have seen lizard people, and rock people, and something that I'm pretty sure was, like, a great big stick insect person. I have been placed in a bizarre picture-postcard version of a concentration camp, but honestly, Ryn, what you just told me may actually be the most disturbing piece of information my brain has processed since I've come here."

"I'm more disturbing than a stick insect person? I'm flattered." I smile weakly.

"No, it's not that. It's just, I guess because we're human we think we've achieved some kind of pinnacle in terms of evolution. It's so disappointing to know that when it comes right down to it, we'll eat our young in order to survive. I thought we were better. I thought, in the face of something as miraculous as The Rift, we would *be* better."

"Well," I say as I lean back into the couch, acutely aware of how close Ezra is to me. I have to be very careful now. "Wasn't it Maya Angelou who said, 'when you know better, you do better'? Or maybe it was Oprah. You do have Oprah on your Earth, right?"

Ezra laughs. "I think it was Maya. And yeah, we had Oprah, too. I'm sure she is a kind of quantum fixed point, like Jesus or *Catcher in the Rye*." We sit there. Time races. There isn't any way we can cram the amount of conversations we need to have in order to get to know each other into the short time my plan has allowed. My mind scrambles to try and pick out what's most important. Ezra must have the same idea, because we both start talking at once.

"No, no, you go ahead," he offers.

"I was just wondering how it happened. How you came through. Alone. From what we know of The Rift, it opens on another side randomly, but rarely in places where there is a single person. It seems to be attracted to, well, we're not really sure, but energy of some sort. That usually means multiple, uh, beings."

Ezra scrunches up his face. "I'm not so sure about that," he says hesitantly. I look at him, intrigued. "Well, I go to MIT. I'm actually a senior there, but I'm only eighteen."

"Ahh, so you're a supergeek. Me too. But I can only claim the title by default. It seems that you come by yours naturally."

Ezra laughs again. He is even more gorgeous when he smiles. It's a lopsided grin, and his entire face, especially his eyes, lights up.

I'm in trouble.

"I suppose you could say that. Child prodigy, blah, blah." Ezra waves his hand away, as if being a genius is nothing. "The thing is, I was working in the lab on our quantum computer model. We are pretty close to actually creating one. My field of study is quantum cryptography, which means—"

I interrupt him. "You use qubits instead of binary to break ciphers. Like code breaking on steroids, to the bajillionth power. But, if your Earth is anything like our Earth, you still have to deal with quantum decoherence, right?" I can see that my statement impresses him, and he just shakes his head and sighs.

"I think you may have just become the woman of my dreams. Wow. I would ask you to marry me, but with me being in a prison camp and you being a bionic guard and all . . . it's very CW."

"I'm not bionic. I told you, I'm enhanced. I'm not like Wolverine; I don't have metal inside me."

"Oh, God, comic book references, too? You're killing me." Ezra reaches out to touch me and I move my knee away. I hope he doesn't catch it. I think he does, though. "Okay, the thing is, I'm almost one hundred percent certain the Rooms—"

"Roones," I correct him. I have to get out of the habit of contradicting people who aren't under my command. Actually, I have to get out of the habit of contradicting everyone, friends included, unless they are under my direct command at the time. It must be incredibly annoying.

"Roones. Right. Well, I think they've solved this problem. I think they are so ahead of the game that something is going on."

I eye Ezra, not sure what he's getting at. "What do you mean?"

"The Rift opened right outside of the lab. I can't explain it, but I'm almost sure that I felt it—a good while before it opened. I know it sounds crazy. But I felt this weird thrumming inside of me. A pull. I got my stuff together. I grabbed my bag. I turned off the equipment, even though I had planned on being there for another couple hours. I walked out, and as soon as I got a decent distance from the building, The Rift opened and I was sucked right in. Can it do that? Choose someone?"

"No," I say quickly. "It doesn't choose. It doesn't have a consciousness. It's a thing that takes, randomly, which is part of its quantum deal. What do you think? That just from working on research, quarks jump off you and attract The Rift like a magnet? That theory *might* make sense if you had dark matter somehow floating around your lab. But just a computer program? A model? Doubtful."

But the way Ezra jumps up, excited, it's clear he doesn't think it's such a dubious theory.

"Doubtful but not impossible," he says. "Because nothing is impossible when it comes to quantum physics. Not really."

I don't know what to say. He's trying to make sense out of fate. I went through this phase, too. It's not like I have peace of mind or anything, but I have a sort of peace knowing that why this happened to me won't change what has already happened. I so want to reach out to him. I want to hold him and tell him to let it go. I understand Zaka now, when he said that hope only led to pain. Ezra has picked up the matchbox. He's very close to striking something that could set us all on fire.

"Listen," I say softly. I raise my hand to touch his, then think again and place it gently on the back of the couch. "I know you want to figure this out. But there is no shame in surrendering to something as huge as The Rift. It's not just bigger than you and me—it's bigger than the world and an infinite number of other ones. You work on a subatomic level, so you get that it's a never-ending loop of chaos."

"Ryn," he says a little more sternly. His eyes are intense and I have to look away from him for just a second to collect myself. "You—"

"No, don't interrupt me. I don't know much about this place. I do know that the rest of your life can suck or be only sort of sucky. You screw with these people. These people who took— *who still take*—a random selection of the most ordinary seven-year-olds they can find to use as weapons. And when I say ordinary, I mean that we were as average as possible. Not just so that we wouldn't stand out as much when we became Citadels, but because they didn't want to take their best and brightest out of the gene pool. That's how calculating they are."

Ezra stops and looks at me stonily. "Wait." He holds up his hand to get me to stop talking. "Just stop. You have to talk me through this because right now it sounds like you're explaining a plot to a science-fiction movie. Where did they even *get* a random selection of seven-year-olds?"

I sigh. I don't blame Ezra for wanting as much information as possible, and I did promise myself I wouldn't lie to him. I'm just not sure that the truth is going help him accept being here. But whatever, I guess I have to.

"Okay," I begin slowly. "We were tested. They used the tests they give to all kids in elementary school. The tests that are required for schools to get funding and awards and shit. They looked at kids within a two-hundred-mile radius of Battle Ground, because any farther would be suspicious in terms of physically getting the kids to move here. After they selected one hundred of us—they select a hundred a year—we all got the same strange rash."

"What kind of a rash? How?" Ezra's brows furrow.

I can only shake my head. "Look what they are covering up! You think they can't give us a rash? They probably drugged us or touched us with some kind of other-Earth slime, I don't know. The point is we were all referred to the same specialist. When the specialist saw us, we were biopsied and that's when they implanted the chip. They tried to implant normal, grown-up soldiers, but they all died. Apparently, only a child can tolerate the chip. We grow with it or something."

Ezra's shoulders sag. "Oh, God," he says in barely a whisper. "This just gets worse. And it makes no sense. How did they know that you were all going to see the same specialist? I mean, how did they ensure that?"

"I don't know," I say, suddenly feeling defensive, like I've done something wrong for not knowing. "They don't answer those kinds of questions. They don't even tolerate them."

"What do they do when you ask? Beat you or something?" Ezra's eyes are as wide as dinner plates.

"No, they don't beat us," I try to assure him. "They ignore the questions outright or they give you an extra round of training if you get mouthy. Very hard, very annoying training. So it's easier to just go along with it. And then, in the eighth grade, our parents were told we were chosen for this highly prestigious gifted program that basically guarantees an Ivy League acceptance and a whole bunch of very tempting promises about our futures. Like I said, the chips were fully activated when we were fourteen. We got all the superpowers, but instead of going to high school we became Citadels. ARC is a perfect cover. Our parents believe that we are doing twice the work of other kids our age, which explains the stress, the long absences, the maturity level . . ."

"And when they told you what you would be doing, did anyone just say, 'peace out, no thanks'?"

There's a moment of silence as I consider his question. I think long and hard. "No one says no. No one ever says no. We have to protect our families and the country and the world. You can't just turn away from that."

Ezra leans back in the sofa. He crosses his arms and looks directly at me. "Let me just tell you," he says with clear agitation in his voice, "from an outsider's point of view, that story is bullshit. There are more holes in that story than, I don't know . . . something with a lot of holes. It makes no sense. At all. *No one* has told their parents? *No one* has given away this huge big secret? You're telling me that *no one* says no to this life of deception and violence and killing and death? That the entire world is protected from monsters by children? Right. *Of course* that makes sense. I mean, who can't count on a fourteen-year-old? I know how reliable and honorable I was at fourteen in between marathon jerking-off sessions and playing Xbox. There is something else going on. You're not seeing that?" he says frantically.

"I know it sounds crazy," I counter, trying to keep my voice level. This conversation is getting away from me. "But once you've fought a Moth Man—like, an actual moth person with wings and big bug eyes and scary black claw things, not to mention fucking velociraptors and a bunch of other terrifying *Island of Dr. Moreau* monsters—the *why* you are there becomes so much less important than staying alive and using your training."

I dip my head down. I've never tried explaining this before and I know I am doing a crap job. It does sound like bullshit, but how can I convince him that it doesn't matter? I stand in front of The Rift and fight because if I wasn't there, something terrible could be let loose in the world and *kill* a bunch of seven-year-olds. So, if it's death or being implanted at seven, I choose the chip. "There are many children who have to grow up quickly," I say, using a different tack. "Refugees fleeing war, kids with cancer, kids who are orphaned. Teenagers who go to college instead of high school." I point a finger at him and cock my head because I can guess that as an eighteen-year-old senior at MIT that's exactly what he did. "A thousand years ago, all of us would be married already with kids of our own. Nowadays, parents are ridiculous. A kid can't even take a public bus or walk home from school without a mom or dad texting to make sure they aren't being followed by a pedophile. Yes, we're young and we have an insane amount of responsibility, but I've got to tell you that despite all the helicopter parents out there desperate to prove otherwise, teenagers are not little children."

There is an uncomfortable silence as Ezra glares at me. In that moment he seems impossibly tired. "You sound like . . . ," he begins, but his words seem suddenly remote, as if they are trying to get as far away from his mouth as they can.

"What?" I shoot back, annoyed that I am trying my best and it's still not working.

"Someone who's in a cult. That's what you sound like to me. A cult member. Unreasonable. In denial."

I jump up, off the couch, unable to contain my impatience. "You know what?" I let my arms fly around my head. "Maybe you're right. It could be a cult. Or aliens. Maybe I'm an angel sent by God. Or maybe Captain America recruited me. But I'm telling you it doesn't matter. You cannot beat this system. You cannot kick this hornet's nest. You have to be cool. That's it. You start nosing around and asking too many questions, they will lock you in a room and *throw away the room.* Do you get what I'm saying? You need to stay safe. Be smart. Smart enough to make a good life here but not too smart to threaten anyone."

Ezra nods his head slowly and sets his jaw. He stands up, too, and sticks his hands in his pockets. "How do I know they didn't send you to try to test me or throw me or convince me?"

I almost want to laugh. Just the idea that I would cooperate with ARC on that level with this boy is ridiculous. Then again, he doesn't know me. All he knows is that I'm the girl he saw when he first came through The Rift. I'm the girl who beat down a bunch of Vikings without breaking a sweat, and I'm the one in the prison guard uniform. I cannot touch him, though I ache to do so. I feel like my fingertips on his skin could say everything that my mouth can't. Since that is impossible, I stand as close to him as I dare, noticing every detail of his face. The arch of his eyebrows, the lock of hair that flops down around his left eye. His mouth, so full and pink, his lips parted just a millimeter . . .

Jesus, Ryn—get it together.

"You're right to be wary of me. I am a liar. I'm a killer. I am not a particularly good person." I feel a lump in my throat. Tears are beginning to well. I cannot cry. It will freak him out. I'm useless at emotions. I wear them so weirdly that it will only increase his suspicions. Once again I have to thank ARC for teaching me how to keep my humanity from seeping through, and I suck the sadness down. "But," I continue, "I am *not* lying to you. I can't explain why or what it is about you. From the first moment I laid eyes on you it's like I couldn't. Like I was totally incapable of being dishonest with you. I don't know what that means. But I know that I'm asking a lot, given the circumstances, for you to trust me. But I swear you can. I snuck in here. I'm not even supposed to enter the Village until I turn eighteen. I only did it because I promised you I would and I didn't want my word to be meaningless. Not to you."

We stand. Inches apart. We are so close that I can feel his breath, which is minty and sweet all at once. He steps forward and I step back. Ezra narrows his eyes in misunderstanding. To his credit, though, he respects the boundary I have placed between us.

"All right," he says finally, and I sigh in relief. "I will trust you. But you have to promise me that you'll think about what I've said. All of you are so smart and none of you are demanding the answers to questions that *anyone*—'super soldier' or not—would ask and it's *really* making me anxious."

I don't generally like ultimatums, but this seems fair enough. It's not like I could *not* think about this conversation, anyway. I'll probably replay it a thousand times in my head.

"Okay, I will consider everything you've brought up," I tell him as neutrally as possible.

"Great. Can you stay?" he asks. "We can . . . I don't know,

I'm binging *Game of Thrones*. We can just sit here and not say anything and watch it. No conspiracy theories. I swear."

"HBO really is a thing here. Crazy," I say, raising my arms in a gesture that speaks to how much I don't understand the way things work here in the Village.

"Not that crazy. It's *Game of Thrones*," Ezra jokes. "Come on."

"I can't. I really have to go." I back away and head to the door.

"I don't know what you had to do to get in here. But . . . can you do it again? Things seem so much more . . . I don't know—*manageable* seems like the least romantic word ever, but it fits somehow. And the word *better* just doesn't cut it." Ezra puts his hands back in his pockets. He looks so vulnerable. If I was smart I would stay away. The thing is, I *am* smart and so is he, though he doesn't understand the full implications of what spending time together could mean.

So of course I say, "I will. I will come again."

Clearly, when it comes to Ezra Massad, I am a dumbass.

CHAPTER 9

Beta Team takes point position at the rock again, right beside
The Rift. It has been four days since my trip to the Village. Each
morning I've woken up and hoped that I would get some sort
of perspective, but my days have been full of Ezra. Not him,
actually, but the thought of him. I wonder what he's doing,
how he is doing, and if he is getting any closer to accepting
where he is. At night I've climbed into my bed, closed my
eyes, and imagined scenarios where we might be together. I
get as far as a posting in the Village, maybe even a rotation
or two nearby where he ends up working. That is the closest
we will ever get to a life together. I've allowed myself brief,
fleeting flashes of him taking my face in his hands and kissing me deeply. I cannot allow myself to fall completely into
this fantasy. I've felt the violence sweep through my fists as I
picture our mouths colliding, and don't want to destroy my

room—and possibly my family—by going any further. If I am to see him again, safely, I can't even daydream about something physical happening between us, or it will be the first thing I think of when I see him in person, and even though physical touch is required to set off the Blood Lust, I would not want to risk it. What if I'm close enough to feel the touch of his breath? Would that count? We've always been so overly cautious when it comes to the Blood Lust (Levi excluded, of course) that in truth, we don't even know where the limits actually are. So we all keep our hands to ourselves and our thoughts as PG-13 as possible because it's just easier that way, safer. Which I'm sure, no doubt, is exactly how ARC wants it.

This is why I feel I can innocently imagine us in The Menagerie, walking hand in hand through the grasses of the pasture where they keep Merle. His hand in mine does not feel sexual in this little mind trip. The unicorn's presence cancels out lust. Ezra's hand will fit perfectly into my own and both of us will stare into the inky black of Merle's eyes. We will see ourselves reflected there as we could be: two kids, normal, stripped of the craziness that is our lives.

I miss him. It's illogical. I keep trying to dismiss him. I can't. He is a bruise I keep pushing, a scab I keep picking. My inability to see Ezra, let alone touch him, is painful, but I know later on down the road it will be agony. Eventually he will find a girl, someone else in the Village, to share his life with. I will have to watch them with a rifle in my hand as they walk down the street, go out to eat, head home together from work. I will become invisible to him, just another guard keeping him trapped in a world that isn't his. I do think about all those questions he asked, as I promised. I haven't come up with any other answer than ARC has probably lied about a number of things. But like I told Ezra, it doesn't matter. I've gone too far down this road already. I don't want to end up like Levi, angry at everyone every minute of the day.

I have been trying not to let any of this affect my job, but of course it has. Violet seems to know that something is up. She has been unusually touchy-feely with me today. Her hugs last longer, she's rested her head on my shoulder twice, she even insisted on braiding my hair this morning, and now it's pulled back so neat and tight I'm getting a headache. Boone hasn't cracked a joke, and Henry, well, Henry is the same. I want to tell them what I've done, but I can't put them at risk.

I was so afraid the first day I came into work after I went to see him that somehow I had been found out, but I hadn't. Things went forward as usual and no one said a thing. It seems I have done it, broken into the Village. I couldn't have done it without Levi's help. He reminded me of this when we drove away from Ezra's apartment. He also explained that we are now even. The debt has been paid. It was the only thing he said as we made our way back to The Menagerie and I was beyond grateful for the silence.

The thing is, I'm pretty sure I can do it again without his assistance. I now have the ever-chipper Audrey to get me into the Village. Before I left, I asked when she would next be on Menagerie duty. She told me that she wasn't on until the following Sunday night, but that she would be working grave-yard, twelve to four A.M., and would happily let me in. I don't relish the idea of sneaking out of my house, nor do I love the fact that I would be showing up at Ezra's apartment in the dead of night, but what could I do? He knows I basically have to break into the Village to see him. I can only hope that he understands I am working with what I've got, and not assume it's some kind of booty call.

I hear the various teams checking in. It's been two hours

and The Rift has been blessedly silent. But then, of course, right after I think that, I feel the hair on the back of my neck stand on end. I look at my team and let them know silently that The Rift is about to open. I close my eyes and focus. I concentrate on the air around me. There is a strange pull and a sort of thrumming. Ezra was right about that; it's possible that his body is simply sensitive to the subatomic changes in the atmosphere, as mine is. There is no way that it chose him or singled him out, though. I have to get that idea out of his head.

I look through the rock and see The Rift begin to shimmer.

"Command Center, this is Beta Team. We have a visual confirmation. Stage one."

"Copy that, Beta Team."

"Finally. Christ," Boone says, rolling his eyes. "My ass has fallen asleep and you guys are about as much fun today as a teeth cleaning." Boone lifts himself up and puts a hand on Vi's leg to maneuver over her so that he can see through one of the rock portals. His hand lingers for just a couple seconds, but it's enough. Violet reaches out quickly and grabs his wrist. Her breath begins to quicken. It's the Blood Lust. Immediately, I turn off my mic.

"Henry, take my spot."

Henry obeys the order and begins reporting back to Command on The Rift's progress. Boone isn't moving. He understands that if he tries to jerk his hand away it will only make things worse. I can see Violet fighting it. Her lip is trembling, she is scrunching her eyes shut.

"Vi, sweetie, let go," I say softly. She opens her eyes and looks at me, pleading. "It's okay, it's fine, babe. We're at work. The Rift is about to open, so we have to do our jobs, all right?" I can tell she is gritting her teeth. She is not in control, so I have to take control for her. "Vi, just listen to the sound of my voice. You don't feel anything. Everything is calm." I see Boone wince—Violet has clamped down harder. From behind me, Henry is telling Command that The Rift is at Stage 3. There is no time. Suddenly, from out of nowhere, I get an idea.

"Violet!" That gets her attention and she looks me straight in the eye. "Martha Graham's Night Dance!" Everyone turns and looks at me funny, including, I think, Violet. "Dachshund puppy dogs, turkey Bolognese, *The Gilmore Girls*, Cherry Garcia ice cream!" Her head jerks back and she lets Boone's wrist go. Boone stays crouched and massages the place where Vi had him. I see a purple bruise forming in the shape of her slender fingers. I can only hope it's not broken.

"What did you do?" he asks in disbelief.

"I just thought of all the things that make Violet happy. I was trying to distract her. I guess I just sort of blurted out all the things that give her pleasure but not, you know, sexual pleasure." I smile wide and Violet smiles back.

"I don't know, I've lusted pretty hard-core over a pint of Ben and Jerry's," she says, "but thanks. I'm so sorry, Boone." I'm sure Violet would have loved to reach out and at least pat him on the shoulder, but she won't dare now.

"It's all good. I'm fine. No real harm done." Boone is lying. The physical pain is nothing compared to how he hurts when the reality of the two of them becomes so dangerous. I don't know how I know that—I've never had the Blood Lust hit me full force—but when I think about Ezra, and how close I've wanted to get . . . I just do.

He moves his wrist back and forth so I can see it's not broken.

"You guys want to sit here and talk about puppies, or do you want to work?" Henry says grimly.

"I *was* working," I say as Boone says, "Puppies." *Good—if he's joking, at least he's trying.* "Stand down, Henry." I turn my mic back on and see The Rift is open fully. "Stage four. Expect incoming, Command."

"Roger that, Ryn." It's Applebaum. He wasn't helming Command before. The fact that he's taking lead now has me paranoid. Does he know about the Village? Or is it just because he didn't like what happened the last time I was in charge out here? I shake off my annoyance. It is time to go to work, and nothing else matters now except for what is about to happen in the next few minutes.

The Rift spits out about twenty Sissnovars from its jet-black hole. I hear Applebaum start the countdown for The Five. I watch the Sissnovars through the rock. They are bewildered, they stare . . . then they begin to yell at one another in their own language. Even though the time I spent with Zaka was brief, I am seeing his species in a whole new light. There are about a dozen males, five females, and the rest are much younger, children. My heart sinks when I see them. Their speech is not unpleasant. It isn't guttural but, as you might expect, sibilant. Their voices are raised in panic, but their language is actually quite soothing. The children hide behind their mothers. A few of the Sissnovars are crying, a few are racing around looking at trees, touching them, even licking a couple.

They might look fearsome, but I know that they are just terrified. The Five are almost up. I radio back to base. "We are going to make first contact. Do not order the Citadels down from the Nests or bring any forward until I give the okay. Copy."

"How about you let me give those kind of orders, Ryn?" Applebaum says with superiority.

"Not today, Applebaum," I answer vaguely and with obvious annoyance in my voice. He and everyone else is wondering if I mean that I'm not going to take his crap today or if I am actually taking complete command of the mission.

I press the mute button on my mic. "Leave your weapons here, on safety," I order my team.

"Are you insane?" Henry says, clearly baffled.

"No, I'm your team leader. Do it." They all look at one another then back at me. Violet puts down her gun first, followed by Boone and then Henry, reluctantly. "Now, follow my lead."

Usually in situations like this we go in with our guns. We show immediate authority because we believe it's actually safer for our opponents to see they are obviously outmatched. I have decided on a new tactic.

I think it's starting to become a habit for me.

I stand; my team follows. I slowly walk toward the clearing, toward the Sissnovars with my arms wide. For a minute they stop and look at me. I take my right fist and bring it up so that it crosses my heart, the gesture I saw Zaka make as I was leaving The Menagerie. I bend at the waist and bow twice.

"What in the good goddamned hell are you doing, Ryn?" Applebaum yells in our ears. "Where are your weapons? Gamma, Delta, and Epsilon Teams—prepare to jump from the Nests on one . . ."

I unmute my mic. "Nobody move," I whisper sternly. "I mean it. Let me try this, or somebody is going to get hurt." I look at my team and raise my eyebrows so they know to copy my body language. All in a row we repeat the same movement. A female Sissnovar bravely comes forward. A male is yelling, but she silences him with a choice word and a look. She returns my greeting and begins to speak slowly. I quickly hold my hand over my lips and shake my head, hoping that she will understand that I don't speak her language. I point to

The Rift, and make a kind of scary face and vigorously whip my head back and forth in an obvious "no/bad" charade. The female nods her head in understanding.

I hope.

I move even closer to her. Gently I raise my hand. She winces slightly and is near shaking with fear. "It's okay," I whisper. I give her my warmest smile as my hand lands on her shoulder. She takes it and examines it closely. I am far more alien to her than she is to me at this point, with my pink, smooth skin, blue veins, and smattering of freckles. She smells my skin and then gently rubs the back of my hand on her cool, scaly cheek. I wonder if she can smell aggression or fear, of which I have neither. It also occurs to me that I should *know* that. That kind of information should be included in our briefing seminars about the different species we have encountered and housed in our Villages.

I point my finger away from The Rift and then gesture for them all to follow. They talk for a minute among themselves, but there is decidedly less tension. The woman nods her head and surprisingly wraps her arm around my own and allows me to escort them all away with us in the lead. We don't say anything—we can't. There is only the sound of twigs and pine needles crunching beneath our feet and birds chirping from the trees. She leans on me, still shaking, but I am in awe of her bravery. I am also ashamed. Sissnovars are gentle, as Zaka had said. They are also now prisoners here, forever, and about to be humanized. I am taking them on the first steps of that journey. There is no denying my part in this.

My only consolation is that no one got hurt. It might be enough.

The vehicles are waiting for us in the safe zone. The Sissno-vars look at the jeeps and vans in an odd kind of way. They don't seem surprised by a motorized coach, but they do seem intrigued by the design. I have no idea what they are used to, because I know nothing about them. I see Kendrick again, and another of his colleagues, Greta, whom I don't really like at all. She has about as much empathy as a diving board. I give Kendrick a pleading look, hoping he will take charge. Immediately, he jumps forward and puts his hand on his chest and says, "Kendrick." And again, "Kendrick." Then he points to the female who has taken her arm and unwrapped it from mine. "Liseth," she says with a smile. Kendrick repeats her name and nods. His smile is broad, genuine, and unthreatening. He points to the open door of one of the vans. Liseth looks at me, uncertainty clouding her face. I nod and point once again back at The Rift, shaking my head. She stops for a moment and looks at her people. She wears her apprehension and worry softly, like a veil, but it is there. I see it. She looks once more behind us, toward the green mouth that had swallowed her people, and narrows her small yellow eyes. Finally she nods her head in resignation.

Liseth walks into the van and tells her people to follow. They clamber up into the separate vehicles. Kendrick looks at me, holding his electronic pad close to his chest.

"That was nicely done, Ryn," he says with approval. "Good job."

Before he can turn to go, I ask, "When they get to base, will there be another Sissnovar there? Someone who can speak their language at least, to reassure them?"

Kendrick's neck jerks back slightly. He tilts his head. "I'm surprised to hear you ask. Usually you guys just sort of dump them with us and go back on duty."

"Yeah . . ." I begin, aware that I don't want to come across as sarcastic or even overly curious. Who knows how anything

I do will be interpreted? But I also don't know what else to say. "Well, today I'm asking." I realize that I am doing the very thing Ezra asked me to do and not just to myself, but to someone else at ARC. He got to me. I was the one who was supposed to be doing the getting to. I realize with a sinking heart that things have changed.

Shit.

That seems to satisfy him, though. "They will watch a recording of a very well-adjusted and confident Sissnovar, who will explain all about The Rift and what they can expect if they cooperate and what will happen if they don't. All their testing will be done in their own language. Sissnovars tend to adjust pretty quickly. It's usually only after they've just come through when there's any sort of problem." The motors are running and I can tell that he is in a hurry to get out of there. Greta taps on the window and then her watch. I wonder how someone's face alone can be annoying, but hers is.

"Okay, thanks, I was just wondering. That's all."

Kendrick is smiling, but his smile is signaling something else: caution. "That's good, yeah."

I step back and he gets in one of the vehicles and they all slowly caravan out.

"Seriously, Ryn?" Boone asks. "Did you just watch that little arm move on an episode of *Star Trek* and hope for the best?" He isn't mad. None of my teammates are, but they are wondering. I kick the ground a little bit with my boot.

"Actually, it was *Doctor Who*," I say innocently with a toothy grin. Before Boone can respond, a jeep comes barreling down the unpaved road.

"Applebaum," Henry says with no emotion. I wish I had Henry's detachment. I feel like I'm about to need it.

"Ryn!" the colonel screams at me, and hops out of the car

before it comes to a complete stop. I watch as he comes toward us and I swallow hard when I see Christopher Seelye slowly climb out of the passenger seat. My team and I look at each other. It's one thing to piss off Applebaum, but the president of ARC? The most powerful entity in the world? It's not looking good for me.

Damned if I'm going to let that show, though.

"Yes," I respond coolly, though my pulse begins to race as Seelye casually makes his way toward us.

"No weapons? No backup? And of all the days, Ryn! When Mr. Seelye is here. *Jesus.*" Applebaum starts to pace in front of me. He's holding his arms so rigidly behind him that they look shackled. "What were you thinking? It's not just that you put your entire team at risk, but those poor snake bastards, too. Had they attacked, well, I don't need to tell you what would have happened." His hair, military short and streaked with silver, is unmoving in the light breeze and his steel-gray eyes are sharply condescending. Seelye is saying nothing. He's just watching and staring. It unnerves me more than I'd like to admit. "Well?" Applebaum demands.

"But they *didn't* attack, sir. I believe I handled things quite diplomatically, so what's the problem?" I say, crossing my arms. Regardless of who is in front of me, I refuse to be intimidated. Sometimes things aren't black and white. Sometimes there is no clear right or wrong, but in this case, I know I'm right.

"Let me ask you a question: Do you *think* you're diplomats? Is that what you think?" Applebaum barks.

"No!" I bark back, and he retreats just a fraction of an inch. *Oh, yeah. He* should *be afraid of his freaky Frankensteins.* "Let me ask *you* a question." I hear Boone whistle. I look at the rest of my team. They are shocked. I'm so far in it that it doesn't matter anymore, so I press on. "Because of the little black box you guys shoved in my head, I can speak fifteen languages, so why not Sissnovar? Or Damalla? Or Ter-Kush or even Karekin? Are we thugs? Assassins? Because it seems to me we might be able to get a whole lot more accomplished without violence if we spoke some more languages."

Applebaum's body shifts in an instant as he lets out a menacing chuckle. Seelye's face, on the other hand, gives nothing away.

"You're soldiers. You follow orders. *My* orders. That is all you need to know. And if you don't like it, I can happily yank out that implant of yours and take all of your superpowers away."

I stifle a laugh of my own. "Oh. No. Please. Don't," I respond robotically. *Is he for real? Is that his threat? That I get my life back?* What a joke. He is bluffing, and we both know it. I am a soldier, and because of that, I understand strategy. I know you never start an intimidation tactic with your worst possible outcome because then there's nowhere to go. I don't actually know what their worst is, so I think it's best, for now, to keep my mouth shut.

"You're this close, Citadel," he says as he shows me the fraction of a space between his thumb and pointer finger. "Maybe a week doing survival training at the Siberian Rift might help you remember how to do your job."

My face does not change. His threat does not register. I have nothing against Siberia and seven days near the Arctic might not be the most fun, but it would get me away from all of them. When he sees that I am not going to give him anything, he tries a different tactic.

"This is a system that works, Ryn." Applebaum's voice

becomes softer, though it scrapes in a tone of condescension. "It works because people a lot smarter than you have figured out the best way to deal with the Immigrants. Now, I know you believe, as a teenager *and* a Citadel, that there is no one smarter than you, but trust me, there is. I'm warning you officially to follow procedure. Are we clear?"

"Yes, sir," I say with just the barest hint of a shit-eating grin on my face. He turns and immediately walks to his car. Seelye remains. He smiles and looks at me with those cold eyes of his.

"You really are a special girl, Ryn," Seelye says, emphasizing the word *girl*. He has an edge to his voice that's peppered with affection.

The effect is nauseating.

"A Citadel like you, who's so smart and capable, needs special attention. I'm going to give that to you. I'm going to watch you more closely, help you navigate all that talent of yours." He squeezes my bicep and I feel it tense. Coming from anyone else, his words would have been validating. Out of Seelye's mouth, I know it's a threat. He casually walks over to the vehicle and it speeds off. I let go of a breath I didn't know I was holding.

"Oh, that's just great, Ryn," Boone says with an eye roll. "So it's not enough to piss off the people here, but you have to go straight up to the top of the food chain. Well, at least we'll know the reason if you go 'missing' all of a sudden. Don't you get it?" Boone says, switching his tone to a more serious one. "They want you to be smart but not too smart. They don't like it. It makes them nervous." I know exactly what he's saying because I said the same thing to Ezra.

"You're such a weasel, Boone," Henry says with disdain. "Ryn is who she is, and it's what makes her such a good leader. She'll put her neck and everything else on the line to make something right that isn't." Henry puts a hand on my shoulder. "It's good that you spoke up. We *should* know the languages and some of the customs of the Immigrants. More peacekeeping, less blood."

I'm a little surprised that it's Henry and not Vi who says this. Henry always seems down to fight, but then again, we're all liars. How well do any of us really know each other?

CHAPTER 10

"Audrey," I whisper as I come closer to the metal fence that she is guarding. Her back is to me. She's standing in a metal alcove at a computer hub, presumably double-checking that the electric fence is up and running again. With her help, I was able to break in much closer to the entrance. The pen I jumped into was filled with huge mounds of dirt. I thought at first it was a type of prairie dog hab until I saw one totally emerge from a hole in the ground. Up top, cutesy furriness; bottom half, earthworm. I had to check my gag reflex.

Getting to the gate was easy enough, but I wanted to give her fair warning it was me. It's never a good thing to sneak up on a Citadel. Audrey turns away from the computer and runs over to me, kissing me on both cheeks.

"Salut, chérie, Ça va? Aucune problème, non?" she asks cheerily. I thought all French people were supposed to be

supercool and act bored all the time. Not Audrey, though. She's . . . chipper.

"No. No problems," I assure her.

Audrey makes a little *tsk* sound with her mouth and arches an eyebrow. "You are sneaking in to see a boy?"

"Umm." I don't know how much to tell her. I fear the more people I speak to, the more danger I put everyone involved in.

"*Ça ira*, it's okay," she whispers conspiratorially. "I remember the first time I kissed a boy, he got ten stitches in his cheek and a broken ankle. But I'm sure he would agree that those few seconds we managed to . . . what do you say here? *Make out*, was well worth it." Audrey is smiling broadly with a glint in her eye.

I am sort of shocked at her admission. Citadels in general do not offer personal information of any sort to others.

"And how bad were you hurt?"

"Pffft, not me." She waves her hand away like she is shooing a fly. "He was a civilian. I wouldn't risk taking a Citadel away from his duties because I am tingling between my legs."

I think for a moment I've misheard her, but no, she seems genuinely nostalgic about beating a boy senseless for a little kiss. Audrey's bizarro vibe is creeping me out.

I can feel my heart thump a little faster in my chest. She is off, this Citadel, and I need to get out of here without giving her any additional information or showing any wariness. I need for her to think we are both still totally on the same page. "No, that's not in the cards for me. I wouldn't . . . I'm not going to . . . uhhh . . ."

Suddenly, Audrey grabs my elbow, just a little harder than I would like her to. "No girl should go unkissed. It's not natural. You should at least try. Maybe you won't hurt him too bad. If you do, come tell me. I can dump his body in with the dinosaurs. It wouldn't be the first time an Immigrant got curious, ha!"

I stare at her in silence. She's serious. I think? Shit, she is full-on crazy. Is that what happens to all Citadels once they reach their twenties?

"You know," I say, walking toward the gate, deliberately keeping it cool, "if I ever need to move a body, I think you would be the first person I would call, Audrey. Thanks."

Audrey pulls out her swipe card. "Of course, we're friends. We do each other favors. I'm helping you now, then one day, I will ask you for a favor. Maybe you move a body for me, or maybe I save that favor for something really hard. Ha!" She is well and truly cackling now. I seriously can't tell if she's messing with me or is totally out of her mind. She swipes the card and I hear the metal latch on the gate. As I run away I can still hear her laughing. Now I owe her. Great. I could kill Levi for involving this unstable person. What was he thinking?

Then again, what am I thinking coming back here?

I run swiftly past the habs. It's dark, so there isn't much in the way of sightseeing. I begin to push it. I am speeding down the pavement. I know I am running faster than the golf cart took Levi and me, but it feels like it's taking longer. Eventually, I end up in the Village proper and slow down. I expect it to be deserted, but it isn't.

The first thing I notice is that the entire town is decorated for Halloween. There are black and orange berry garlands running up every streetlamp. On each lamp is a basket of dark-petal dahlias and marigolds. The main street itself has staggered strings of plastic ghosts and witches hung between the buildings. There are pumpkins in front of every business and each window has a creative display of some spooky yet vintage-looking Halloween scene. The graphic *Humanity* posters have taken on the orange-black of the season. One of them has a Sissnovar in a mask with the word *tradition* in the same bold lettering. I love Halloween, but why should the Sissno-vars? It's not their tradition. It's one thing to ask a culture to tolerate another peaceably, but to ask them to feel the same way about the things we love? That we grew up with? How can they? It's not logical.

I take my time to slowly walk and look at the shops that Levi sped through before. There are cute clothing boutiques, a Mexican restaurant all decked out in fairy lights and sugar skulls. There's a hardware store, a furniture store, a garden center, a knitting store, another restaurant—a fancier-looking one. There's even a candle shop. On top of everything else, there's a Starbucks.

Mind.

Blown.

There are people and other species wandering the street. The weather is still mild, and I suppose when you can't leave your town, staying home on a Saturday night has a whole other meaning. There are more than a couple bars. One is open air, and I see folks seated at tables around a few outdoor fireplaces that I can smell burning from the street. There's another bar that looks to be more of the dive variety. The front is covered in hubcaps, bottle caps, and twinkling lights embedded in the exterior stucco walls. Music blares from the entrance. People party in the Village. Wasn't expecting that, either.

It all seems so perfect. Too perfect. I think it would piss me off after a while. Are people happy here? From this vantage, it seems like it. Maybe they are all just making the best of their situation. Maybe it's a hell of a lot better than wherever they came from—there's that idea, too. I notice two other Citadels on patrol. I duck into the dive bar entrance. I get a bizarre look from the guy at the door, and by *guy*, I mean a Maribeh. I wait for the Citadels to pass, and try to look official while I'm inside listening to what I think is a Beyoncé impersonator. I look at the walls, covered in notices and flyers, and then nod gravely to the Maribeh and run out.

Once I get into the neighborhood district, I assume it will be quieter, which it is, but only marginally. Through open windows I hear laughing and music. I suppose because there are so few children here, the adults have the freedom to stay up late and entertain their friends.

What is it about the Village that seems so wrong? People and other people-like beings are interned. That's not ideal, certainly, but it's more than that. I place myself in their shoes for a minute. What if I was sucked into The Rift and ended up on an Earth totally unlike my own, like, for example, a Hobbit Earth? Sure, the meadows and glades would be lovely and those cute little Hobbit houses would be cozy and all, but it might as well be a different planet. Which, okay, technically it would be. I wouldn't be able to speak English or celebrate my own holidays or have my own traditions or eat my own food (what do Hobbits eat? Pizzas? Tacos? Dandelions?). Then I imagine a Village that is a great, big, loud town made up of all the different cultures and foods and languages of all the species that come through The Rift. What would that look like? Less boring, for sure, and also less fake. And I think that's what bothers me so much: So what if it hurts to keep your own identity knowing you can never go back to the place where you got it from?

Because wouldn't it be better to feel like you're home in your actual home? Or at the very least have a choice in the matter? What is it that scares ARC so badly about the Immigrants that makes them insist on humanizing? What's so great about humanity? We caused The Rift in the first place, and history has proven time and time again that humans can be the most terrifying monsters of all.

I think about all this stuff as I walk into New York and all the way up to Ezra's apartment. It dawns on me that I've been justifying my coming here because he asked me to, because this is what he wanted. I lie and lie, to myself most of all. Standing here in front of this door, I cannot escape the truth of it. Ezra has only an idea of who I am and what I'm capable of doing, but *I know*. It costs me, spending time with him. I exert more energy keeping a safe enough distance and my mind in a platonic place than I do fighting a horde of Kare-kins. If all goes well tonight, and he doesn't take my hand or brush up against me too hard, triggering the Blood Lust, then I shouldn't come back. I don't want to hurt this beautiful boy. This will be the last time . . . but his beckoning door keeps getting in the way of my own delusions. I can tell myself that I won't see him again, but it would only be another lie. I'm awful. I should walk away right now, but I can't. My feet won't turn around. My hand knocks on the wood in front of me before I can stop it. My body wants what it wants, despite my best intentions. I hope he's awake. And wearing clothes. The door opens swiftly, and thankfully he's dressed.

"Ryn, hi!" Ezra is surprised, and extremely excited. "This is great. I didn't know when you would show and there's a ton I need to talk to you about." He does a quick sweep of the hallway with his eyes and then pulls me inside. I have to spin around quickly so that he makes contact with only my uni-form for a millisecond. I grit my teeth. I have to find a way to warn him without scaring him more and leaving him feeling even more betrayed. It's just . . . he *cannot* do that again.

"Yeah, sorry it's so late, it's just . . . I had to wait for this girl to come on duty. Audrey. By the way, she is French and probably a psychopath so, like, don't engage if she tries to talk to you. Especially if she's flirty. No *bueno.*"

Ezra looks sideways and tilts his head as if I'm the crazy one. He walks to his kitchen and lifts up a plate of chocolate chip cookies. "Got it. Want some coffee? Tea? Cookie?"

"Did you . . . make those?"

"I did, yeah. Baking calms me down and also helps me think better. Many great men have been bakers, so don't judge." He grabs a couple cookies and puts them on a paper towel.

"I get it. I myself am a knitter. So. Yeah. It makes sense to me. I'll have some coffee, if you're making it." I sit down on the couch and angle my body so I can watch him in the kitchen.

"You knit? Really? No offense, but it's hard to picture you knitting. Do you knit in your uniform? Or ⁄ . ." Ezra bangs around, opening cabinets. He runs the faucet and then after a couple minutes he joins me on the couch with the cookies. I choose to ignore his judge-y knitting comments.

"Okay, don't freak out, but—" he begins.

I shoot out my hand. "Please don't start a conversation that way. It never goes well when someone starts a conversation that way."

Ezra bites his bottom lip and pauses. "All right, I'll just jump in. I'm going to escape and I need your help. Or rather, I would like your help . . . please." Ezra grins.

I remain stone-faced. I don't say anything, but I do stare.

"What?" he asks finally. "I asked nicely."

"Are . . . are you *insane*? Are you medicated on your Earth and need more here? You cannot leave. You will die. What part of this whole experience are you not getting yet?"

"Actually, I think it's you who's not getting what's going on . . ." He lets the last word trail off.

I am probably wearing my resting bitch face, which can and has shut down many a conversation. I open my mouth to say something, but he gets a new, fixedly determined look on his face as he holds up his hand. So I sit back, arms crossed in front of me.

"Listen," he begins slowly, knowing that he is walking on a thin sheet of verbal ice, "I won't die. Or at least, I probably won't with your help. But even if you don't help, with enough time, I won't actually need it. I've been working in the admin building here. It's the main hub that runs the entire show. The whole place is filled with computers that *aren't* quantum ones, just normal binary." He gives me a knowing look. "Binary ones that are totally easy for me to hack into." Now he's smug. He even crosses his arms.

I just stare at him.

The smell of coffee begins to swirl around the room, and Ezra's satisfaction turns into incredulity, like one of us is a total idiot—and I don't think he means him.

Obviously he's wrong about that.

"You still don't seem to understand," I say. "You cannot get out of here without a retinal scan. So unless you're planning on gouging out someone's eyeball, you can't leave."

"That's not the only way out or in. That's not how you got here." Again with the smug look. I almost want to punch him, he's being so dense.

"I jumped down, over a massively tall electrified fence. I'm the one with all the crazy superpowers, remember? You're . . . well, normal," I insist.

By way of an answer, Ezra scrunches up his shirt and shows

me a bandage on his arm. "Please," he says dismissively. "I may not be able to catch an ax being flung into my face, but I am far from normal. I've already started. See?" Again he lifts up his arm.

"Are you going to dress up like a mummy and scare open the doors? What is it with the bandage?"

"No, but that would be amusing. Look: I took out my tracking device."

They tag them? Just one more thing I didn't know about Immigrants.

As if reading my thoughts, he confirms them and says, "I've been in the room where they track all the thousands of Immigrants. It's got this massive flat screen with red dots superimposed all over a map of the Village. Including one that used to be mine." He walks over to the kitchen and leans back against the counter, waiting for the coffee to finish.

My heart starts to hammer. I wonder what the punishment for something like that is when he gets caught. Because the thing is: He will get caught. Maybe he thinks because I am being so nice that all the other Citadels and the brass at ARC are as understanding as me. Oh, God. If something happens to him, it will be my fault.

"You took it out? By yourself?"

"I did. All I needed was a paring knife, tweezers, and a copy of *Gray's Anatomy*. It was easy." I raise my eyebrows at him. "Okay, no—that's a lie. It hurt like hell, and the stitches were crazy painful. But I did it."

I press my hands into the back of my neck and rest my elbows on my knees. I'm impressed and yet horrified. How am I going to get him to stop this? "That is gross and hardcore—kudos. But, Ezra, *come on*." I lift up my head and look at him. He's so handsome and brave. Stupid but brave. But mostly stupid at this moment. "Even if they can't track you, they'll find you. That is, if something doesn't eat you in The Menagerie before you can get out, on your way to being electrocuted to death."

Ezra takes out a couple mugs from the cupboard and sets them on the counter. I hear him pour the coffee and the little hiss of the liquid as it continues to percolate out. I wonder if he's even listening to me. He's clearly an impatient guy, and I get it. But there is no escape from this place. He *has* to see that.

"Listen, don't let my extraordinary good looks fool you into thinking I'm some sort of a bimbo," he says with a laugh. He's joking, playful. I stare him down. I don't think any part of this is funny. "Ryn, okay, honestly. I can do this. I already got my hands on a blank swipe card. I can program it to get me through the main gate of The Menagerie. I can also disable the electrified fence from there. Citadels are posted at those entrances, but they do patrol the area every hour on the hour for ten minutes. That gives me ten whole minutes to get to the alcove, turn it off, and run to the closest pen with the least terrifying creature and the shortest fence. That's obviously where you come in." Ezra returns to the couch and sets down the coffee cups, into which he has put cream. The last thing I need right now is caffeine. I will bounce off the walls. I'm already close to bouncing on his skull.

"And then what?" I ask. "I draw you a map that you are able to follow in the dark? You *are* planning to do this in the dark, I hope. So, you wander for miles in the forest, in the dark, with no GPS, and emerge in Battle Ground somehow, where there is a full battalion of Citadels, and probably regular troops as well, to hunt you down?" I shake my head, getting madder.

He is eating a cookie.

I don't smack sense into him right then and there, but I'm

sorely tempted to. And after he finishes chewing, he says, "No. I leave my tracking device here and go on a night when I have a solid two days off. They won't know I'm gone for two whole days. Do you know what I can do in two days? You might be able to kick ass from here to kingdom come, but get me on a computer and I am a very dangerous man." The smile is off his face. Finally. Ezra angles his body so that he's fully facing me. "With the right equipment—and by equipment, I mean a computer, a Wi-Fi network, and a printer—I can create an entire new identity for myself. I can access money that isn't mine and make it mine. I can book a plane ticket. I can book *two* tickets, Ryn. We can both get out of here."

My breath catches, and I pause to let the words he said sink in. He wants to rescue me. *Me.* I have never thought about running away. As much as I hate my job and the overall suckage of my life, I have a duty. I have to protect the world. It sounds so melodramatic in my head, yet I truly believe it. I just don't think I can say this to Ezra out loud without sounding like I have an ego the size of the entire country. I try anyway.

"Ezra, I can't leave. It's sweet that you want to help me." I reach my hand out, then snatch it back again. He's so close. Too close. "I hate what they did to me. It's wrong and messed up on a hundred different levels, but that doesn't change the fact that I need to be here—to protect this town, my family, my friends. I can't just go. This isn't a job, it's who I am. You just don't get it. I'm dangerous . . . I'm . . . I hurt people," I blurt out. Immediately I want to suck the words back in. I'm so unused to this level of honesty, I almost feel sick. My God, what must he think of me? I search his face, but instead of shock, he looks baffled.

"You're right. I don't get it. I'm sorry. You hurt people, I get *that*, but you don't seem to understand, or you're in complete denial about, how much you can actually control and how much power you actually have." Ezra shifts in his seat and runs his fingers through his hair. "You're absolutely right—you are dangerous, but I don't think you're dangerous in the way you think you are. Your implant? Your chip? You don't know anything about it. You don't even know the basic truth about how they managed to pull off implanting the little fuckers in all your tiny second-grade brains. What if it does something else that you don't know about? You've gotten the majority of your education downloaded through that thing. What if went in the other direction? Wiped out your memories? Your personality? Made you do things that they wanted but that you would never agree to. Can you honestly say that ARC would never go that far? Please, you know they would, so we should both get out now."

If Ezra's words had been weights, they would have landed at my feet with a thud. What he said is not only reasonable but obvious. So why don't I—Miss Contingency for Everything That Could Ever Go Bad Ever—know that already? Why don't I think about what else the implants could do or make us do?

My head starts to buzz. My body feels suddenly wrong, like my skin's been put on too tight. All I can think is that it must be the job. I spend so much time fighting and worried about the next fight that I don't think about who's actually sending us in there because the truth is right here in this room. He is absolutely right. Still, no matter how much validity there is to his argument, he still isn't grasping the scope of ARC. He seems to understand all the bad they do (*while completely ignoring the good, thank you very much*), but it's clearly not clicking that however we got here, here we are. That there is no beating this system. "Look, this is not about me," I try to explain. "This is about you. Dying. Badly. Or worse, and yes, there are

worse things than dying. The people in charge here think they
are being benevolent and good and progressive, but one look
around this place tells you that they have one agenda for all
of you: Be human. Accept the program. I think it would be far
less scary if they just treated you like actual prisoners, right?
It's . . ." I search for the right word and look around Ezra's
cute little apartment, which is as fake as everything else. "It's
sinister. And if they can make this fake Utopia feel shitty, you
can bet they know how to make things ugly, too. If you try to
get out, there is a good chance you won't make it, even with
my help."

"Yeah, maybe," Ezra concedes. Then he leans in closer to
me. I can smell the sugar on his hands from the baking. His
skin looks golden in this light. I close my eyes and open them,
hoping to shake myself loose from the pull he has on me. It
doesn't work, and I realize he's going to get us both hurt—one
way or another. "I swear, though," Ezra says, "I would rather
die than live my life in this gilded cage."

"A gilded cage is better than a pine box!"

"But it's more than that, and I think you know what I mean.
It's not just my life, Ryn. There is something going on here.
Something I don't understand yet, but it is major."

"Really? More major than a portal to the Multiverse opening in my hometown or me being turned into a super soldier
or you being in a prison camp that looks like a Thomas Kin-
caid painting? *Please*—we are literally living inside a show on
the SyFy network."

Ezra laughs that same easy laugh that disarms me and I
work to pull myself together. I sit up straighter. I focus, trying
to find something unappealing about him that I can concentrate on. There is nothing. Even his hands are beautiful.

"But what kind of show is being produced?" Ezra asks. "Do you ever think about that?"

"I was just saying . . ."

"Yes, but keep going with it. Consider: Did you know there are over fifteen thousand Immigrants here? Of those fifteen thousand, almost five hundred are physicists, cosmologists, chemists, biochemical engineers. People—or, you know, beings or whatever—who are highly specialized scientists. It's a statistical impossibility. It's like they're using The Rift as a STEM casting call. There is something much bigger going on. And I want to know what it is."

"Why?" My voice is rising. I rub my hands on my pants out of frustration. "Who cares? Maybe The Rift just attracts people who are working with subatomic energy. Maybe it's a coincidence. It doesn't change anything."

"It changes everything."

"It's not worth risking your life over!" I sound shrill. I hate the pitch of my voice. I am not the cool, calm, collected Ryn who can handle a life-or-death situation. I am suddenly a nag.

And I'm not sure I even agree with myself anymore.

"Ryn," Ezra says. His voice is low, almost a purr. His eyes lock on to mine, and I start to tremble. With so many emotions flying around the room, my resolve is crumbling. I dig my nails into my palms as he says, "Listen to me. This is important. I'm not just saying this to be dramatic. I am telling you that this is *huge*. They let me work on individual algorithms, so obviously I'm only allowed a peek at one tiny piece of the big picture. But from what I can suss out, and based on what I've heard from the other people I'm working with, I am troubled." Ezra's face is serious now. I think about what I sacrifice, the risks I take to make everyone safe. It occurs to me that it's condescending of me to dismiss Ezra for wanting to do the same. It also makes me like him even more.

Damn it.

"Okay, well, you must have some kind of a working theory, some kind of an idea if what's going on is enough to disturb you so much. So tell me," I coax, relaxing my posture.

"I do. But let me start by asking you a question: What do you think the number one priority of all the research we are doing is?"

"Closing The Rift," I answer.

"Right. *Exactly.* And yet . . . that isn't in the data. It doesn't tell that story. It seems like more of a . . ."

"More of a what?"

"I don't know. Like I said, this is just a theory based on the programs they asked me to code. We were in a meeting yesterday, and from what I put together from my job and what they asked of others, I'm pretty sure they want me to start on a quantum key distribution to *hide* something. I mean, you only use a QKD to hide something with infinite variables. Add that to the algorithms I've already looked at, and if I had to guess, I would say they are working on some sort of a map. Do you know what that means?"

"A map . . ." I whisper. "A map of the *Multiverse?*" I shake my head. "That's not possible. That's like drawing an atlas of the world using only a single grain of sand as a reference."

"But what if it isn't?" Ezra counters. "What if instead of wanting to close The Rift, ARC wants to use it? Pull out people like me or more species like the Roones? They could gain control over not just this Earth, but any Earth they wanted. What if navigating The Rift was possible? Tell me, who do you think they would send through it to do all the dirty work?" he asks, giving me a significant look.

I can't help myself. I practically leap off the couch. *Who is this guy?* This guy who has been in my life for, like, five minutes, is now sitting here trying to tell me what's going on? I don't like his version of the truth. It's cutting me up from the inside out. It's too much. He presses on anyway.

"Ryn, I have a photographic memory, but I physically don't have the time to look at every piece of data coming out of all the labs here. I need time and space and—most of all—data above my pay grade to get some kind of proof. That I can get. I can hack in and steal it from here. But once I do, the clock is ticking, and I can no longer stay here. Given a few months, I might be able to make sense of what's happening, but not if I'm in the Village. That *would* be suicide." Ezra stands up and walks over to me. After the heart-racing pace of the information he's thrown at me, suddenly I feel like everything is shifting to slow motion. I see his hands raise. I see them reach out and land gently on my shoulders. I feel his thumb stroking my clavicle. We are inches apart. "Ryn—I don't want to die. And I certainly don't want you to get hurt. I . . . I care too much about you to ask you to risk everything without having thought this through. I was being an ass before—I really can't do this without you. I don't *want* to do this without you." His voice is almost a whisper, and I worry the pounding in my heart is going to drown out his words. His head moves forward.

Oh, God, I think he's going to kiss me . . .

The fury sweeps through me like a lightning strike. I begin to pant. Without being able to stop myself, I push him back with the palm of my hand. Ezra lifts into the air and lands on his right arm, skittering past the kitchen.

"What the hell, Ryn!" There's an edge to his voice. I've hurt him already. At the moment, though, I'm not really sorry. I literally don't have it in me to be sorry. Quite the opposite.

He said he understood. He has no idea.

"Get into your bathroom and lock the door," I say through clenched teeth. It's taking everything I have to keep myself still. I feel my foot step forward, but I did not make the choice to start moving toward him. My body is no longer mine. "Now!" I scream.

There is genuine fear in his eyes as he scrambles up and hops the few feet into the bathroom. I hear the door slam and lock. I close my eyes. I plead with myself to stop. I can't think. I can't breathe. I want to hurt him so bad that I am in agony. I whimper. I bite my lip and I can taste blood. I see a flash of images in my mind. Naked bodies touching, kissing. I use my last bit of free will to force myself down on the ground. I smash my head into the hardwood floor. The pain gives me a moment of reprieve. I take this moment, away from direct contact with Ezra, and stretch it into two. I claw at the floor, my fingernails trying to gouge tracks in the boards; I feel some of my nails cracking and ripping. That pain helps, too. A little. The Blood Lust begins to ebb. It's not immediate. It pulses, like a throbbing ache that eventually winds down after a sharp pain. It's not localized. It's as if I've been stabbed with a thousand needles, deep and repeatedly. I lie here, a quivering, sweating, bloody mess. I'm afraid to move, afraid to bring that pain on again . . . or worse. Eventually, my heart is only pounding—as opposed to being close to exploding— and I exhale slowly. Crawling on my hands and knees, I make it to the bathroom, where Ezra is locked in.

"Ezra," I whisper. "I'm sorry." I hear his hand on the latch and quickly say, "No, don't. Not yet. I'm not sure it's completely safe."

"Tell me what that was" I hear from the other side.

I lean my cheek against the wood and fight back a sob.

"That is what I'm talking about. I can *really* hurt people. Part of it comes from the implant inside of me. The one that gives me all these amazing superpowers, and could potentially turn me into a cyborg zombie according to you. It does something else, too. It . . ." I trace my finger on the painted grain of the door. It's probably the closest I will ever come to touching him again. This is my version of intimacy, and already I can tell it might be too much, so I jerk my hand from the wood. "It sends a signal to my brain so that any time I feel attracted or aroused, I go into attack mode. It's sick. It's pretty disgusting, actually. What's even worse is that, as a soldier, I actually *see* why they put this fun little safeguard in here. I get it. You can't have an army of teenagers who are more concerned with their boyfriend cheating, or getting laid instead of being on duty. Kids our age, not so great at prioritizing when hormones take over."

"Jesus. I'm . . . sorry? God, that sounded trite. I don't know what to say to that. I'm okay, though. You didn't hurt me," Ezra says with a soothing tone in his voice.

"But I could have. You . . . you can't ever touch me again. Not a pat on the shoulder. Not a hug good-bye or peck on the cheek. You shouldn't even get too close to me." My cheeks burn. I can't believe I have to admit this to him. I don't want to, but I have to, to make sure he's safe. Especially since it doesn't look like I'm actually strong enough to stay away from him. I'm hoping that his sense of self-preservation will kick in hard enough so that he listens to me. That as horrible as that moment was, it showed him enough to override *his* hormones. "Ever since I saw you at The Rift, I've been half-crazy. I like you. I . . . Oh, God, this is embarrassing. I really like you. I can't stop thinking about you and I'm putting you in more danger than you already are."

"Ryn, enough," Ezra says sharply. I give the door a dirty look. "Although this latest tidbit about the brave new world I'm in is disturbing, it's also motivating."

"What do you mean?"

"I mean, I like you, too. A lot. And if your problem really is technical—I mean, if it involves circuitry and code breaking and hacking . . ."

"What?"

"If it's an engineering issue, I can fix you. Do you understand what I'm saying? I can undo what they've done to you."

For a moment, I *don't* understand what he's saying. But then it comes at me in a rush. Can he really rewire me? This is Roone technology, after all, so what if he tries and something worse happens? But then again, what if he really can fix me and Violet, and Boone and Henry and Levi? And I realize that ARC has said something that indicates it *might* be possible: the opt-out when we turn thirty. So now I start thinking less in terms of "can it be done" and more "can *we* do it." In other words: Can we pull off something so major without getting caught?

Clearly Ezra thinks we can. "All you need to do is get me out of this place, Ryn. Will you help me?" I hear the lock, and the door swings open. We are both on our knees. It almost looks like we are praying. Maybe we are. The word pops out of my mouth before I can catch it.

"Yes."

CHAPTER 11

"Okay, so you have the number of the villa we are staying at, and our cell phones will work, too. Daniel, you made sure that they activated our international data plan, right? You called them?" my mom asks my father in front of the waiting cab. I had offered to drive them to Portland, but they insisted on getting there themselves. They always feel so guilty about leaving. I try, even in my own minimalist way, to let them know that they shouldn't stress, but they claim the airport good-byes are too tough. I don't see how it's any worse than the one here in our driveway, but who am I to understand their weird parent logic?

"Oh, and you know the country code for Spain is thirty-four; you have to dial that before the phone number of the house we're staying in, but not our cell phones. I don't think . . ." Mom looks at Dad, who is trying to be patient. He knows that if I need to reach them, I can do so quickly. He understands my efficiency. I know my mom does, too, but this dance she's doing is, again, all about guilt.

I can't give my parents very much. I certainly can't give them the truth, nor can I give them much of myself. So instead, when I was fourteen, I decided to give them Thanksgiving. That makes me sound noble when, in fact, it was kind of the opposite. I was a new Citadel. I hated being around my family. The lying was so much harder back then that I almost never spoke (which was saying something) and when I did, I was rude and angry. I suggested that they take the time off to spend alone together. As a couple. I offered to spend a week at my grandparents' house with Abel, helping them look after him. I told my parents I didn't care about Thanksgiving and neither did my brother, which was a super bitchy move on my part because the truth was I had no idea how my brother felt, nor did I particularly care. My reasoning was that we would have been with my dad's family anyway. At first, they waffled. What kind of parents leave their kids alone on a holiday? Even when one of them is a jerky asshole teenager. (To be fair to them, they didn't say that out loud, but I'm pretty sure they had to be thinking it.) I assured them they deserved time off and it was no biggie—that was *my guilt* talking. Eventually, I convinced them and they've been going away ever since. For this vacation they will be gone for a little over two weeks, coming home just a couple days after the holiday, which will give me almost the entire time here alone before I have to worry about any family obligations.

Abel will stay with his best friend, Dylan, while my parents are gone, just like he did last year. Since they basically do everything together anyway—including football, and they have a game that Friday—everyone agreed it would just be easiest for him to stay over there. I will drive us down to Portland for Thanksgiving dinner, but I have ages before I need to worry about that. If things go sideways and I can't take Abel, well, I'll either have to make up the world's best excuse or it'll be so bad that ARC will step in and solve the problem for me. I *really* don't want that to happen.

"I understand how the phones work," I assure my mom. I stayed on my own last year, too. It was such a relief to have the house to myself. To come and go without lies or bogus explanations about what I was doing. I think I probably look forward to this vacation more than they do. My mom pulls me into a hug and tells me she loves me. I tell her the same. My dad follows and I hold on to him for just a fraction longer than I usually do. I realize why: I am about to do something dangerous. I am probably putting my whole family at risk.

And I am downright terrified.

But I know this has to happen. Ezra needs to find some answers. *I* have to find some answers. It's the right thing to do even though I know it's wrong to put the people I love most at risk. Things seem to be getting more complicated by the minute.

I watch my parents drive away. They will drop off Abel on their way out of town.

Our house has white clapboard; it's a two-story farmhouse set well back from the street behind a row of high hedges. I have always felt safe here. There is something about this property that makes it feel different from the rest of the neighborhood, magical almost. It's probably only been projection on my part, but now I am hoping that it will truly protect us from the world outside its walls. A citadel for a Citadel. I let out a nervous laugh at my lame wordplay and move quickly up the long path that leads to the front door. I maneuver around the bizarre three-tiered stone fountain that was here when we moved in. It's never worked, but I've always liked it. Probably because it doesn't quite belong . . . just like me.

I walk in the front door and close it. I lean my head on the frame. I have a lot to do before Ezra gets here, but I feel overwhelmed. I wish I could bring my friends in on this. I trust them with my life, but I don't know if I can completely trust them with *more* than my life. Because that's what this is—something much bigger than simply making sure we aren't killed by Immigrants. Besides, the more people who know, the more likely someone at ARC is to find us out. For now anyway, this will just be another lie.

Ezra and I made the plan three weeks ago that night in the Village. We didn't talk about our feelings or the future or airplane tickets or fake identities. We discussed strategy and logistics, conversations I navigate well with words that wouldn't potentially kill him. I drew a map of The Menagerie. I remembered where all the cameras were that Levi identified. I made notes of the ones I had seen in the commercial part of the Village and the ones around the habs. Ezra doesn't have my speed. It will take him a while to get not only to the metal gates of The Menagerie, but through The Menagerie itself. Once he's deactivated the fence, he'll have ten minutes to get to it. Not a lot of time at all. He'll have to locate the Prairie Dog Worm pen and scale its twelve feet. He swore up and down he could manage it, but I gave him some exercises that would increase his upper-body strength. To his credit, he paid close attention, though I caught him checking out his biceps with a frown when he thought I wasn't looking.

We both agreed that it would not be wise for me to meet him in the forest. Our connection was known to Levi and possibly Audrey. I'd need an ironclad alibi when they started the search for him. It's bad enough that it was me, alone, who met him when he first came out of The Rift. I know that every move I make once they figure out he is gone will be scrutinized, and since he is staying here with me, I will need more than my usual awesome poker face to sell the lie that I have no idea where he is. Which means the safest thing for both of us would be for me to go out with the gang the night he breaks out.

The one thing we haven't quite figured out is *how* he's going to make it to my house. Even with the three weeks he's had to figure out a way out of the forest and then into town, the Village is still miles and miles away from me. I gave him the exact longitude and latitude of The Menagerie, but I didn't have time to teach him how to use those numbers to navigate a way out. He said he would take the three weeks to learn. It might take him a while to get to me, but he promised he would have a plan and be prepared. Since he is technically a genius, I figure he'll do his homework and then some.

Regardless, I worry.

Vi is expecting me in an hour, so I don't have much time to get the last bits and pieces ready for Ezra's arrival. I race through the house and to the back door to my dad's office. Ezra will need all of my dad's gear. I wince a little as I unplug his monitors and hard drives. It feels wrong dismantling my father's private space, but what else can I do? Go to Best Buy and spend thousands of dollars on equipment? I have to provide the hardware, and Ezra is providing all the data in the form of top-secret files he's stealing from the Village. I think, in the big scheme of things, Ezra's got the shorter straw.

That said, I, too, had put the three weeks we had to good use. I couldn't build a secret lab, but I was able to reconfigure the attic to hide a workable space for Ezra. No one in my family really goes up there because it's such a pain in the ass to access. The entrance is hidden in our upstairs linen closet, which makes it even more ideal. I start taking Dad's stuff up to the second floor. I pull down the ladder from the concealed panel in the top of the closet and begin to climb up. In the weeks leading up to this day, I have already spent every spare second alone in the house preparing this space. I bought bookshelves and shelving from Ikea, and I modified two of the bookshelves to sit on wheels. I then constructed paneling around the bottom so that the casters couldn't be seen. When I finished, anyone just glancing would see a tiny space filled with Christmas decorations and clutter enclosed by a long wall of books.

In reality, I had cut the room in half. The bookshelves can swing out, and behind them I had put an old desk (one that was already up there, thank God) and a camp bed. I found a rug and a small table—a lamp, too—just to make it look less dingy. It isn't much, but it doesn't have to be. We'll only have the days my parents are gone and then Ezra has to take off and use his crazy computer skills to pull off his disappearing act.

I hope he's the technical magician he says he is . . .

I plug in the equipment and arrange it as best as I can on the small desk. I turn around and tug gently on the blanket on the bed, making the fold crisper. I run my hand up and down the soft fabric of the duvet so there isn't a wrinkle in sight. Ezra will sleep here, far away from me . . . but all too close. There is only one small window in this section of the attic. It makes the lab that much safer but far more claustrophobic. I hope Ezra doesn't have a problem with things like that. If we knew each other better I might know if he did. I realize at that moment, though, that we are still relative strangers. We are two people drawn together because of chemistry and a secret. It doesn't sound like much of a solid foundation for anything.

I quickly leave the room. In my own, I throw on a pair of leggings, a T-shirt, and a cardigan I knitted myself. I throw up my hair in a messy bun and look at myself in the mirror. Whatever the opposite of sexy is, that's what I see in my reflection. I plan on looking my absolute crappiest for these next few days. I consider that I might not even want to shower, then I think again. Ezra will at some point have to get close enough to my implant to decode it. It's one thing to want to dampen our mutual attraction, it's another thing to make his eyes water.

I run downstairs and out the door. I have to be happy but not too happy. I have to remain calm and not look distracted. I have to act like there is nothing especially interesting going on when *everything* is going on. I have to monitor my heart rate to remain at a steady pace because my team will hear it race if I think too hard about what's happening. I have to play this part with Meryl Streep–like perfection because there is so much on the line.

So . . . no pressure.

I gather myself and drive to Violet's. I knock on the door and she opens it quickly.

"Hi!" I say with a bright smile. Immediately her brows furrow.

Shit. Too happy.

"What's going on with you?" she asks as she closes the door behind her.

"Nothing." I rearrange my face to appear more passive. "I'm just excited to see the movie tonight. *Sorry,*" I say sarcastically.

"Really? *Transformers Five?* Big fan?" Violet chuckles and makes her way toward my car.

"Yeah, I love explosions and robots and exploding robots. Optimus Prime is very spiritual."

We both get into the car.

"He is a *truck*, right?" Vi asks jokingly.

I am going to have to do better. I bite the inside of my cheek. It's getting dark. Ezra will be heading off any minute. I make some small talk. I calm down. I should be able to do this, no problem. I am a liar, it's what I do. We pick up Boone and Henry, who both live in a cute little development called Battle Ground Square, then we head off to the movies.

I physically have to stop myself from checking my watch every five minutes. I purposely only look at my phone every half hour. I am grateful for the loud, obnoxious, mind-numbing movie. It has little to no plot and lots of action, which is about all I can handle. In the dark, my friends cannot see my fidgeting. After the movie, we eat at the North Wood Pub. I am extra careful to come across as normal. Since none of my friends are shooting me weird looks, I must be succeeding. Ezra should be clear of The Menagerie and in the forest by now. When we get outside, the boys walk home to their own houses, which are just across the street from the restaurant. I stare up at the stars. It is a moonless night, a blessing and a curse for Ezra.

Violet and I head back to Meadow Glade. She comes over to my house and watches a TV show I've recorded. When it's over, she asks if she can just spend the night.

"Oh," I respond neutrally. "Would you be super annoyed with me if I say no? I just . . . I haven't had the house to myself, you know . . . haven't gotten a chance to be alone in a really long time. I know that sounds selfish . . ." I trail off.

Violet stands in front of the couch and folds her arms. "We're best friends, right?" she asks softly.

My hackles are up. Why would she ask that now? "Yeah, of course we are," I answer genuinely.

"I would do anything for you. If something is going on, you can talk to me."

I look away, glancing at the clock above her head that's in the kitchen. I look back at her. I am careful not to rush my words. I absolutely cannot be defensive. "Why? Does it seem like there is something going on?"

"Not really. Not in a way that someone who didn't know you so well would pick up on. But you're acting different."

I breathe out slowly. *Heart rate!* I pause to keep it steady. I should have known Violet would sense something. She does know me better than anyone.

"Different how?" I respond as casually as I can. I purposely begin walking to the door, and she, taking the signal, begins to follow.

"I don't know—softer? Less conflicted?"

Well, I wasn't expecting that. I'm just happy she didn't say nervous or distracted. The idea that I am coming across as more easygoing is only going to help my case if Vi is questioned. I mentally curse myself for going to such a dark place.

"Oh. I guess I'm just happy to be on my own. There's always so much pressure with my family, to be normal. I think what you're picking up on is just . . . relief, really. Now I have fourteen whole days to let loose and not have to . . ."

"Lie?" Violet interrupts.

"Right. Exactly." There is a bit of an awkward silence. We are at the door now. It's past midnight. I know I should offer her a ride home, but I am reluctant to leave. Besides, if Vi hustles, she'll make it home before I could even fish out my car keys and lock up the house.

"Space. I get it. In theory, anyway. My parents are so wrapped up in their own shit all the time that I don't mind the double-life thing so much. Your mom and dad are really cool. I know how tough it is for you. But it will get easier once we graduate. Or lie about graduating, that is," Violet says with a laugh. She hugs me tightly.

I feel a pang, but I have to remember I am protecting her. I am doing what's best for her. Except that's not true, either—I'm lying to myself now. If I was to involve her in any of the Ezra business, it would only be because it would be better and easier *for me.*

I am a horrible friend.

I close the door behind her and turn off the lights. I sit back down on the couch. There is nothing to do but wait. I cannot sleep. I barely sleep on a good night. Tonight, it will be impossible. I am paranoid. I don't even bother turning the TV on. If anyone was to drive by my house they would see that almost every window is dark except for a hall light I've left on upstairs.

Time pulls and drags. Each minute stretches out like a rubber band, then snaps back and smacks me when I realize that only one has passed. As a Citadel, I am often asked to simply sit and wait in silence. In fact, I would even go as far as to say that I'm pretty much an expert at it. This is different. I don't feel like a soldier. I feel like a girl waiting for the guy she likes to show up. I throw my head into a cushion. This is absolutely the wrong thing to be thinking. I have to somehow rid myself of these feelings I have for Ezra. Stupid. I might as well wish for an invitation to Hogwarts. *Why do I always go to Harry Potter when I'm feeling stressed out? It's not like Harry Potter's world is peril-free. . .*

Great, now even my mind is rambling.

The hours pass. I see the first flush of gray in the sky. I start to worry. I try to calculate how long it should have taken him to get from the Village to my house: It's about ten miles from the Village to the base. It's another ten from Camp Bonneville to my house. Twenty miles in the dark with little to no survival skills. Twenty miles without my endurance or speed. But if he left when it first got dark, and it's now five A.M., that's almost twelve hours. It shouldn't take that long.

Should it?

An hour later, I begin to pace. I have to go to work at seven thirty. I can leave the back door open, but really, I don't know how I'm going to get through an entire day of not knowing. I don't have a choice, though—Citadels don't get sick days, because we don't get sick.

I go upstairs to shower and change. This time I switch it up with jeans and a T-shirt with a different cardigan. Man, my wardrobe is lackluster. I guess that's for the best, given the circumstances. I make some coffee, eat some oatmeal. It's almost seven now—shit. Where is—

Then suddenly, I hear a slight tap on the kitchen door. It's him. I practically trip over myself to open it and there he is. I let out a breath I didn't know I was holding.

"Oh my God," I sigh. I pull him in with my thumb and index finger, careful not to touch anything but the fabric on his jacket. The magnitude of what we've done makes me momentarily dizzy. It's all well and good that he wants to rewire me, fix me, but if I break his neck or slice open one of his arteries before that can happen, it will all have been for nothing. He could be on his way to living a whole new life right now. Instead, he's here.

Why did I agree to this?

I search his face for trepidation or fear, but all I can see is a look of excited defiance. I realize that he wouldn't be anywhere else. In the same way that I won't remove my chip when I'm thirty, he could never lead a normal life now. He's seen too much. He's a scientist. He wants to know why and how. He wants to know it all. Even though I have to be even more careful of every move I make now, I ache to put my arms around him. I can't. He won't. We just stand there like a couple of morons. "You did it," I finally say.

He drops his knapsack and I can see he's exhausted. "I can definitely scratch 'break out of a prison camp' off the bucket list."

"Go sit down and I'll make you some coffee." Ezra doesn't argue. Instead, he falls backward into the couch with a whoosh. "Tell me how it went, but I don't have long. I have to leave for work in half an hour."

"It went totally as planned. I left my tracker in my bed. I walked out of the house. I jogged to The Menagerie. I have been jogging every morning for the past month, by the way, so my endurance isn't terrible."

"That was smart," I tell him while pouring out coffee into a cup. "I'll let you make your own breakfast after I leave, unless you're starving. I just want to hear what happened, and there isn't much time."

"No, I'm fine for now. I grabbed something when I was in Portland."

I walk over to him and hand him the coffee. I put one hand on my hip. That wasn't part of the plan. *Be cool, calm down.* I can feel the screechy voice coming on. I have a sudden urge to put my hands on him, but there is *nothing* sexual about it this time. "Portland? Are you crazy? Do you know how many cameras there are in Portland? And cops? Why did you go there? *How* did you get there?"

"I stole a car and drove there." Ezra smiles at me. Smugly. *He's proud of it. This stupid son of a—*

I try to take a deep, cleansing breath. "You . . . stole a car? Did you manage to run over any hookers or shoot a drug lord while you were at it?" Apparently the cleansing breath didn't help. "I mean, you *do* get that you aren't actually a criminal, right? Why would you take such a risk?" I sit down in a chair, not beside him on the couch. I am far from pleased.

I am also apparently the queen of understatements.

"Okay," he says, "first of all, just back off a little, all right?"

I bite my lip. I am not used to anyone besides Applebaum telling me what to do. It feels weird and irritating.

Understatement. Again!

"Second of all, in order for this thing to work between us"— Ezra gestures with both of his hands back and forth, implying the connection—"you are going to have to trust me and you are going to have to let go of the notion that you are always going to be the smartest one in the room. Admittedly, there are things that you are going to know that I am not going to have a clue about, but there's other stuff that *I* am going to be the expert in. That's why we are going to succeed. Our strengths and weaknesses balance each other out. But if you start second-guessing everything I do, without even giving me time to explain, then we are fucked. Got it?"

He's being bossy and domineering. I find this to be simultaneously rude and totally hot. Well, of course. I'm me— I wouldn't fall for some spineless guy. An alarm bell mentally blares in my head. I am not *falling* for Ezra. No way. I have feelings for him, lusty ones, and obviously there is a connection. But it's a connection that cannot be explored in any way, shape, or form. Unless, of course, he can get my implant rewired—then, whew . . .

No. I can't go there. Not yet.

"You're right," I concede. "I'm sorry. Go ahead."

"So we have limited access to the Internet at the Village. I hacked into the system, but not very well. I wanted them to find all my search histories about survival skills and orienteering and auto theft, but I wanted it to look like I was hiding those searches." Ezra pauses and takes a long sip of coffee. "I got through the forest. Wasn't easy, got turned around a bit, but I made it. Then at the first sign of civilization—a house, actually—I stole the car. It was easier than the forest part."

"Great," I mutter, looking at my watch.

"Then I drove to Portland, dumped the car at the bus station, and bought three different bus tickets to three different destinations."

Again with the smug face. We are going to have a talk about that if we are laying ground rules. It won't do if half the time I'm slapping that expression off of him.

"No one asked why you were buying all those tickets?" I wonder.

"I just said I hadn't made up my mind yet. They really aren't that curious at the bus station, funnily enough."

It's almost time for me to go. "So how did you get back here?"

"Good old public transportation."

I clench my teeth. I am not going to freak out, but taking public transportation was a seriously dumb move. "You realize there are cameras on those things, right?" I say it passively, though it is taking a fair bit of my willpower not to turn into the incredible screeching woman again.

"Of course." The way he throws that out, so nonchalantly, it's almost as if he's exasperated with *me*.

It's not like I was the one gallivanting through public places just days before a massive manhunt starts up.

I force myself to focus on what he's saying.

". . . bought the tickets I made sure the cameras at the depot caught me. I was wearing a coat and a very bright red baseball cap. When I exited through the back of the depot and came out on the street again, I gave that coat and hat to a homeless guy and put on this very dapper knitted cap and a different jacket when I got on the train. I got up here. And then walked to your house. Ta-da!" Ezra is smiling, but he looks exhausted. I have to hand it to him. He did it. He also left a false trail, which might actually buy us some more time.

Whole hours, in fact.

But there isn't much to do about it now. And we still—hopefully—have a day or so before anyone even notices he's gone. So I'll let him have his little victory.

"That was good work and smart thinking. Let's go upstairs and I'll show you your room." Ezra stands without saying anything. In all likelihood it is all catching up to him now. He needs rest and some time to adjust. I show him the bathroom and give him a towel. I'm sure he'll want a shower before he gets into bed. Then I pull down the metal stairs from the linen closet. He looks at the narrow opening and then back at me.

"If you're going to make an Anne Frank joke, please don't because I really, really love Anne Frank," I say before he can say anything.

"I wasn't going to. I think I was going more toward a Hunchback of Notre-Dame thing. But no, this is good. Scary, but good." We climb the stairs and I show him the bookshelf. He is duly impressed and it's my turn to be just a bit smug.

"I hope this stuff of my dad's will be okay. There's a lot there and I did buy a one-terabyte drive, which I didn't think would be too suspect." We stand facing one another in the small space. I am acutely aware of the bed. Of *him*. He smells like the forest, loamy and just a little smoky, as if some far-off bonfire had found him somehow in the woods.

"I'll have a better idea once I start working. Thanks, Ryn.

Really. I would hug you, but . . . well . . . you probably need to go, right?"

I nod slowly and cross my arms. Things are strained between us. He's had a glimpse of the monster inside of me and he is wary, as he should be. I am relieved and heartbroken all at once.

"Are you ready for what you've got to do?" he asks tentatively. His eyes change. He looks pained. It dawns on me that this is his worry face. He's worried for me. For what I have to do today.

"I am. And if nothing happens when I'm on duty, then I will make something happen during training." I begin to walk down the stairs and Ezra follows me so that now we are both on the landing.

"All right, well, I'm going to use your facilities." He gestures toward the bathroom door.

"Have fun with that," I respond with a bit of sass. I turn to go, but Ezra stops me.

"Hey," he says with that same worried look. "Make sure you get hurt, but don't get hurt so bad that . . . well . . . I don't know. Just be careful getting your ass kicked."

CHAPTER 12

We've been on duty for an hour. The Rift has already opened and dumped out a few alligator-type things. Violet tranqued one from up here in Nest 6. They were dragged off by the Zoology Team and now we are waiting to see what else will come through today. Actually, it would be more accurate to say the rest of the team is waiting; I am trying to work out which part of my body will be the least useful over the next few days.

When Ezra and I discussed the implant—or, more accurately, *rewiring* the implant—I told him everything I knew about it. It took speaking about the chip with a civilian to make me realize how little I know about the thing that is responsible for who I am. In a way, the implant is like a bizarre, electronic parent.

When I explained about the magnetized disks they put on the chip to run diagnostics, Ezra told me that it was imperative we get one. Although I am fairly sure they store the disks in Medical, I don't know exactly where they are kept. That night in the Village I reluctantly admitted to Ezra that the only way I could get close to a disk safely was to get an injury. He didn't get it. How could getting hurt be safer than sneaking around an infirmary? Ezra doesn't know the layout of the bunker or how insanely guarded it is. I just told him that I was going to do it. End of story.

I couldn't tell him how I really felt. That I would take a hundred blows and kicks and punches—a thousand, even—just to be able to touch him, to kiss him, to lay my head down on his chest. I'm not a masochist; I don't enjoy pain, but I would take more than my fair share if it meant even the slightest chance that things could be different. A concussion is nothing compared to struggling against the Blood Lust. Ezra thinks he understands it because of what happened that night, but he has no idea how little of it he actually got to see, how deep it runs. We destroy, but we can't love the way people are really meant to. There is no balance, and so I think each of us, in our own way, is going slowly insane.

How do you explain that to someone who hasn't experienced it?

"*Come on*, Ryn, you have to play."

It's Boone, snapping me from my reverie. For the past ten minutes he has been at me to play one of his favorite games. I keep hoping that if I don't say anything or change the subject he'll let it go, but there's no way. Boone is like a dog on a fetch loop when he wants something. "Henry is no fun. He ends up choosing to kill everyone."

"That's because we would kill everyone, no matter what. It's pointless," Henry snaps back.

Boone lifts up a knee and casually rests his arm on it. "It's a *game*, Henry. You're supposed to use your imagination. I don't understand why you don't have one. It's like a birth defect."

"Well, I'm imagining all the ways I could beat the shit out of you right now," Henry tells him with a stony face. "Does that count?"

"That was a joke! Ryn, did you hear that? Henry made a funny!" Boone seems to be the only one laughing, but still he continues. "And if Violet goes first we'll be here till next week. She always takes too long to decide."

"That's only because you bring inappropriate names into the mix, like Jesus or Buddha. You can't do that. If you could be less sacrilegious, then maybe I wouldn't take so long," Vi counters. She crosses both her legs and her arms. She's not pouting exactly, but it's close.

"Fine, no gods. But you're still going last, Vi." Boone rubs his hands together like a Bond villain. "Okay, here we go, Ryn. Fuck, Marry, Kill: Gandhi, Eleanor Roosevelt, Christian Bale. Go."

I have about as much desire to take part in this game as Henry does, but I have a part to play. Violet has already noticed a change in my behavior. I can't afford any more inconsistencies.

"Are we talking *American Psycho* Christian Bale or *The Machinist* Christian Bale?" I manage to answer with a little smile on my face.

"Ohhh, that's a good question. And I like how you didn't bring Batman CB into the mix, 'cause it's so obvious. You're really thinking about this. You're *committed*." Boone draws out the last word while looking directly at Henry, who just rolls his eyes. Before he can elaborate, though, we hear the voice of a team leader down on the ground. The Rift is opening. With-out saying anything further, we all jump up and stare into the shimmering green light, watching it morph and change. We have a fairly obstructed view with the trees, but we can see it well enough to know when it gets to Stage 4.

I can sense the change in the air. That same sweet pull down toward my abdomen. I have goose bumps. The hair on the back of my neck stands up. Out of the gaping, black center comes a large number of people. By a quick estimation, I would say at least thirty. Upon first glance, they look human. I grab the binoculars to get a better look. Yes, human men and women, but they are disproportionately good-looking. I wonder if The Rift opened up at Paris Fashion Week. They are all insanely, weirdly, gorgeous. Yet while their hair is all different shades, their skin is the same: alabaster, smooth, and fair. The clothes they are wearing are modern, but there is something about them, something not right.

"*Unde Sutem?*"

"*Ceea ce sa întâmplat?*"

"*Este toată lumea în condiții de siguranță?*"

We hear them speak calmly to one another. Too calmly. It's unnerving. They are speaking a language I don't know. Some of it sounds familiar, like Latin, but I don't understand the words. I look at my team. It's The Five—we can't speak—so we keep a whiteboard up here for situations just like this. Henry grabs the board and begins to write. He holds it out. It says *Romanian*. Then he writes that they are just asking where they are and if everyone is okay. He is straining to listen.

"*Simt miros de sânge,*" one of them says quite loudly. The rest of them go still. Henry gets an odd look on his face and starts to translate on the board. "*Am auzit batai de inima, multe, nu-i așa?*" Henry scribbles furiously, then holds up the sign:

I smell blood

I hear many heartbeats

Boone gets the same look on his face that a ten-year-old boy would on Christmas morning with a new bike under the tree. He mouths slowly so we can all understand him:

"Are those motherfucking vampires?" We all look at each other. Baffled. Before any one of us gets a chance to answer, one of the supermodels scrambles up Nest 3. She moves fast, as fast as any one of us. We hear a scuffle and then one of the Citadels plummets to the ground. I had a plan to get hurt today.

I think this qualifies as a "be careful what you wish for" scenario.

We wait to get the Go signal from base. The four of us are standing, ready to attack. Vi has her rifle aimed. Henry's fists are curled up, his back is tensed—he's about to pounce. Boone, on the other hand, is practically squirming. I can tell he is dying to crack a joke. He opens his mouth.

"Don't," I hiss.

"Oh, come on," he whispers forcefully. "It's vampires, *I have to.*"

I roll my eyes and sigh. Each of us deals with these things in our own way. "Just one," I concede.

Boone grins and nods his head. Finally we get the go-ahead from Command, but Boone gets it in before we all leap off.

"See? This is why I was always Team Jacob." He jumps down. We all follow.

"Twilight? Really? That's what you're going to go with? The entire vampire canon and that's what you choose?" I say as we land. He just shrugs at me. From above, Violet shoots one of them in the chest. The guy startles, but he doesn't seem all that dazed. Now that I'm this close, the elongated fangs that spill out over their bright red lips are unmistakable. I have seen a lot during my time as a Citadel, but this? This is over the top. If we weren't in so much danger I would actually be laughing. I guess it's not impossible that there would be a humanoid

species that lives off blood. But if that's the case, why aren't they burning up in the sunlight? It occurs to me that it's stupid to think that anything about vampire lore on this Earth would apply to a species on another version of Earth. Evolution just doesn't work that way.

The other Citadels have charged, but whatever these things are (and okay, let's call them vampires for lack of a better word), they are fast and strong. We are about evenly matched, and I can't remember the last time that has happened. There are more of us, so it stands to reason that we will win. That doesn't mean that this is going to be easy.

Suddenly, I am face-to-face with a super sexy vampire guy. He has dark brown hair and violet-colored eyes. His features are chiseled enough to remind me of Superman. He has a cheeky kind of a smile on his face, and it takes me a moment to figure out why. Then it hits me.

Oh, God—he's excited. *This is* fun *for him. Great.*

Of course, he probably took one look at me and thought I might be a dainty little morsel, like a finger sandwich or one of those French multicolored cookies. And I realize something: this might actually be fun for me, too. I smile back . . . and punch him in the face. He doesn't move.

Not good.

He responds by backhanding me hard enough to launch me into the air and onto my back. I spring up off my hands to face him again. He lunges, I dodge. I throw a punch, he whizzes out of the way. He kicks me, I manage to grab his foot and throw my full weight into his shin, hoping to break a bone. It doesn't break. I raise an eyebrow and we circle each other for a couple seconds. The thought occurs to me that I actually have no idea how to best this dude. He's stronger than me and a damned good fighter. The only thing I have is the element of surprise.

I leap up and straddle him with my legs. I wrap both arms around him and lick my lips. This wasn't exactly how I imagined this would be, but given my particular life, it totally figures. My instincts were right—he is somewhat shocked, but I can tell by the look in his eye he's not entirely displeased. He smells amazing, an odd mix of blackberries and sea salt. I breathe him in. He slides his hands up my thighs and cradles my bottom in his palms. I have never been this close to a man in my life and I can feel the Blood Lust inside me building, fueling my power.

"Kiss me," I whisper, but I don't wait for an answer. Instead, I touch my lips to his. I would have been more aggressive, but considering he has fangs and all—and I've never actually kissed anyone—I do my best. I hear him growl inside my mouth. God, I am a sick person, but this guy is hot and I can't deny that the whole experience is, in its own way, kind of a turn-on. No, scratch that—a massive turn-on.

Which is exactly what I am hoping for.

The fury explodes in my limbs and I squeeze harder, my mouth still on his. I feel his body tense and then scramble to get me off of him, and he manages to throw me. I feel like nothing in the world can stop me. I've never let this anger run its course and it feels wickedly good. I am panting now. I want to rip him apart. I ache to kick him in the chest so hard that his sternum breaks. My strange behavior has thrown him off balance and he is not prepared for the solid punch I land to his temple. He staggers a bit. I punch him again with an upper cut and he tries to shake it off. He looks at me with narrowed eyes. I see desire and rage.

Perfect—I feel the same way.

He runs at me, and I leap up over him, somersaulting in the air and landing behind him. I could take out my knife or my gun, but I don't want to. I want to kill him with my bare hands. I have never felt so strong in my life. I know I could crush his windpipe if I get close enough . . .

And then I remember Ezra, the implant, the disk. I have to let him hurt me. I feel like that's impossible. I can't let the Blood Lust go. I'm on fire. The vampire uses my momentary distraction to pick me up and throw me as if I was nothing but a rag doll. I land in the soft peat. He hasn't hurt me. Not even a little. I spring up again and then jump to a low-hanging branch above me. I use the momentum from swinging to hit him hard in the stomach. It works. Finally he's down.

My rational mind is screaming to get injured. My body is literally trembling to hurt him. I scramble over to where he is in a flash. I am straddling him again now, me on top. I hear him laugh and say something in his own language. He's not scared of me. In fact, if I'm not mistaken—and based on what I am feeling beneath me, I'm not—he's pretty excited. It must be so simple for him. He wants blood and sex. I want everything. I want to hurt him, kill him, kiss him, undo his pants, press his eyeballs back into their sockets, lick him, strangle him, and let him hurt me. It's too much. I try to pin his hands down, but instead he rolls me over so that he's on top of me.

I have never felt the weight of a man this way, between my legs; it's foreign and strange. He absolutely should not be here, but I can't help the feeling that this is exactly where I want him to be. I don't know if it's my screwed-up wiring, or his exotic strangeness, or that finally, somehow, I am getting this kind of physical contact. He grinds against me slowly. It feels so good, and I am ashamed and furious. I buck my hips to try to get him off of me, but since I have zero experience in the sex department, it takes me a few seconds to understand that I am only making things worse. I stop and stare into his deep violet eyes. There is only one way I am going to win today. I go perfectly still. While my body is retreating into opossum mode, however, my mind has other plans. I close my eyes and turn away from his beautiful face, exposing my neck. I can feel my jugular beating from the exercise and the adrenaline. He sees it. I know he does. I feel his mouth on my skin. His breath is hot, his lips are almost gentle at first. He kisses me and the only thing stopping me from raging against him is that my base instincts have strategically retreated and are waiting for another opportunity to fight back. My brain knows the truth of it. When his teeth sink into my vein, I involuntarily groan. It's painful, yes, but it's something else, too. It is dark and savage and . . . hot. Nice girls don't want to be hurt this way. I am not nice. Maybe this is all I deserve in the end. I could take out a weapon, shoot him in the forehead or cut his throat. The only reason I've engaged him hand to hand is so that I could get injured. The only reason I want to get injured is so that I can do this for real, without the violence. The irony of this is not lost on me as I feel the sticky blood he is sucking out of my neck trickle down behind my ear. I am suddenly very tired. It all seems pointless now. The edges of the forest blur and darken. The tension I've been holding in my body evaporates completely. If I was all alone I know I would be dead soon. I don't even really care that much.

"Jesus, Ryn, what the hell?" someone says—Boone, I think—from somewhere behind me. I hear a thump, and the weight of the man who was between my legs is gone in an instant. I struggle to look around, but it's impossible with my eyes closed. I want to open them, but I don't have the strength. I feel pressure on the wound on my neck and some other loud voices. I want to tell them all to shut up so I can sleep, but my mouth isn't working, either.

I drift in and out of consciousness. I feel myself being lifted off the battlefield and onto a stretcher. The medic shoves a needle into my arm, I assume to replenish the blood that has been taken. I feel the movement of the van. We are speeding back to base. The momentum of the car makes my body sway. It's almost like being rocked. I manage to open my eyes once I am in the infirmary. I catch a glimpse of Edo. When I hear the click of the disk over my implant, I smile weakly.

"Do not try to be brave, Citadel Ryn. You have lost much blood."

I see the concern on her face. I don't care about the blood. I don't care about whatever pervy thing just happened out there by The Rift. The first part of my plan has worked—not, I'll admit, that it was much of a plan. Edo and a doctor begin repairing the vein in my neck. I don't even feel the sutures they are sewing. There's nothing more that I can do at this point. I know they have drugged me to keep me from moving. This is part of my plan, too. I give in to the blackness that has wanted to take me ever since the vampire first put his mouth on my neck. I sleep.

For hours.

It takes only a few seconds for me to get my bearings once I wake up. Loss of blood is not the same as a bump on the head, which is good—I need to be on my game. Edo. She looms over me; her eyes are so blue they look neon. It is hard to read the face of someone who has so little expression. Edo's features are set somewhere between exasperation and worry. I think.

"Citadel Ryn, you were injured most grievously," Edo rasps. The gorgeous face of the vampire flashes through my mind. I shift my body uncomfortably. He's probably dead now. "Why did you not use a weapon? Why did you try to fight him with nothing?" Edo's small, childlike hands flutter around her.

"Let me *ask you* a question," I say, staring directly at her, "where do you live?"

She pauses for a moment and then cocks her head to one side. "I live here, at Camp Bonneville. Seventy-three Roones came through all those years ago, and we are scattered equally among the fourteen Rift sites. Why?" She has taken a step back. The concern, or what I may have taken for concern, has left her face.

"Why don't you live in the Village?" I ask her directly.

Edo sighs impatiently. "Because our talents are needed here. Why are you asking these questions when you should be resting? Why does it matter where I live?"

"Because you're a person. Because we did something—us, *perfect* humans that ARC is trying to turn every sentient Immigrant into. We sucked you out of your world and put you in this place, this prison, where you aren't even allowed to speak your own language. Doesn't that piss you off? Why do you even help us?" I hadn't meant to say that. I basically just admitted that I'd been to the Village. It must be the drugs. My words are embers, like shooting sparks. I shake my head. I need to shut up, but when I look at Edo, I feel unsure about everything.

"I am surprised, Citadel Ryn, to hear you speak this way. It was the Roones, after all, who placed the device in your body that made you what you are. Made you into the kind of girl who, for a few short seconds of intimacy, would wrap her legs around a blood-sucking creature who might well have killed her. In the face of that, what difference does it make where I lay my head at night? I rarely sleep."

I turn my head away, wincing slightly at the pain in my neck. I feel the tears well up, but I keep them pooled beneath my lids. Clearly I am sensitive right now—I guess the pain, blood loss, and drugs will do that. I have to keep it together. I have to get home today.

"Ryn," Edo says, and I feel a slight weight on the edge of the bed. "We all have our parts to play in this. The Immigrants in the Village give up their customs and beliefs. Citadels give up their adolescence; sometimes they even give up their lives. We Roones give up every spare moment we have to find the best solution to each new problem The Rift presents us with."

I clench my eyes shut and then rub them with my thumb and index finger. Does Edo really care about me? I want to believe it so bad. I want to believe that all of this is for the greater good. And since she's not lecturing me about the Village, it must mean she doesn't care that I broke in there. But if Ezra is right, then the Roones must be helping ARC with whatever it is that they are hiding. Because clearly the biggest problem with the Rifts—the fact that they exist at all—isn't being worked on by anyone, let alone the Roones.

"Well," I concede quietly, "I guess the Citadels are a necessary evil. Emphasis on *evil*. It's torture. But I am not convinced that every other species that comes through The Rift should have to give up who they are to feed into some grand delusion ARC has, or that by doing so they'll become less threatening. Why are they so afraid of everyone who's different? It doesn't seem smart, not if you're playing the long game."

Edo stares off and looks past me, as if she can see through the wall behind my head. "Fear can be good, Citadel. Fear drives the instinct to run from a fight you cannot win."

"Agreed," I say as I sit up. "But fear creates monsters. Fear created me. Fear fuels angry mobs, starts wars, and lets the powerful keep the powerless down. Ethically . . . wait, do ethics even apply anymore?" I huff out my breath in a single laugh. "I'm not sure we're the good guys. I don't think what we are doing with the Immigrants is right."

"The Village is not a bad place. Humanity has its flaws, but for the most part, you are a good and honorable people. I have seen far more of the other species, in much more detail, than you have. I have studied them at length, and so my opinion on this matter is based on both observation and research. The concept of humanization creates community and cohesion. It allows an Immigrant to focus on our shared similarities instead of highlighting our vast differences. Humanization is the best solution." Edo is smiling without showing me her teeth.

"You're lying," I tell her abruptly, because suddenly I don't feel like dancing around some version of the truth. For some reason, I want her to know that I see what others can't or won't. I don't know why. Maybe I'm testing her. Maybe I'm just tired of hiding so much of myself away. When I think about it, it's probably a version of both.

Edo stands up and backs away from the bed. "What?"

"You. Are. Lying. Your super-ninja box-chip thingy has given me many gifts, but the ability to lie and to catch the lies of others—that's my own special talent based on both *observation and research*, not to mention years of fieldwork. You aren't being honest with me, and that's okay because it doesn't really matter what either of us thinks. We can't change anything. We can only do our jobs."

Edo looks away and with a single finger taps the electronic pad she is holding. She is making it clear she no longer wants to have this conversation, which works for me. "I need to go to the bathroom." I sit up fully and swing my legs over the side of the bed.

"I can help you, or I can get a nurse."

"No." I cut her off harshly. "I can manage on my own. Take the IV out. I don't need it."

Edo looks me up and down, studying me as I stand here. She walks over and removes the tape from the skin on my arm and then slowly slides out the needle.

"Thank you," I say, and I mean it. It really doesn't matter if she is being honest with me. Edo has always been good to me. She has always been kind when the other Roones have only been cold and condescending.

I walk to the bathroom and close the door. I sit on the toilet and start to pee. I reach back and grab the disk from my neck. I was hoping that maybe I would have been injured just enough to keep my uniform on. No such luck; they must have removed it in my sleep. I am in a hospital gown. There is nowhere for me to hide the disk. Thankfully, I had a contingency for this, too. I take some toilet paper and wrap it around the small silver piece of metal. I relax and shove the wad of toilet paper up inside of me. It feels like a tampon, sort of. I am annoyed that I have to resort to this. I wait a few seconds, flush the toilet, and open the door with a contrite look on my face.

"I'm so sorry, Edo," I say genuinely.

Immediately she is suspicious. "Why?"

"I forgot I had the disk on my neck and I went to feel my wound and it went flying. I looked all around for it. I heard it drop. I thought it dropped on the floor but I think it flew into the toilet. I flushed it while I was looking around the bathroom. I could be wrong, but I don't see it anywhere." This is a good lie. I am calm. I am genuinely sorry because I don't like lying to Edo. But I'm good at it regardless. I maintain eye contact. I make sure my facial expression matches my words. I do not blink rapidly or look away or fidget.

"That's all right, Citadel. We have many. Do not worry your-self about it." Edo really doesn't seem to mind at all. There is something, though, a look in her great big luminous eyes, that doesn't sit well with me. Maybe she knows I'm lying and is happy to cover for me. Maybe it is something else entirely.

"I'd like to go home," I tell her.

"That's fine. I have recommended to Colonel Applebaum that he should give you and your team the day off tomor-row. It was a particularly difficult fight this morning." Edo is checking her pad; she has a small frown on her brow.

"Is everyone else on the team okay?" I ask, mentally chid-ing myself for not asking sooner.

"Bumps and bruises. Citadel Boone was distraught when he saw the parasite sucking on your neck. He was quite afraid you would become 'a creature of the night,' whatever that is. I requested the time off for psychological reasons, not phys-ical ones."

I walk toward the small wardrobe to the left of the bed. When I open it I see that my street clothes have been put inside.

I grab the pants off the shelf and quickly pull them up, under the hospital gown. "Oh, yeah. I guess I *could* turn into a vampire. But wouldn't I need to have had some of his blood? I mean, I don't feel any different, but given what I'm already capable of, maybe I wouldn't even notice."

"The species you encountered today was born with a chro-mosomal deficiency that requires them to ingest the addi-tional white blood cells found in blood to boost their immune system. There is nothing supernatural about them. We tested your combatant's body for several diseases that could be transmitted via saliva and found none. I do not understand the mythology around this species. I apologize."

I quickly throw on my sports bra and T-shirt. The first guy I ever kissed and now he's dead. I hope it's not some kind of an omen.

"Great. Thanks for checking and sewing me up and everything." I walk toward the door.

"Ryn," Edo rasps softly, and I turn. "Be careful."

"Be careful with what?" What *exactly* is she talking about?

"You aren't completely healed. That's all. Try to rest."

She smiles at me. I walk out of the room. Edo has just lied. Again. I can't say how or why I know, but she wasn't talking about my injuries.

CHAPTER 13

I walk through my front door in the late afternoon, and even though I am not remotely hungry, I remember that I am sharing my house with someone. I will just order a pizza. I don't have the energy to reheat something, let alone cook. My phone has been going off since I retrieved it from my locker. The team wants to know how I am, wants to know if they can come over. They also want to know if I have a sudden aversion to crosses and garlic. That's mostly Boone. I have put them all off, as nicely as possible. They cannot come here. They also cannot know why.

I lock the door behind me and climb up the stairs. I go to the bathroom, remove the disk, and then go to my bedroom to change into sweats. I pull down the ladder to the attic and make my way up loudly enough to let Ezra know I'm coming. When I get to Ezra's room he looks up at me and smiles with obvious relief. There are papers everywhere. The whiteboard he asked me to get him is already covered with formulas. He is so beautifully disheveled that I have to clench my fists just to fight the urge to touch him somewhere, anywhere—I've lost too much blood already today. I manage to keep a safe distance.

"What happened? Are you okay?"

I can see that he, too, is having a hard time staying in his seat, not getting up to check me, hug me. I flush when I see his concern, but of course, I have to ignore it.

"I'm fine." I show him the bandage on my neck. "So . . . it was vampires. Today. I mean, I'm pretty sure they don't call themselves 'vampires.' But that's what they looked like. One of them bit me."

He immediately gets up off his seat and folds his arms. Then he cranes his own neck to look at mine. "Seriously?" He doesn't even try to hide his amusement. I can tell that he is struggling not to laugh.

"Yes, and if you call me Sookie I will hit you in the face."

Ezra does nothing but raise his eyebrows. "Were they like Nosferatu vampires, or Count Dracula types, or eeesh . . . Were they sparkly?"

"They were extremely good-looking, pale-skinned people with fangs. And I don't want to talk about it. *Ever*. I got the disk." I open my palm and he walks over to me and grabs the quarter-sized object. He holds it up and squints at it.

"Huh," he manages to say.

"Well . . . *That's* a super-encouraging observation. Please tell me that I didn't let some guy suck me off for nothing." I wince as soon as the words leave my mouth. "That came out wrong. You know what I mean."

Ezra grimaced. "Unfortunately, yes. I know exactly what

you mean and, also unfortunately, there is no way that I can unhear that sentence or unsee the lovely visual that accompanied it." Ezra circles the silver disk with his thumb. "I'm going to need some time with this. I have to find a way to take it apart and run some diagnostics. It's a good thing I asked you to get all those 'nerd tools,' as you called them." Ezra takes the disk back to his desk and begins examining it under a large magnifying glass, the round kind, with attached lights.

"No, I think it was actually *you* I was calling a nerd and a tool."

"Ha, funny. I want to get started on this right away. Why don't you take this flash drive with all the Immigrant languages files you asked me to hack? I know you'd probably prefer me to just download them into your brain *Matrix*-style, but since you have a photographic memory, it might actually be quicker for you to go the old-school route. I also printed out that list that you wanted, which I kind of wanted to ask you about. But first, should I sharpen this pencil into a stake?" he says, holding up a no. 2. "Just in case you don't like my line of questioning?"

"Aww, honey, if you want me to break your fingers, all you need to do is run them through my hair," I say with a sadistic grin on my face.

Ezra pales.

"Too much?" I ask, only half joking.

"Yeah, a little."

"Sorry. It was a weird day. Ask me whatever you want."

Ezra gets up once again and walks toward me with some papers and the flash drive.

"You wanted all the names of the Immigrants in the Village who have been charged with at least one violation of non-cooperation of the humanization agenda. I just want to know why. I mean, I think I know, but I also think it's important for us to be absolutely clear and up front about everything."

I take the papers from his hands, as well as the flash drive. "I'm not going to free them, if that's what you're wondering. At least not yet." There are a few seconds of silence as Ezra eyes me warily.

"Come on, Ryn," he sighs. "People like me—actual people— okay. But snake people? Praying mantis guy? Out in the world they would create absolute chaos. I'm not saying I agree with how the ARC is handling this, but I don't think the species in the Village should just be let out to fend for themselves. They wouldn't last five minutes out in the real world."

I stare at him in disbelief. "Wow. Stockholm syndrome much?" I shake my head and put out my one empty hand as if to stop him from speaking further. "So only 'actual people' deserve freedom? On one hand humans are supposed to be the pinnacle of evolution, but on the other we can't trust them with the idea that there are other species on this planet without them all turning into KKK members? Which is it? You've spent time with other Immigrants: Do you think you're better than they are?"

Ezra's lips disappear into a thin, firm line. "I never said that. Don't put words into my mouth."

I'm frustrated and tired. It occurs to me that I am taking this out on Ezra. I have to stop making assumptions. I have to start being more empathetic but somehow stay unemotional. How am I supposed to do that? At the moment, everything feels impossible. "Look, I'm sorry . . . I don't know what you think. I don't even know what *I* think for sure. Relax—I'm not going to go all freedom fighter tomorrow and throw open the gates of the Village. But I don't like it there. The whole thing feels wrong, *instinctually*. And seeing as their best hope is a map to the Multiverse—which, let's be honest, could be years away, if ever—all I'm looking for is intel. If you get caught, if you have to go back, it might be nice to know that there are people there who we can trust."

Ezra nods his head slowly and then goes to sit back down. It's not good for us to be so close when the discussion is this heated. "Good call," he concedes. "Strategy. You're a soldier and I get that's what you do. I also know that you aren't used to people questioning you, but I'm always going to speak up if I feel like you're making a mistake. I don't follow orders. I take polite suggestions." Ezra grins charmingly, immediately lightening the mood.

"Great. I'm going down to my room. I'll bring up some dinner in a couple hours, so get cracking. *Please*." I start to move the bookshelf and then I turn away again to face him. "We've only got about fifteen or sixteen hours left before they realize you've gone. Ticktock, Ezra." I know I am being brusque, mostly because he's right. I'm not used to being questioned. I'm not used to feeling like I don't know what's going on. And I'm especially not used to feeling powerless.

I retreat into my room, put some music on, and look at the list. I don't recognize any of the names, except one: Zaka. This makes me smile. I knew there was something about him I liked. In honor of him, I start with the Sissnovar language. Ezra had been right. Although I would have preferred a direct download into my chip, I do have a photographic memory and an excellent ear. This will take time, but all things considered, maybe it should. Lately I've been thinking that I take entirely too much for granted. It's immature.

I start with the simple translations of nouns. I work up to verbs. I order the pizza and deliver it to Ezra, who has opened the disk but is so absorbed in it that he barely looks at me when I drop off his food. I work on the reptilian language through the night. I listen to the pronunciations included in the lexicon, saved as an endless stream of MP3s. I wonder about how this information is coded onto our chips and then routed through our brains. How does it work? It's so complex. How in the hell is Ezra going to figure it out in just a few days?

After about six hours, I have a solid grasp on the language. I could start another, but I decide to close my eyes for a bit. I think about what a crazy day it's been and mentally run through it. I stowed a hot guy fugitive in my attic, had my first kiss, was bitten by a vampire, got stitches in my jugular, and learned a new language. Impressive. I spend so much time being annoyed at having to lead a double life that it is only just recently occurring to me that it is actually twice as full as a regular person's life. I didn't choose it, but maybe it's time to start enjoying the things I can choose. I fall back on my bed and close my eyes. I am asleep in seconds.

I GUESS I MUST HAVE gotten a couple hours of sleep in when I hear Ezra's voice at my door. Wisely, he has chosen not to enter my room. He has not shaken me awake. I guess he's seen those movies, too, the ones where the war veterans always almost kill someone whenever they are awakened abruptly. I wouldn't have done anything—unless I was having a really saucy dream, which I'm pretty disciplined about not having. It's good that Ezra is following protocol with the not touching, although it might just be a few short hours until that's a thing of the past.

I know—I shouldn't let myself hope. But I do just the same.

"Ryn, wake up and come upstairs. I'm ready to run a diagnostic with the disk." I hear the exhaustion in his voice. I can only imagine how sleep deprived he must be. Once we're done, he has got to get some rest. I'm going to insist he gets at least ten hours. He probably won't listen to me, though. I'll have to ask nicely. Hey, if this works maybe we can get in bed together. Not for sex or anything, just holding and cuddling . . .

I roll my eyes. Not even I believe that one.

"Okay, I'm coming." I go to the bathroom and brush my teeth. I quickly examine the bandage on my neck. My super-stellar healing powers have kicked in. There is more suture than wound. Good. I know Ezra wants to get started, but we both need some coffee and food. I yell up into the attic that I'm going to get some and then I go down to the kitchen. I quickly assemble some toast and cereal. I put it all on a tray with the coffees I've made. I notice that Ezra has been down here at some point because little things are out of place. I check the dishwasher, where he has dutifully put his plates and cups. I'm so relieved he's not a slob. I had never really imagined what it would be like to share my life with a guy. Now that these odd circumstances have made that happen, it's hard for me to believe that I would even notice something as mundane as dirty dishes, but I'm a neat freak. I suppose your basic personality doesn't change even when you're thrown in the deep end of life-altering change.

It's not easy to manage the tray on the tiny ladder. I get near the top, then put the tray on the floor and shove it forward with my hands. I get the rest of the way up and retrieve the tray, backing into the bookshelf so that it swings open. I place the breakfast on the bed and notice that Ezra has set up the desk chair away from the monitors. Immediately, I wonder what it is that he doesn't want me to see. I have been happy this morning, hopeful. Now, looking at that chair, scuffed and wood worn, I realize that I might not like the answers

Ezra finds. There is a secret in my brain and it could reveal itself to be much darker than I ever imagined. I shouldn't be happy. I should be nervous as hell, and suddenly I am.

I say nothing as I sit down. I take my hair and scoop it up in my fingers, twisting it into a bun so that it's perched on the top of my head. Ezra stands in front of me. He's grabbed the coffee and is holding the mug in his hands. He looks worn. The purple smudge of bags beneath his eyes makes them look even bluer.

How is that even possible? How can exhaustion make this guy look even better? I'm supposed to be the superhuman here.

"First of all, I want to manage your expectations," he begins grimly. "I don't have an MRI machine or medical equipment. I won't be able to see the actual synapses firing in the exact locations inside your brain. What I have been able to do, though, is write a very basic program that will allow me to see—in binary only—the information that is being transferred from the disk. It will take me a while with that data to understand it enough to write more code. Nothing is going to change today. Baby steps."

I sigh. Of course. I don't know why I let myself get so excited. I look at Ezra, and the way he's looking back at me, and then I remember why I let myself get so excited. I sigh again. Ezra's going to need to hook me up several times to understand the complicated software in the chip.

"But you did manage to figure out how to use the disk to get my chip to talk to your computer. That's impressive, Ezra. It must have been difficult. Thank you." I hope he can't tell exactly how disappointed I am.

"It's a pretty complex little system, but what I'm going to do now, in layman's terms, is kind of like a jacked-up Bluetooth. Okay?" I nod. "Good—here we go." Ezra puts down his coffee and then picks up the disk off the desk. I know his first instinct is to attach it to me, but that would be a very bad idea. I don't want Ezra anywhere near the back of my neck. I hold out my hand and raise my eyebrows. He nods silently and I attach the disk. I hear the magnetic part of it make a little click. I sit very still.

Ezra moves behind me. I hear him typing. Over and over again his fingers tap on the keyboard. I wait five minutes and then ten. Ezra mutters to himself. His finger strokes seem to be more aggravated.

"Well," he says finally. "Shit."

I turn around. I wrap my legs around the front of the chair and put my arm on the back of it so that I can rest my chin there.

"What is it?" I stare at the monitors. They are blank.

"Pick up your foot," he commands.

I do so and we look at the screen. Nothing.

"Punch something in the air."

An odd request, but I do it, and still the screen remains blank.

"Okay, I'm going to try to get you to do something Citadel-ish. Can you do, like, a handstand on that chair?"

I don't say anything. Instead I move the chair away slightly and I grip the sides of it with both hands. I carefully lift myself off the floor, raising my legs as slowly as possible so that I don't knock anything over.

"Balance the other side, will you? With your arm or foot," I ask. I begin to slowly lift up a hand and quickly Ezra grabs the chair so that it doesn't tip over. I figure anyone, really, could do a handstand on a chair, but a handstand with only one hand—not so easy.

"You can come down now," Ezra says quietly.

I gently lower my hand and feet and then stand up. I push

the chair back to Ezra and he sits down on it. I sit on his bed and look at the toast. I am not hungry anymore. I know that something is wrong.

"It's not working, is it?" I manage to say softly.

"Ryn, the program works. The code is solid. I'm going to say something to you, and I'm going to need you to stay calm."

I narrow my eyes. I thought we had this discussion before. The worst thing you can say to someone is "stay calm." It never works. It just adds unnecessary drama.

"Fine."

"There is no signal emanating from the implant in your head. Well, there is, but it's not linked to your brain."

I lean forward in frustration. "I don't understand. There has to be a signal. You've seen what I can do. So, obviously, the Roone technology stumped you. It's no biggie. You need more time with it. Maybe I can even swipe something else from medical that will help," I offer. He's tired. After he gets some rest, he'll figure something else out.

"I am not *wrong*. I am telling you—I am linked to your implant. It is sending out a signal, but that signal is registering in a way that is not consistent with brain activity. There is nothing in your implant that is controlling a single one of your impulses."

"That can't be right."

"That's what I'm saying. But I started with basics. I should have been able to track your blood pressure or heart rate. Not in actual vitals, but in a binary that should have come up immediately. When you move, when you did that awesome thing with the chair—nothing. There is definitely a piece of hardware in your skull, but whatever it is, it's not giving you superpowers. It's not giving you anything."

I jump up off the bed, take off the disk, and put it back on the desk. "I don't get it," I say. "I think I would have remembered being bitten by a radioactive spider. Or how awesome it was being raised on Paradise Island with my Amazon sister Wonder Woman."

"This isn't funny," Ezra says with a groan.

"No," I say, all flippancy out of my voice, "it really isn't, Mr. MIT, Mr. I Can Fix You. *You* messed up somewhere. Obviously. I'm a cyborg, not a superhero." I fold my arms. He's wrong. He has to be. "Okay, then. Let's just, for arguments' sake, say that you're right. Explain how on Earth—and I mean literally, on this particular Earth—I could possibly do the things I do."

Ezra paces for a few seconds, then sits on the bed. He runs his hands through his hair and looks up at me. "Here's what's interesting to me about this. Your whole life is one giant lie. It's not just that no one in your family or your other friends know what you are, but they don't even know about the most significant scientific phenomenon in history that is just miles away from their own home." Ezra drums a single finger on his thigh. He's agitated, but he's playing it as cool as he can. I don't blame him. I wouldn't want to piss someone like me off, either. And he's certainly doing a better job at it than I am. "And then you have ARC," he continues, "your bosses, whose acronym alone sounds like a super-evil society. They put people in internment camps. They modify the prisoners' behaviors in an attempt to make every species they encounter human. They create teenage super soldiers who guard a portal to the Multiverse on the sly, but your first instinct is that *I'm* wrong."

I look down. I process what Ezra is saying. He is totally right. I've been sold on the whole idea of the implant for so long, I take it as a given. The most logical explanation is that it is, in fact—in the face of the evidence before us—a lie.

"So what did they do?" I ask, knowing that my voice sounds desperate and small.

"I don't know. Drugs? Gene therapy? Demonic posses-sion? I have no idea. I don't even have the equipment to try to figure it out. I'm sorry, Ryn." He *looks* sorry. He looks devastated. All he wants to do is help me. He's told me this incredible news and he can't even hug me, which right away makes me think harder.

I start to pace now: three steps forward, three steps back. "Wait—wait a minute. If there isn't a chip that's controlling my body, then why can't I, or we . . . How is it possible that we can't touch?"

"Again. I don't have the answer. But if it's not technologi-cal, then it's psychological. If it's psychological, then ARC did something . . . they—"

"Don't finish that sentence," I say quickly. I can't bear the thought of him saying what we both suspect. "Oh my God," I whisper. It's too terrible a thought. It's so ugly I almost want to faint.

"I am so sorry, Ryn." Ezra gets up off the bed. He reaches out to me. "Just. Let me . . ."

I jump back from him, my arms out, ready to push. "Don't," I say softly. "Don't even think about coming near me right now. If anything happened to you—now that I know it's not some evil thing in my head, but it's actually me, I couldn't live with myself. Not that I'm doing such a stellar job living with myself right now." I put my hand on the bookshelf. "I have to go." There is an ominous tone in my voice. I don't care.

"Where? I hope you're going to say 'Downstairs to my room,' because you need some space. That's what you're going to say, right?"

I turn to face him. I swore I would never lie to him. I am not about to start now. "For now, until it gets a little later. Then I'm going to the base. I'm going to find out the truth. For once."

"Hey," Ezra says worriedly. I turn and see that he is obviously afraid. "They'll know soon, that I'm gone. And that signal your implant is sending out? I'm almost positive it's a tracking signal."

"So what? I'm going into work. I know I got the day off, but I can say I don't feel well and want to get checked out." I'm clenching my fists. Why does he keep questioning everything I want to do? Does he not understand that I'm a soldier? My entire life revolves around strategic decisions, and quick ones at that. I know what I'm doing. I weighed the risks the moment I realized that Ezra was right about the implant.

"It means they know where you've *been*. It means they know you've been to the Village, to *my* house. Besides, what are you going to do there? Who is going to tell you the truth? We need to think of another plan. You need to steal files or I need to find a way in to their mainframe." His voice is calm, but his body language is rigid and tight.

"Ezra, it doesn't matter if they know I've been to the Village. If they can track me, they'll figure out that I wasn't anywhere near there when you left. I just don't have it in me to sit on my fucking hands and find out what I am from some damn file. I'm going back to the base because I want to confront the person, *the thing*, that did this to me. I want her to have to look me in the eye and explain. Try to get some rest. I'm serious, you need to sleep." I push the bookshelf open and make my way down to my bedroom.

It takes all my will to not look back.

I COLLAPSE ON THE BED and stare at the ceiling. What am I? A monster? A hero? A mutant? When I first saw the images from The Rift at basic training when I was fourteen, when I saw the Karekins literally tear apart soldiers, rip their limbs away as if it was nothing, I was frightened. But I was also angry. I could feel the power building inside of me. I knew I could do something. I knew I could save peoples' lives. I wasn't born special. I wasn't chic and mysterious like my mother. I wasn't cool and artistic like my dad. Abel, well, he was always good at everything. Me? I wasn't particularly pretty. I wasn't really good at anything except for reading. I sucked at math and sports. I couldn't sing or dance. I played the cello, badly. I didn't have a single thing that set me apart from anyone. I would mentally line up the lame-ass jobs I could have had as an adult. Desk clerk. HR middle management. Executive assistant. Although they wouldn't have been lame to me. They would have just been normal, because *I* would have been normal.

Maybe I've been blindsided by the power. I am a badass *and I enjoy it*. I do hate the lies. I hate seeing the fear on people's faces when they get dumped out of The Rift, but I really loved knowing that I was helping them. Little did I know I was packing them off to Martha Stewart World (with all the throw pillows and jail time that implies). I couldn't have known when I gently escorted them away from what I thought was the biggest danger, that I was actually sending them to be stripped of their lives, their identity, and of everything else that made them who they were, so that they could become more like me. Except that was a lie, too—they could never be like me. No one is like me, except the other Citadels, but even there, I am a team leader. I am one of the stars at ARC.

Everyone wants to be special. I want to be special. Maybe that's why it's taken me all these years to ask the questions I should have asked that very first day I found out what I was. I bitch and moan and complain about what they did to me, but would I really change it? I can't get laid. Big deal. Nuns don't get laid, you don't hear them whining about it. The truth is now I *have* to walk toward the truth. I *have* to face it. I wouldn't change what I can do for anything. I have to accept it and honor it. What I don't have to do is take a payment of total bullshit in return for the absolute loyalty I've shown ARC. I won't. I'm going to find out how exactly they turned me into what I am.

Even if it kills me.

CHAPTER 14

I tear into the parking lot of Battle Ground High and fly out of my car before the tires can shudder to a complete stop. I whip open the front doors of the school, noticing that the students are milling around. It's just before first bell. As I walk toward a couple of boys, I hear one of them say something about my ass. While I find this flattering, I have to say I don't appreciate the tone. I pick him up by the shirt with one hand until he's a couple inches off the ground.

"Do. Not. Objectify. Me." I let him go and he staggers but stays on his feet. "It's rude." I breeze past them. I know I don't need the added attention right now, but teenage boys, Jesus. If you want to talk about my body, at least say something smart. Something sexy. Internet porn has ruined everything.

I walk into the ARC section of the building and I wonder: Can I break in here if I have to? Why would I, though? If I really needed to get to base and/or The Rift, I could just drive and easily maneuver through the Camp Bonneville defenses, which are much more complicated than they look, but manageable. Yet that's how my mind works: assessing potential threats. And walking through the school, I'm realizing I now think of this place as a potential threat.

I go through the metal detector and then the eye scan. I wait for the train with many other Citadels. A few of them talk to me and I talk back, but I don't really engage. That's the thing about Citadels, though—we are supergood with boundaries, so I am mostly left alone. When the train stops, I follow everyone up the steps and watch them branch off into different directions, most headed for their locker rooms. I wonder if it wouldn't be a good idea for me to put my uniform on, or at least my training one on. Not only would it make me less conspicuous, but if I get into trouble, it could save me. Defiantly, I decide against it. If I'm going to do this, *face this*, then I want to be me—Ryn—and not a Citadel.

In order to get where I'm going, I have to walk past Applebaum's door. We all front and say we aren't intimidated by him, but on some level, we are. He is the patriarch of this place and no one likes disappointing Daddy. At the moment, I despise him, but still, I can't help it that I want to make him proud. It's just another sick thing I hate about this place. I wait for more than one or two troops to walk by. Then I hit the jackpot: four soldiers barreling up the hallway in a straight line. I quickly join their ranks at the far end. I'm so small compared to these guys that even if Applebaum was to look out of his glass office at that moment, he wouldn't see me.

Once I make it past him without discovery, I turn twice. I am now in front of the medical facility. I know there will be doctors and nurses there. Occasionally, there is another

Roone there, named Wyk, but he is more of a surgeon than a general healer like Edo. He rarely makes an appearance unless it's life or death. You'd think that might give him a severe case of the God complex. But Wyk rarely speaks, never smiles, and seems to have no emotions at all, let alone vanity.

I enter the double glass doors of Medical. There is no reception, just several exam rooms and two operating theaters. There are also several offices, none of which I have been in before, but I figure one of them has to be Edo's. I check the exam rooms first, all of which are empty. It's early; The Rift action must have been fairly tame last night and so far this morning it seems to have been the same. I peek my head through the glass windows of the operating rooms, and they are empty, too. I notice a sign that says EMPLOYEE LOUNGE over a single door. There's no way Edo will be in there. Roones don't socialize.

I begin to check offices. I walk into each one without knocking. The first two are empty. The second and third have doctors, but I quickly close the door before they can even say anything. In the fifth office sits Edo. She is behind a desk, working on a laptop. When she sees me, she keeps her face passive. Who knows what she could be thinking? That my neck is bothering me? Or maybe I have more questions about where she lives and the treatment of Immigrants. After I'm done with her, I'm sure she's going to wish that either were true.

"Citadel Ryn. Are you feeling all right?"

I like Edo. I really do, but in that moment it is taking everything I have not to pick up the chair closest to me and throw it at her. I must, at all costs, remain calm in order for this to work. In order for me to get the answers I want, each question must be absolutely precise and leave no room for vagaries.

I sit down in the chair across from her. "No," I answer stonily.

"I am sorry to hear that. Would you like to go to an exam room? I can call and have one prepped."

Edo picks up the phone, but before she can put in a number, I speak—in a low, threatening tone. "Put down the phone. Now." She clearly isn't scared. Rather, she seems curious. I don't know if this is a good or bad thing. Regardless, she hangs up. "We are going to have a conversation. In this conversation, you will answer every one of my questions. You will not lie and you will not reveal to anyone in ARC what we discuss." She gently clasps both hands together on the surface of her desk. "Before we begin, I am going to warn you: If you tell anyone about this, I will hurt you. If you somehow manage to get to me before I can do so, another Citadel will do it for me. You will never be safe around another one of us again. Are we clear?"

Edo blinks once, slowly. It is in this moment that I will see where she stands. I have laid my cards on the table and I have not been subtle. Roones are stronger than they look, but we both know that she wouldn't stand a chance if we fought. I'm not giving her much of a choice; she has to answer me, but that doesn't mean she has to tell the truth. I have to watch every single thing she says and does now, with total scrutiny. I am a master liar, but is she?

"You don't need to threaten me. I will help you." Edo's voice rolls out in a steady rasp.

I narrow my eyes. She's making it easy. Too easy. Since she isn't afraid, that means she really does want to help, or she's planning to lie. Her flawlessly smooth face remains impassive. I'm going to have to rely on her tone, the way she answers my questions, and on my gut instinct. In theory, I have the upper hand, but it doesn't feel like I do. I need to give her something. I need to let her know that I am in control. "In return for your cooperation, I will promise you that our deal goes both ways. I will not reveal to the other Citadels what I learn today. But I have made provisions if something happens to me. If I don't check in, then every Citadel will know what I've already figured out, and believe me, you wouldn't want that." I actually hadn't done this, but given how thorough Ezra is, I know he's likely done something along these lines. He probably rigged some e-mail alert the second I left the house. If I don't return, I know he won't hesitate to send it out.

"I told you that you need not threaten me. I understand your paranoia, but I am willing to answer whatever questions you may have."

She seems so serene. It's unnerving, which I imagine is her intention. I don't know what her motives are, but I do know one thing for sure: I am not leaving this office without proof—actual, tangible proof.

"The disk you placed inside of my brain. It's useless, isn't it? It was never the source of our abilities." I am perfectly still now—watching, waiting, listening. How fast will she answer? Will she blink? Will she show remorse? Will she deny it?

"Yes and no."

"Not good enough. Try again."

"I was going to explain. This will be easier, Citadel, if you don't interrupt me."

My first instinct is to widen my eyes, but I keep them level and stare her down. "Do *not* give me orders."

My hearing is so exceptionally good that I can easily hear another person's heartbeat in a quiet room. The Roones, of course, have molten bodies, which means everything about them is thick except their intellect. I wish in this moment they were built differently. I wish I could hear her blood pumping so that I could check its speed. If there was any justice in the world, her pulse would be racing. Edo would be afraid of me. She *should* be afraid of me—indeed, she *might* be afraid of me, but there is no way to tell.

She nods slightly. I can't tell if this is a gesture of respect or the complete opposite. I am going to have to get better at reading her body language for this to work. Edo clears her throat and continues. "When the chip was first implanted, it housed several thousand nanites. This nanotechnology rewrote specific strains of your DNA. It took several years for the process to be completed, which is why you were only a child when implanted. You have been genetically altered. Your strength, speed, and mental acuity is wholly a function of your own biology." Edo says this casually, in the same tone a person might use to talk about a movie they watched on TV or the paint color on a wall. I know in this instant she is not lying. This is the truth.

"And the nanites, where are they now?"

"Flushed out of your system long ago."

Damn. If they were still in my bloodstream, maybe Ezra could isolate one and we could use it as proof.

"The chip still serves a purpose, though, right? It's a location device?"

I see a slight movement in Edo's eye. She takes longer to answer this question, which means that whatever she tells me has been carefully constructed.

"It is, yes."

Ezra was right and now I know that there is something about the tracking aspect of the chip that Edo is more reluctant to talk about. I file that information away.

"So let's get down to the fun stuff, okay?" I lean forward. Edo doesn't like me being so close to her, I can tell. She is sending me subtle signals. It's in the way she stiffens and looks away for a brief flicker of a second. Maybe I was hoping to scare her, but it's not fear I'm reading. It's an odd mix of distaste and guilt that would probably be imperceptible to anyone else. These micro-gestures are making my jaw clench. My body seems to know the truth that Edo's cues are hinting at, even if my brain doesn't. "If there isn't a chip inside me controlling my . . . impulses, how is it that I can't touch a boy . . . or a girl, if I played for that side?"

"That part is more complicated," Edo tells me, her voice box grinding out the words.

"So, uncomplicate it," I volley without any emotion. These are dangerous waters and I have to be careful now.

"I want you to know . . ." she begins, and then lifts a single hand to finger the blue fabric of the scrubs she is wearing. Edo is nervous now, and we both know she can't hide those nerves from me. Although I am grateful for this small victory, I know the answer must be pretty bad to put her so obviously ill at ease. My own heart starts beating faster. "I want you to know," she repeats, "that I voiced my opinion very loud and very often against what they did to you. I felt it was cruel and ultimately unnecessary. So please understand that what I am about to tell you is just as disturbing to me as it will be to you."

"I doubt that," I say sarcastically, betraying the first hint of emotion that I quickly rein in. "I mean, Roones aren't passionate, but you can hold someone, right? Kiss them? You can have sex?"

"I can. I do, regularly." Edo sits up a little straighter.

I know that Roones are known for their candor, but I wasn't expecting that level of honesty. "How great for you." I'm pissed off now. She's so cavalier about something her people made sure I would never experience. I want to stay on track, but I can't help it. "I'm just unclear as to how your presence on this Earth has really benefited mankind beyond making a bunch of X-Men to deal with The Rift. With the knowledge you possess, your grasp on chemistry and physics? I mean, you could cure every disease known to man. But you don't. You sit around here and play God. You decide who lives, who dies, who gets to have sex, who doesn't . . ."

"There is a compelling argument that you have far more freedom and power than I do, Citadel Ryn. You may come and go as you please. You can fight. Your basic personality is commanding. I'm not much more than a prisoner here."

I notice another twitch in her eye and she's started talking faster. Edo is lying. But why? Why try to make me believe she's a victim? She has to know I would never fall for that.

"We have helped humanity. We solved the mystery of dementia and Alzheimer's for your people, but we can't suddenly cure everything. It would be too suspicious. And also—unless your governments are willing to put a cap on reproduction—potentially devastating to the continuation of not only your species, but all the resources on your planet." Well, I couldn't argue with that. Still, that last bit of information just proved she's hardly powerless. What is she playing at?

I let it go. "Fine." It's not the information I came for, but I know there is more to this. I'm not prepared. I don't have the intel or the backup to deal with this whole other truth. It's like Ezra said. Baby steps. "So tell me. What did they do? Did they molest me?" Oh, God, I feel myself getting emotional. I cannot be emotional right now. I can process this later, at home. I can show Edo only strength, but that feels impossible. "Did they . . . rape me?"

Edo looks down into her lap and then up again at me. There is something there. She is feeling something, too. "You were not raped and you were not molested in the way that other children are violated. However, you were"—Edo pauses for the right word—"abused."

I let out a long breath. I had been ready to hear just about anything, but I have to admit, I might not have been able to take it if she had told me I had been subjected to a worst-case scenario.

"So what, then? What did you do?" The conversation is distressing her. I see that. I don't care.

"The same drug that helped us cure Alzheimer's has a twin. Instead of helping one remember, it makes sure that one forgets. We also developed another drug that leaves the mind totally open to suggestion. Are you sure you want me to continue?"

I sit up straight. I look her right in those luminescent eyes of hers. She is not going to get away with not telling me the full extent of her complicity. "Yes."

"When you were brought here at fourteen, the summer before you became a Citadel, you stayed a week. Your families were told it was an ARC prep camp. That was a lie, of course. It was when you were told what you were and what your life would become. You were given an inoculation the first day, the first hour of your arrival. The shot contained an antidote to the genetic suppressor that the nanites had built in when they recoded your DNA. You were told the chip was activated. It wasn't. The shot turned on your altered genes in the controlled environment of the base for obvious reasons. It also contained the drug that left you open to suggestions. When Mr. Seelye spoke, you listened, you believed, and you obeyed. You think it was willpower alone that let you keep the secret of the Citadels and ARC from your loved ones? Let us not mince words. Teenagers would be incapable of such a feat."

I had always known something about that day was weird. Seelye had basically taken away our free will and we let him, without argument or question. I had always wrestled with keeping my life as a Citadel a secret—we all did. But they must have really done a brainwashing number on us all, because if I was being honest, I would literally rather die than tell my family the truth. Even now, the idea of telling them makes me anxious. A drug that makes us believe anything and then another to make us forget what they wanted us to. It made perfectly disgusting sense and Ezra had been right this whole time. He had seen clearly what I could not because of the drugs and what I can only assume was brainwashing of some sort.

"Most of the memories you have of that experience at the camp are false. For four of those days you were under total control of those drugs. We showed all of you many images, some very romantic and lovely. Some images—well, most of the images, actually—were movies that were sexually explicit. You were monitored to see which of the stimuli affected you most. By that, I mean the sex acts and the acts of romantic love that each of you personally responded to. You were shown a loop of those movies and pictures—and then you were hurt."

Silence. I look at her. To Edo's credit, she does not look away. "How was I—how were we—hurt?" I'm getting angry again.

"Sometimes you were electrocuted. Sometimes you were beaten. With our medicine and your altered DNA, the bruises and broken bones healed quickly enough so that there was no evidence." Edo breaks eye contact. Is she ashamed? She damned well should be.

"Broken bones, huh?"

"It was that bad. And we—"

"Damn it! We. Were. *Children*." I grip the desk. I want to

pick it up and throw it at her. I want to pick her up and throw her through the desk. I want to hurt so many things, and it hurts even more knowing I can't.

"Tell me how to undo it. Tell me there is a way to fix this. Because I am not going to go through the rest of my life without ever being touched. Not when it serves no other purpose than keeping me a perfect soldier. Not when it was done by torturing and abusing me as a child. No—I'm not going to let you do that to me."

"It's psychological damage. It was done through behavioral therapy. Presumably, it can be undone the same way. In that regard, your research is as good as mine."

I let that sink in for a moment. *I can* be rewired, just not in the way that Ezra originally thought. But the fact that they had no process to reverse it themselves spoke volumes about what ARC really thought of us.

Something suddenly occurs to me. "Speaking of research," I ask, "if the implant isn't viable, then how is it we know so much? How are we so smart? How can we speak so many languages? I watched you—you personally—download them into our brains."

"Again, we used a combination of the drugs. What you thought you saw, you didn't. If you'll recall, we made you study, made you read a number of textbooks on each subject, including foreign languages, that we had already 'downloaded' under the guise of reinforcement. We said we had to test you to make sure the downloads weren't corrupted. Your genetic enhancement gave you an eidetic memory. In the end, we didn't do anything more than encourage you. You are all self-taught."

I can't help myself, but I laugh at this point. "Yeah, but learning isn't the same as knowing. Citadels operate within the parameters that we are experts at things that we aren't. I thought I had the equivalent of a PhD in applied physics. All I have are formulas."

Edo sighs and the condescension is audible. "I know. That's why all you really ever do is fight." Her head is so smooth, so flawless and mesmerizing. I wonder if it would break into a thousand pieces if I smashed it hard enough against the desk. I close my eyes briefly to center myself. She has basically accused me of being a thug. I won't give her the satisfaction of being right.

"I am finished with my questions now. I appreciate your . . . honesty. But I need two more things from you."

Edo's eyes narrow. Her version of the truth is one thing; physical action might well be another. "If it is in my power to give them to you, I will." She takes her tiny hands and folds them together, propping her elbows on the desk. It's an oddly human gesture, which might not bode well for my requests.

"First off, I need an ample supply of the drug you use to leave people open to the power of suggestion. When I say 'ample,' I mean a lot. I have no idea how long it's going to take me to recondition my brain and I don't want to have to come here and ask you for more."

Edo cocks her head to the right as she considers. "Done. And the second thing?"

"I want you to remove the chip from my head. Now. Today."

Edo blinks. I stare her down. She lowers her arms and places her hands on her lap. She does not like this idea. "That would not be wise, Citadel Ryn."

I start to nod. I bear down on my jaw. "I know you think all I'm really good for is fighting—"

"That is most certainly not what I think—"

I slam my hand down on the desk and Edo flinches ever so

slightly. "Don't interrupt me. You don't get to interrupt me. You don't get to choose what I think or what I say or when I say it. Are you clear on that?"

Edo does nothing. She just sits there. She doesn't even give me the satisfaction of agreeing.

"You understand that we are much smarter than you give us credit for, don't you?"

Edo shrugs her shoulders. "Some of you are smarter than others."

I let out a little chuckle. "Maybe so, but *I'm* smart enough to realize that you aren't telling me the whole truth about the implant. I guess you never thought, being built the way you are, that your body language could give you away, but it does. So what could you be lying about? What else could the implant do besides act as a tracker?"

Edo looks down and to the side. In this moment I know that I am right. I had been running possible scenarios since Ezra told me the truth about the chip. What *would I do* if I needed to control a bunch of killer teenagers? Psychological castration, that's one way. But knowing how strong we are, and the damage just one of us could do alone, I would be afraid of what would happen if ten or twenty of us lost control. I would need a way to stop us immediately—*remotely*. In a flash, it hit me.

"It's a fail-safe. It's a kill switch, isn't it?"

Edo doesn't answer me.

"Isn't it?" I yell.

"It is," she says finally.

"So how *wise* would it be to keep it in my head?"

"It doesn't work like that. There are very few people who have the authority to use the fail-safe. There are protocols, a quorum—"

Fury sweeps through me like a tornado on an open plain. I can no longer resist. I'm literally shaking with anger, so I take my unsteady hands and finally let loose some of this rage by lifting the desk and slamming it down on the concrete floor so hard I can actually hear the metal warp. Edo jumps. "I don't give a fuck how it works. I don't want to know about the *committee* that gets to decide whether I live or die. I want it out. *Right now.* And if you really feel bad about what you did to us, then you will help me. But maybe you don't feel bad. For all I know, the kill switch was your idea."

Edo says nothing, admits nothing. She sits there a moment. I can see her thinking. She may well be afraid of me, of what I know, but I am an asset. There is the possibility, and of course I can't be sure about this, that she may even care for me. She also knows that I'm not stupid enough to tell the other Citadels, at least not yet. I won't risk the safety of Battle Ground. Maybe it's the conditioning, or maybe I actually believe, but I will keep the secret. Probably. It's probably the part that has her hesitating.

I realize I'm holding my breath.

"Fine," she says finally. "I will remove it, but you will have to promise to keep it on you at all times. ARC cannot know that it has been removed or think it is defective."

"Agreed. But you won't put me out. I want to be frozen locally and I want a mirror. I want to see everything you're doing in there."

Edo stands and shakes her head, which is so shiny and smooth that it catches the fluorescents above us. Pinpricks of light dance on her skull like a prism in the sun.

"If you are thinking of performing this procedure on your fellow Citadels, I highly recommend that you do not. The implant is extremely volatile."

I roll my eyes. "At the moment, what I want is to make sure that you don't kill or paralyze me. I don't trust you, Edo, or anyone else in here."

She gives the briefest of nods and then walks to the door. She opens it and gestures for me to go through to what I can only assume will be an operating theater. My answer seems to have mollified her. But in this moment I know that she isn't as smart as she thinks she is, because I'm lying my ass off.

CHAPTER 15

I am desperate to get home. I think maybe I feel desperate in general. For once, I wish my parents weren't out of town. Pretending that everything is fine would be harder than usual, but just being around them makes me feel safer, more normal. I can't see them . . . but I can see my brother. He's basically in the same place my car is, and I've never slacked in memorizing his schedule. Right now he's in his science lab—physics. I walk up a flight of stairs and go down a hallway. I look through the leaded glass of the door and see Abel at his station taking notes. I open the door and walk over to the teacher.

"Hi, sorry to interrupt," I whisper to her. "I'm Ryn Whittaker, Abel's sister. I just need to have a quick word with him. Our parents are out of town and I'm in charge. Nothing serious, but time sensitive."

"Okay. Abel, your sister would like to speak to you." She

gestures with her hand. She looks young for a teacher. I wonder briefly if she's an ARC employee. I wonder, with a not unrealistic amount of paranoia, if ARC secretly runs everything in Battle Ground.

Abel gets up and I smile a big, fake smile so that he knows right away that nothing is wrong. I walk out the door and Abel follows, closing it behind him. "What's up?" he asks.

Instead of saying anything I just hug him. I hang on to him for dear life. *My sweet little baby brother, you are too close to all this craziness. How can I ever really protect you when I have no idea who I'm really supposed to be fighting?*

"You're freaking me out, Ryn, and also maybe breaking my ribs. God. Is that, like, a kale thing?"

I let him go and look at him oddly. "What?"

"You know, because it's a superfood. And that hug felt uncomfortably strong."

"No, I haven't been eating kale. No. I just really missed you. I know it's weird. I guess I had a bad dream last night," I lie, "and I wanted to see you this morning. Make sure you were okay."

"You could have texted," Abel says, clearly unconvinced.

"Yes. I could have done that," I admit a little awkwardly.

Then Abel pushes through his average teenage boy obliviousness and reaches around to hug me. He doesn't latch on to me like I did to him, but it's a genuine hug—it's got love in it, if not tenderness. He *is* only fourteen. "I'm fine. I miss you, too. I'll see you in a few days at Grandma and Grandpa's house, unless you . . . want me to come home?"

I hear the hesitance, and I know it's because he's having the time of his life over at his best friend's house. Dylan's parents have a lot of money and are rarely home. It's probably like *Lord of the Flies*, except maybe with weed and an XBox.

"No. I'm fine. I'm being stupid. But I'm happy to see your face." I grab it and give him a kiss on the cheek. "I'll see you later."

"Okay," he says, putting his hand on the door. "Just, you know, text or whatever if you need me or want to talk or are scared of something. I can be home in, like, ten minutes from Dylan's house."

"Thanks, bud. You're a good guy." I turn and practically run down the hallway. It was a stupid thing for me to do. I'm too raw. My head hurts. I'm confused. I guess I panicked and needed something familiar. But it wasn't cool. Now that I have the implant out, things are more dangerous. Edo could tell Applebaum. Anyone close to me is at greater risk. I drive home with a feeling equal parts dread and terror. *I have no idea what I've just done.*

CHAPTER 16

I make my way home and drag myself up the stairs to see Ezra. I push open the bookshelf and stand there. We stare at each other. I can't take it anymore. There is something about being around Ezra that makes me feel strong and weak all at once. At first I cover my face with my hands. I don't want him to see me crying. Not because I'm afraid of being vulnerable in front of him, but because I know it must be so hard not to be able to comfort me, to have to just sit there and watch me hurt. Still, once I start crying, I don't know how to stop. I fall on my knees. I weep. My head hurts, my neck, there's an ache I have that is so deep inside of me, I feel like every cell in my body is eating itself alive. Ezra stands. He walks toward me. I see his bare feet and I look up at him.

"This is going to sound crazy," I manage through the sobs, "but I sort of wish you would just hit me or kick me. I don't know how else to touch you. We can't kiss or hug, but if you hurt me, I could feel something besides my feelings. I hate my feelings right now. I can barely breathe. It's like I'm drowning . . ."

I keep crying and it is getting harder to catch my breath. I keep trying to fill my lungs with air, but it's as if there isn't enough in the room. Ezra crouches down and sits on the floor in front of me. "I don't know what happened out there. But don't *ever* ask me to hurt you. Ever. Because it would kill me."

I curl up into a ball. I get as close to Ezra as I possibly can without actually touching him. He does not tell me everything will be okay. He doesn't offer me any bullshit. He doesn't say anything. I just cry. I cry for what feels like hours and still we don't move. When I finally sit up, all puffy eyed and red faced, I see that Ezra's eyes look even bluer. It's not because they are bloodshot. I think he may have been crying, too. Not like me. I just won a gold medal in hysterics. Ezra is also hurting, and not just for me, but because he might not ever see his family again. He might be a fugitive for the rest of his life. He might have to go back to the Village.

He might get hunted down and killed.

The invisible wall between us somehow feels thinner after that. I can't explain it exactly, but something has shifted. I still want him, but now I want more from him. He's seen me go to a place no one else has and he's still sitting here. In our own way, what we've just experienced feels closer than sex, more intimate than two bodies scrambling in the dark.

"Ready to talk?" he says, his whisper breaking the silence.

"You were right." I very ungracefully wipe my nose on my sleeve. "The implant does nothing. It did, at first, when they put it in. It was nanotechnology. They recoded my DNA so that I can do all these nifty cool murder tricks now. But the implant has nothing to do with my abilities. I'm always going to be like this. There is no going back to normal like they promised. Here's the kicker, though. The not-touching thing? That was good old-fashioned brainwashing chased with a fun cocktail of drugs that make you totally open to suggestion and then erase your memory. Basically they made us watch porn and then beat us during the parts we liked the most."

"Oh."

I know he wants to say more. I can hear the slight edge in his voice. But he understands, just like I do, that there is little point in raging against something that happened years ago. We are both practical in that way. We have to look forward, not back, if we want to get through this. "That's awful, but it isn't something we can't fix. We can undo that damage. We can fix that. Together."

"Yeah, well, you should probably start pulling all the research you can on behavioral cognitive therapy. I guess the only good thing is that Edo gave me a lot of the brainwashing drugs they use, so it won't take as long as it probably should. Apparently it only took them four days to make us like this. Which is—obviously—terrifying and gross. But the bad part, or maybe the part that has me worried, is that she gave the drugs up so quickly. I don't know if that was her guilt or something else. I just can't think about it right now. I have to lie down."

He looks me over, checking for bruises, for blood. "Why? Are you okay? Did they hurt you?"

"I made her take it out. You were right about that, too. Except it's more than a tracking device. It's also, wonderfully, a kill switch."

"Jesus."

"Yes—that was a fun discovery." I take a deep breath, hoping not to lose it laughing at the absurdity of the situation.

"Anyway, I also made her put a mirror up there when she did it so I can see how it's done. You know, just in case I have to perform an emergency chip-section on my friends." I reach into the pocket of my flannel shirt and take out a small black box, about a quarter of an inch by a quarter of an inch. I put it into his hand. "You can take a look at it, but whatever you do, don't disable it. If it goes dark, they'll know I figured it out, and that would be very, very bad." Ezra gently takes the implant from my hand. He squeezes his fist around it and looks at me. With his other hand, he reaches up, like he's going to touch my hair or maybe my face. I shrink back from his would-be touch.

"Listen," he says, "I don't know what it's like to be a super soldier, or a killer. I don't know how to do a somersault in the air or what it's like to fight vampires." Ezra takes his hand back and closes his eyes, shaking his head. "And you don't know what it's like to go through The Rift. To lose everyone you love or care about or to have the thing that you feel like you understand best—for me that would be physics—turned on its head so that the basics no longer make sense. It doesn't matter what we don't know. What matters is that, for whatever reason, you chose to help me that day and I am so grateful. However much time we have together, let's make the most of it. Let's focus on the things we have in common. Let's just be here for each other. I don't know what that looks like, but let's try."

I nod and rise up to my feet. "I'll be back up in a couple hours. It's funny how the whole brain-surgery thing can take the pep out of a girl. Please do what you can to figure out how to counter the behavior modification." I push open the bookshelf. I walk downstairs, take a shower, and slip into bed. Sleep finds me eventually, but it is filled with dreams of sex and bruises—the vampire's mouth on my neck and a gun in my hand. The green light of The Rift is everywhere, and even when I awaken, the scent of pine and sap lingers.

When I walk up to Ezra's room, he's at the computer. He's got my chip in a glass. It doesn't look like he's done anything with it so far, which is good. The thought of him tinkering with that thing fills me with dread. I'm going to have to get used to carrying it with me at all times now and keeping it safe when I'm fighting, like I don't already have enough to worry about.

"Sit down," he says, gesturing to the bed. I furrow my brow. "Don't freak. I'm not going to try to make out with you. I've started with the research and I think I know where to begin. Here . . ." Ezra hands me a pad of paper and a pencil.

"Are we going to *draw* sexy things? Gotta tell you, stick people are about as much as my skills allow in that department." I smile weakly.

"No. You are going to write a list of everything that makes you feel safe and calm. Divide the list into your five senses. And really think about it, especially the things that made you feel that way before you became a Citadel, before you even got the chip. It could be a particular song or singer, maybe you have a stuffed animal that—"

"I don't have a stuffed animal," I interrupt.

"No, I didn't think so."

What the hell does that mean? But I begin to write anyway, categorizing each item by placing them in double-outlined boxes I've drawn according to my senses. When I'm done I hand it back to him.

"That took fourteen seconds, Ryn. This is serious. You could break every bone in my body and that's a best-case scenario."

I shrug and point to my head. "Super brain," I say sarcastically as I hand over the paper.

He raises his eyebrows when he sees that it's filled. "Buffy? The Vampire Slayer?"

I narrow my eyes at his raised eyebrows. *Nobody fucks with my love of Buffy.*

"Clearly Buffy and I have some things in common. I suppose you could make an argument that Angel and I are more similar, considering that every time he has sex he turns into a monster. But no, Buffy and I have a connection." He reads the rest of the list and sighs.

I start to fidget. Suddenly I feel like I've failed some sort of test. "Look, I'm not an intellectual," I explain. "I do read. A lot. But I read things that help me escape. Were you expecting Nietzsche? Or that I write up papers in my spare time about eastern Europe and the rise of nationalism? Or that I love to spend my Sunday afternoons staring at modern art? I'm not a scholar. I'm a soldier. And the things that make me feel safe and calm are banal. *Harmless.* I don't need the extra stimulation." I bite my lip and hunch my shoulders a little. I'm embarrassed and I'm annoyed that I'm embarrassed. Ezra is really smart. I'm smart, too, but I've done nothing, really, to stretch my intellectual muscles. If we're being technical, I didn't go to school past the eighth grade. I don't get to go to lively seminars with amazing professors who help me reframe the world, like he does—or did, anyway. And from what Edo told me, a lot of my knowledge is rote memorization, not actual applied learning.

Apparently Ezra makes that realization, too. "I'm sorry, you're right. This is a judgment-free zone. Besides, you do have NPR on that list. And some cool classical stuff."

"Whoa, easy there, Mr. Snobby. I can also speak fifteen— wait, now sixteen—languages," I say in perfect Arabic with a smile.

"Fine. I won't make a single comment even about the items on your list. The thing is, to me, you're incredible. Sometimes I wonder if you're even real. It's hard for me to wrap my head around the fact that you like *Doctor Who*. It's so . . . normal. Well, normal for a dork ass like me." We both smile at that. "Grab one of those pills Edo gave you and then go and get some of your dad's clothes." It's an order, but he made it sound like a suggestion. I nod and leave.

When I'm back, I look at the red pill in my hand. Edo could have been lying. This could be poison. It could even make me more violent. I don't remember taking any pills that week when I was fourteen, so they must have dosed our food or water. I suppose they could still be drugging us that way. It could be in our protein shakes. Shit, for all I know, they could be pumping it through the ventilation system at the base to make *everyone* there more compliant. This cluster fuck just gets bigger and bigger. But I can only solve one problem at a time. I quickly swallow the pill. Maybe it will kill me. Right now I'm more afraid of living my entire life without ever being able to be close to anyone, about what that would do to me. That scares me way more than dying. I wait ten minutes. Nothing happens. If it was going to kill me it probably would have by now. I feel the pile of sweaters I took from my dad's closet. They're on my lap, and I pull one up and put my nose into the wool. This smell, this is safety, this is love. With my face pressed into this sweater, I am a little girl again.

Ezra holds out his hand, and for a moment I think he wants me to take it. But I realize he wants the sweater. I give it to him and he puts it on but doesn't say anything. He angles the computer monitor so I can see it from the bed. He logs into Netflix—I had given him my account so he wouldn't go out of his mind being alone all day—and chooses *Buffy*.

"Wait," he says before I press Play. "This won't work if you try to fight it. That's what you do, right? You feel attracted or turned on and then you and your brain have an epic fight for control. That can't happen. You might even need to say some of this stuff out loud. In fact, you should, like a mantra. You have to acknowledge that this is who you are, that this is how you're wired, and that you *can* be different. You have to say that nothing bad will happen if you allow yourself to be touched. You can't fight this the normal way. You have to surrender a bit, admit that it's a weakness, and push through it. Can you do that?"

I think about what he's said, and maybe it's the red pill, but I get it. I can't fight. "Yeah."

He nods, presses Play, and the TV show begins. He comes to sit down on the bed, both of us surrounded by pillows. At first all I can think is: *Ezra is beside me.* Close, but not touching. I'm glad he's here. What's more, I don't feel like killing him, which to me is a win, considering that I can feel the heat that's coming off him. We watch an entire episode this way. I can feel myself relax some. Ezra is right here, so close that I can smell him. But of course, it's not Ezra I'm smelling—at least not completely. Some of it is my dad.

"Okay, start talking, Ryn."

I wince. I don't want to say what I'm feeling out loud. It's mortifying. But if this is what it takes to get it done, I'm going to have to buy in.

"I like it that you're next to me. I know that if you try to kiss me, I will hurt you. But I am safe here with you. I don't need to hurt someone I want to be close to. There is something wrong with my brain that makes me lose control when I am attracted to someone. This is a problem only I can fix." I look at Ezra, wondering if I've said enough.

"Go on."

Guess not.

"I'm not going to hurt you. I'm not going to hurt you. I'm not—"

Ezra interrupts me. "Stop saying that, please. I'm worried that it will become some sort of reverse self-fulfilling prophecy. You only have to acknowledge that there is a part of you that is not working right and that you understand that. The key here is to feel close to someone *and* feel safe at the same time. It's not that you might hurt me—that's not the issue. The issue is that *you* won't be hurt."

I nod. Another episode of *Buffy* begins. I watch the slayer, with all her blond, perky cuteness, kick butt and still have friends and a life. I've always been jealous of her in that way. That and the fact that she is awesome with puns.

"I'm safe," I say out loud. "I'm safe and you won't hurt me." I say this over and over again. I watch Buffy. I look down. Without even realizing it, somewhere along the way, Ezra has taken my hand.

"Keep talking, Ryn," he says softly.

"I'm safe and you won't hurt me. I'm safe and you won't hurt me." There is a part of me that recognizes Ezra's hand in mine. It feels good there, *right*. There is another part of me that is detached from this contact. I am focused on Buffy, on feeling safe, on knowing I am not going to experience pain, though oddly I am expecting to. I guess there is just so much going on at once that I can't totally focus on Ezra's hand. But it's there. It's happening. The episode ends. I stop speaking. Ezra lets go of my hand. I feel a tiny ache once he's pulled away. He smiles. It is a bright and hopeful smile. His blue eyes are filled with light. There is nothing but silence in the room. Ezra takes my hand again and I do not flinch. I do not push him away or try to strangle him. I'm also not particularly turned on, either. I try not to think about what would happen if I was. It doesn't matter, though. Finally. I am holding hands with a boy.

"Do you feel up to doing some more?" Ezra asks patiently. "We don't have to if you're too tired."

"No, I'm good, unless . . . do you want to get some rest? Or do some more work? I could go. Or if you need to go . . ." The last thing I want him to feel is obligated. My cheeks flush a little at the thought. And at my total descent into babbling.

Very smooth, Ryn.

"I'm up for it. Maybe you want to take another pill, though?" I nod my head in agreement. "Great. Have you got cake downstairs? Or Voodoo Doughnuts? Whatever those are."

I don't bother to explain. The perfection that is Voodoo goes beyond words.

My parents had gone overboard with the grocery shopping before they left. It's become a kind of tradition with them, to prepare for doomsday with the amount of food they leave me when I'm on my own. They got me a chocolate cake, which they know is my favorite and always on the list. I bring the cake upstairs, along with two forks and some whipped cream, which I prefer to frosting. Ezra wisely says nothing when he sees the can. I spray a generous amount of cream on a portion of the cake.

"Ready?" Ezra says.

"I am, but I'm not even that hungry," I admit.

"It doesn't matter. Just take a bite and keep it in your mouth. Focus on how it feels on your taste buds. Try to associate other good memories with the cake."

I do as he asks. I close my eyes with the chocolate in my mouth. I think about birthday parties, goofy hats, and brightly colored presents. These are home-movie type of memories. I am watching a younger version of myself, with pigtails, laughing, happy. I am not seeing these images through my own eyes.

"Okay, now I want you to sit here," he says, spreading his legs a bit, "with your back on my chest. Keep saying the mantra in your head, or out loud, whatever. I won't touch you. I just want you to lean against me, get used to what it's like to be close to me."

My heart hammers. Holding hands is one thing, but nestling against him is something else. I trust Ezra. I trust that he knows what he's doing, and most important, I trust myself. I will not be hurt in this room. I take another bite and position myself so that I'm kind of tucked into him. I feel his thigh muscles against mine. I hear his heart beating. I smell him, but I also smell, because of the sweater he's wearing, my dad. If I wanted to, I could turn around, put his mouth on mine, grab his hair, seriously make out with him . . . No—too much. I say my mantra. "I'm safe and you will not hurt me. I'm safe and you will . . ."

Baby steps. I focus on the sweet chocolate in my mouth instead. I focus on being safe. Yes, I am basically sitting on top of a boy, but that isn't the point. Like before, this is more than sex. It's literal closeness, and I'm blown away by how wonderful it feels. I take a few more bites and Ezra sits perfectly still. He doesn't seem afraid, which is amazing to me. I sit there for twenty minutes, pressed against him, eating, thinking, chanting. When I get up, we both smile.

"That was really good, Ryn. But I think that's all we'll do today. I've got a bunch of work to do with the data, so you can just do whatever you normally do. Don't let me stop you."

I cross my arms. Is he dismissing me? Seriously?

"I just work better alone," he says, as if he's read my mind.

"I can help," I offer.

"At some point, yeah, I think you can. I'm just collating the data still. I know the patterns I'm looking for. It would be faster if I did this part on my own."

"Okay, thanks for . . . everything. I know this whole thing is really insane and dangerous for you. I want you to know that it means a lot to me that you'd take such a risk." I pick up the cake and forks. I want to say more. I literally don't know how to express my gratitude in words.

"Ryn, I like you. I mean . . . I'm into you. My motives aren't entirely unselfish, so don't put me on some kind of pedestal. Right now, I just want to do as much Rift work as possible, but tomorrow I'm hoping we can actually talk. I want us to get to know each other, like normal people do. I'm hoping our entire relationship isn't going to be based around deprogramming and math equations, you know?"

My cheeks burn a little. "We have a relationship?" I ask hopefully.

"Well, we for sure have something that's a big enough deal to make both of us put our asses on the line in the hugest way possible. We don't have too much time to figure out what that is, but . . . I don't know." Ezra smiles sheepishly and waves his hands around. "Let me get back to work."

I guess neither one of us is so great with the whole talking-about-our-feelings thing, which suits me just fine. For now.

CHAPTER 17

I walk into the locker room at work the next day with a lightness I haven't felt in years. I have a secret, which isn't quite the same as a lie. People my age keep these sorts of secrets all the time. This is ordinary. Liking someone, not wanting to explain it yet to your friends, wanting to keep it to yourself so that it doesn't get picked apart and analyzed in its newness is unremarkable, even if the feelings aren't. I take off my clothes, and just as I do, I feel a tap on my shoulder. I turn and see that it's Audrey.

And I am suddenly deflated.

It takes a lot of work on my part to keep my face indifferent. Why is she here? They must know at the Village that Ezra is gone by now. Did they send her to The Rift to watch me? To get answers? They must have, and yet, I'm not sure that makes complete sense to me. I know Audrey is crazy, but I don't peg her for a tattletale, especially if she could get into trouble, too. Something doesn't add up. Unless they caught her, they figured out she helped me and narking was her Get Out of Jail Free card. She's psycho, but she isn't stupid.

She pulls me into an embrace. I am naked except for my underwear. *Who does that?* It's beyond awkward. Violet's right beside me at her locker and I can see her "what's going on?" face over Audrey's shoulder.

"*Bonjour*, Ryn. I am here!" Audrey says brightly.

"I see that," I say passively as I take a step back from her and grab my uniform.

"Yes, the Village, so boring. Well you know; you've been there. No action. No fighting. Just guarding stupid sheep. Immigrants. It's all dinner parties and karaoke. *Mon Dieu!* I asked them to reassign me to The Rift. I could not get full reassignment, but three shifts a week, better than nothing. Now we can have some fun—together." Violet gives me a second questioning look, but I glance knowingly at Audrey. Vi nods, knowing I'll explain later.

And the thing is that I actually want to—explain, that is. Yes, I could lie. It would be so easy to say she's a friend of Levi's and that he introduced us. But I'm so tired of the bullshit. I want the lies to be over . . . at least with my friends.

Because it's clear ARC has their suspicions. I'm certainly not buying that Audrey's sudden appearance is a coincidence. Not for one minute. Her presence is a game changer, but it's a game I'm confident I can win. "Great, Audrey. I'm sure you'll be an asset in the field. I'm just going to get dressed now. Don't want to be late." I smile in a way that tells her I'm not buying what she's selling, but the French woman is undeterred.

"Of course. See you on the playground, *mon amie*." She turns and walks away.

Violet shuts her locker and looks at me as I'm zipping up my suit.

"Later." I hold up my hand. "I'll explain to everyone."

We are working another Nest that day, and I wait until the entire team is in place and has checked in before I begin talking. I disable my mic. As soon as I do so, Violet jumps in.

"Spill it. How do you know that girl and how in God's name do you know what it's like in the Village?"

Boone and Henry whip their heads around and stare at me as if they've just heard I was going to have a baby, or maybe eat a baby. With Henry, it's always hard to tell.

"She works with Levi," I begin.

"Levi?" Henry says suspiciously.

"Yes." Deep breath—time to start coming clean. "I asked Levi to help get me into the Village. I wanted to see it. I wanted to—"

Violet interrupts before I can finish. "See that guy Ezra."

Boone rolls his eyes and shakes his head. "Holy shit, Ryn. Are you telling me that you broke in there *to see a dude*? You have got to be kidding me."

"Oh, Ryn," Vi says sadly.

"That was an incredibly impulsive and reckless decision—not to mention stupid. You're smarter than that," Henry says quietly, but his anger is clearly rising to the surface.

I hold both my hands up. "It's not what you think. Yes, I *did* want to see him—I had made a promise. But that's nothing compared to what I saw there. It's not like some apocalyptic concrete prison. They call it the Village because it's really a village—well, more like a town. It's cute. It's quaint. It's also creepy as hell and totally unsettling."

My teammates all look at one another.

"What do you mean?" Boone asks. "I don't get it."

"I mean, whatever comes through and isn't hostile—though God only knows what they do to the hostile ones—whatever they were before, whatever they believed, whatever it was that made them who they were, is stripped away. The entire point of the Village is to humanize *everyone*. They have to speak English, they have to celebrate our holidays, dress like us, act like us. They can't have families of their own and even if they *are* humans, they can never, *ever* leave. It's like the scariest propaganda campaign you have ever seen. It's fucked up. Wrong." There is silence among us for a few seconds as I let what I've said sink in.

Eventually Violet speaks, clearly disturbed. "Well, I get not letting some of the more . . . I mean . . . the species that aren't obviously human and could never pass, I understand why they need to be kept in the Village, but I guess I always thought humans were sort of debriefed and then released, with ARC's help, of course. Treated like people in Witness Relocation or something."

A snicker escapes my lips. "Oh, please," I say sarcastically. "We're all so wrapped up in our own drama, about what they made us into and what we can and can't do that we assume we have it the worst of everyone. The fact is, I know I never even actually thought about the Immigrants at all. None of us did. And yet I'm telling you, we're actually the lucky ones, if you can believe it."

"Well, since I've never actually gotten lucky, no, I don't believe it," Boone snaps at me.

"For the record, I can believe it," Henry says. "I've always thought something terrible happens to the Immigrants. I just didn't know what, and now I'm kind of ashamed that I never asked or went to find out the answers like you did, Ryn. It's just, every time I thought about it, I'd get distracted and forget. Which makes me feel even worse about it."

I bite my lip and squirm inside. I have a pretty good idea of why he was "forgetting."

"Don't, Henry," I tell him softly. "I mean, no one talks about it. No one said anything, so it's not like you're the only one. The thing is, Applebaum and ARC, they make us feel like we have no power and no say. Guys, *we* are the most powerful people in this entire system. We need to start acting like it. If we're going to be sending Immigrants off to the Village, then it's our moral responsibility to know exactly how that process goes. We can't put our heads in the sand anymore. We cannot be part of the system in that way. We can't just be good soldiers and follow orders." Instinctively, I put a hand on my rifle and stand a little straighter.

Violet shakes her head. I can see that she's afraid, but angry, too, and maybe a little ashamed. "How do we start doing that?"

"Whatever comes through today? We're going to sit in on their debriefing session. I want to know what lies ARC tells them. I want to hear how it all starts, right from the beginning." I stare at them all intently.

Boone bristles. "And just how are we supposed to do that? Are we going to go up to one of the intake coordinators and be like, 'Hey, where's the brainwashing room?'"

I wince a little when he says the word. I should tell them the whole truth. I want to—and I will—but it's too much, too soon. Let them live with this first.

Just like I did.

"Yeah, no one is going to let us just waltz into an intake room," Violet argues.

"With the four of us asking? I think that's exactly what they are going to let us do." I look over to see Henry nod and give me a tight-lipped smile. Violet looks between us two, and nods as well. We all look at Boone.

"Fine!" he says, throwing his hands up. "I always wanted to Clockwork Orange someone anyway, so maybe this is my chance." He's joking, which means Boone is in, too.

My team is with me. Of course they are.

It's not long after the decision is made that we devise a loose plan. Then, just when we are getting to particulars, The Rift opens. We all tense. I hear Levi. He's on point, down at the rock, leader of Alpha Team. We hear it before we get a visual, a long wail of chirping that sounds like a thousand tiny screams. Hundreds of bright purple and turquoise birds fly out of The Rift, moving together as if they were one body. They are breathtakingly beautiful, like little fairies all rushing together, waving, undulating.

The teams on the ground fan out. I see Audrey on Alpha Team with Levi. Does ARC know that he helped me? Did they put them together to work as some sort of an investigation? Into me? Into each other? Seven ground teams pull out what looks to be a bazooka. I know it's not, but that doesn't stop me from wincing when they fire. A spray of nets flies up into the air around the murmuration of what looks to be a version of starlings. It doesn't take long, maybe five or six seconds, and the birds are captured. Their gorgeous plum wings flap against the white rope of the nets. They crash and flip over each other. Momentarily, they get enough leverage in a few of the nets to actually make it off the ground, but it's pointless. They crash down again and their screaming chirps bounce off the trees and echo up to the Nest. The four of us look at each other. We don't need to say it. We all know what each of us is thinking—that at the end of the day, anyone who comes in contact with The Rift is as trapped as those birds are—Citadels, Immigrants, even Applebaum with his underground bunker life and his lies and the way he hurts children year after year, believing it's for the greater good. Applebaum isn't a monster; I've seen plenty of those. He's just a man with a terrible job. I turn away from the scene below me and sit down against a post. I lower my head onto my knees.

Shit. I don't even like birds.

LATER ON THAT DAY, TOWARD the end of the shift, a group of about ten Maribehs come through. Yes, they do sort of look like they belong in a *Planet of the Apes* movie (the older ones), and I've joked about it, called them damn dirty apes, but never again, not now that I know where they are going and what the rest of their lives will be. They might not be able to speak English, but the least I can do is honor them by calling them what they call themselves in their own language.

Levi's team and another on the ground surround the Maribehs. They are a docile species. Personally, I've never seen one get violent on the ground. They are more of the pee-their-pants-in-fear variety, which, given the circumstances, I might be, too, if I wasn't a Citadel. The Maribehs are crying, arms are flailing. Levi is being calm, giving off an authoritarian vibe, but one that isn't scary. Say what I will about Levi, he *is* good at this. The two teams have the Maribehs circled and are herding them toward the vans that are waiting to take them to HQ. One of the Maribehs trips, and I watch as Audrey yanks him up hard and shoves him forward. Levi gives her a stern look and she just shrugs and smiles. I can't believe there is any situation in which I would prefer Levi's company, but I'd take him any day over Psycho Girl. There are about thirty minutes left of our watch. The team sits it out and when the other Beta Team comes in to relieve us, we make our way back to the base in relative quiet. I know what they are thinking: They are beginning to see the Immigrants in a different light. They aren't just victims and they aren't always enemies, either. They are sentient beings who will now be prisoners for the rest of their lives.

We all change into our training uniforms and meet in the hallway. Collectively, we walk to the intake section of the bunker. I have only been called here a couple times, to deal with Immigrants who seemed passive at first but then went bonkers. It isn't entirely unusual for a Citadel to be in this part of the base, but it is out of the ordinary. Generally, regular military take over from here. As such, we get a couple looks from some soldiers. We look right back at them. It almost makes me smirk—they know to not even try. I see a few coordinators, but I want Kendrick. He's the only one who might just let us go where we want without too many questions. Other than my few times in the Village, I know most of what I know about the Immigrants from him.

So obviously we run smack into Greta.

"Shit."

"What?"

Did I say that out loud?

"What are you doing here?" she demands. "Nobody called in the Citadels. It's just a group of Maribehs—we can handle it."

"I'm looking for Kendrick," I state simply. Greta furrows her brow. She's thinking. Not good.

"Why?"

"That's none of your business," I answer coolly.

"I'm a manager of this division. Everything that happens here is my business."

Wow, is she going to try to pull rank? Or maybe she thinks because she's older than us, she's automatically in charge.

"The only reason you have a 'division,'" I say as I twirl my finger around in a circle, "is because me and my friends risk our lives every day out there in the kill zone. Now, tell me where I can find Kendrick and stop asking me questions." I am not angry when I say this. I am not smarmy, either. She knows what we are capable of. Regardless of her definition of management, we have all the authority we need scrambled into our DNA. Moreover, she's a bully—using condescension and intimidation to get results. When it has no effect on me, she wisely backs down and tells us to follow her.

You are in no way superior to me, lady.

We walk farther up the hallway until we get to a door that requires an eye scan to enter. I wonder if we have the clearance. We must, because ARC can never be sure when it comes to a newly arrived Immigrant, but I have never been in this room. The other times I was in this section, the action happened out in the hallway.

We walk in and see a long line of monitors and double-sided glass. Kendrick is sitting at a desk with a couple other coordinators and a soldier, fully armed. I give a subtle nod, but Henry is already reading her, looking for which vulnerability to go for first if it comes to it. Boone and Vi subtly spread into the room, marking the rest of the people. Perfectly natural, perfectly calm, and perfectly executed.

Kendrick turns and eyes the four of us. He seems surprised, but not suspicious, which is perfect.

"She demanded that I take her here, to you," Greta blurts out, the frustration evident to anyone with ears.

"Ryn," Kendrick says with a smile. "How can I help you?"

It's hard to get a totally accurate read on him. He seems

nice enough, he always is. He's also really smart. He seems to know, while the others don't, just exactly what we are capable of. He is always respectful, sometimes even deferential, but he is never totally authentic. It's both empathy and a mask. Is it just part of his job, or is he good at his job because that's the way he is? It doesn't matter. Right now all that matters is we're all here together, at this moment. And he's clearly "on," treating us like the Immigrants, like invaders to be handled. We are predators and he is right to be wary.

Which means I have to be wary, too.

"Kendrick, I need the room." This is not a question. It's not a demand, either. It's simply a fact.

"You can't just do that, you don't have—" Greta begins, but Kendrick interrupts her.

"No, it's fine. If Ryn and her team would like to talk privately I believe it's the least we can do, considering all that they do." Kendrick says this all while keeping his eyes on my face. He doesn't bother to turn to Greta and address her directly. She might be a manager, but it looks like he's the one in charge. She opens her mouth to say something, then closes it and storms out of the room instead. Kendrick nods at the others—including the soldier—and they all leave.

"Thank you," I say genuinely.

Kendrick taps a pencil on a yellow pad of paper. Weird. I didn't think anyone at ARC actually used paper anymore. "No problem. Greta's a little territorial, that's all. So, what's going on?"

"We'd like to watch the initial debrief with the Maribehs."

Kendrick cocks his head and leans back a little in his chair. "You know, that's not something that ARC generally encourages," he says, keeping his voice level. If he's surprised by our request, he's not showing it.

"Why?" Violet asks quickly.

"Well, I think it's their policy that the Citadels have just enough information about the Immigrants to keep them safe. The fear is—and I mean, this is my own theory; I haven't asked—is that to get too close to an Immigrant, to feel a disproportionate amount of sympathy for their situation, would put you at risk. Take the Maribehs for example—what do you know about them?"

Boone answers. "They are a hominid species, peaceful, docile almost. They have an intellect equivalent to our own but technologically, at least the ones that have Rifted so far, are about five hundred years behind us." Right as he finishes, the lights go on in the room on the other side of the double glass. There are three long benches and a flat-screen TV.

"Right. And what does that imply?"

"What?" Boone asks.

"You said they are docile. Unconsciously, then, you are judging and generalizing an entire species. But you aren't anthropologists—and even anthropologists generally specialize in a race and study it for years. If Citadels start coming to the intake sessions, they might think that they have a better handle on the species they are dealing with. They might let their guards down with one species over another. They might feel a compassion that could weaken a necessary resolve to do the dirty work."

We see the Maribehs shuffle into the room. They are talking to each other, murmuring low, pointing, afraid.

"Let's say that after this intake you watch, you feel that you understand the Maribehs better. You go in less aggressive. You are nice, gentle even, which would be great ninety-nine percent of the time. It's that one percent ARC worries about. Most Maribehs are lovely, but what if one comes through that's a serial killer? Or there's a version of Earth where Maribehs are ruthless and vicious? I think ARC is trying to give you professional distance."

Without being asked to, the Maribehs sit down on the benches. They are waiting for someone, or something.

"Well," I begin, "I think it's the complete opposite. I think that knowledge, any knowledge, means power. And, in the case of the Citadels, that equals a tactical advantage. I'm all about the tactical advantage, especially as I'm a team leader and responsible for making the tough calls. Besides, we don't let our guards down. Ever. Nothing I see in that room will change that fact." I fold my arms.

Kendrick nods silently. "Except—when was it, October? With that kid Ezra Massad. You made an assumption based on how he looked and his body language, but you didn't know for sure. You let your guard down then."

Ezra. I don't like hearing his name in this building, but I don't react. I give nothing away.

"And what about that last group of Sissnovars? Going in without any weapons?"

"I might have acted a bit impulsively with the boy," I concede, hoping that by not using his name I can keep emotion out of it, "but I didn't, not for one minute, let my guard down. I'm not built that way; none of us are. I wish we could because I'm pretty sure it's why so many people think we're assholes. Understand this: I could have had him subdued in under two seconds if things had gone south. And with the Sissnovars, extra knowledge about that culture actually made our job *easier*. But even then, we were completely in control of the situation—I wouldn't risk my people if I thought otherwise." Realizing I've been on the defensive for a while, I try a different tack.

"Maybe you should come and watch us train, or even better, come out to The Rift and watch us work. Then you would really understand how we operate and what we can do."

The room tenses for a moment. That wasn't a threat, but it could be taken as one.

Kendrick holds up both his hands and chuckles softly. "Hey, I never said that I agreed with ARC; I was just trying to give you a working theory. I happen to think that you're right in this case. I think that everything you can learn about the Immigrants will help you in the field. I'll call in the others and you can stay and watch, but just understand that our goal here today is to remove as much fear as possible. The Maribehs can't understand what The Rift is yet. They wouldn't get the truth, so they get something else—for now—that makes them feel safe, okay?"

I thank God he didn't ask about how I *knew* about the Sissnovar customs in the first place and say, "Okay." I step back and Kendrick gets up to open the door. The other coordinators come in, along with the armed guard. Thankfully, Greta is elsewhere. When everyone is settled, Kendrick pushes a button on his keyboard. My team stands back against the wall, ready to watch the show. The TV in the room on the other side of the glass turns on, and the Maribehs make sounds of awe and wonder.

"Hello, fellow Maribeh, and welcome. I know that you are afraid. I know that you are struggling to understand this new and strange place. Please, offer up your fears to the one true Goddess, Akaela-Han, for it is she who has brought you here. From the moment of your birth, she has been watching over you. She has taken note of your good deeds and your hard work. You are special. You were destined for greatness. Yes, it is your destiny that pulled you through the

shimmering green light so that you may live here, in Akaela-Han's paradise. The language I am speaking in to you now is the language of the Goddess. You are reading my words at the bottom of the screen only so that you might understand what has happened to you. It is a great honor and privilege to be able to speak in Akaela-Han's divine tongue. You will learn it in time; do not worry. In truth, friends, fellow Maribeh, you need not ever worry again. Akaela-Han has brought special souls like yours from all the heavens in the universe. You will see wonders. Akaela-Han will provide for your every need, just as the great book of Lrok-M'hain promises. You will never be without food or shelter. You will never be sick. You have a sacred purpose now, to accept this higher calling. Eventually, you will be given a divine task that you will attend to daily. If you can leave your fears and doubts behind and listen well to the representatives of Akaela-Han, you will be granted a great reward: a meeting with Akaela-Han herself who sits in her divine temple watching you right now. But you must let go of your old life. You must embrace this new life with an open heart and mind. You must make yourself worthy every day of this great honor that has been given to you. Go now. Follow the other pilgrims on this road. Heed them well and work hard. Peace be with you."

The four of us look at one another after the screen goes blank. The Maribehs in the next room do seem pretty excited, elated even. I know they aren't a dumb species, but they are naive. Maybe it will be easier for them, but that doesn't stop me from feeling a little nauseated after having to watch that bunch of absolute bullshit. It makes me wonder what ARC tells the other, more advanced species. My team and I, we are all unsettled by this lie, but we keep our faces impassive—no signal is needed for this; we just all do it instinctively. We thank Kendrick and head out to train. As we travel, we try to deconstruct what happened there in that room. What was the worst part? The blasphemy? The fact that they used a god to explain why they are here or that they will use the idea of pleasing that goddess in exchange for compliance?

I keep coming back to the thought that the reason it bothers us so much is that it worked so well.

CHAPTER 18

When I get home, I shower and change and walk up to meet Ezra. He's sitting at his desk with a pencil in his mouth. I see that he's printed up a map of all The Rift sites around the world. I just want to go and hug him. I'm tired of the stupid baby steps. I want to be normal or—well, as normal as someone like me can be. Instead I sit on the bed. I cross my legs and rest an elbow on a knee so that I can hold my head in my hand.

"Hi." I am so happy to see him, but I know that's probably not coming across in my body language or my tone. I had told the truth before to Kendrick: We Citadels don't know how to let our guards down.

Whatever my body is conveying, it doesn't seem to bother him. "Let me ask you something," he begins. "The Rifts."

"What about them?"

"There's the big one in California, which they explained

was an earthquake and which made that town essentially a ghost town. But the others, like the one here—look at them. Look where they are. Notice anything strange?"

"Well, they aren't smack in the middle of any populated areas, if that's what you're trying to say. But statistically, there are only fourteen, and there's far more of the world that is remote than the other way around." I lift my head and lean back against the wall.

"Yeah, but still, not one in the middle of even the smallest little village. All of them—the forest, desert, the jungle. And yet not exactly inaccessible, either. Like, none in the Himalayas, for example. Hell—this one is in the middle of a military base. It just seems pretty lucky for ARC."

I think about it for a moment and concede that yes, it's lucky . . . unless, of course, you're me or my friends.

"It's unsettling to me. It doesn't make sense. The more time I spend analyzing the data, the less I'm comfortable with the word *coincidence*. I don't have any proof yet, but the scientist part of me feels instinctually that it's not likely, all these happy accidents."

I'm not sure what to say to that. He says he's a scientist and then in the next breath he says he's going on a gut feeling. Scientists don't really do that, but it feels combative to point that out. "Hmmm," I say, which feels like a neutral enough answer. "So, how's it going, then?" I ask, leaning forward, looking at one of the monitors on the desk.

"It's going. Nothing new to report, though. Not really. Should we do some red-pill stuff?"

"Definitely." As stressful as today has been, the idea of spending quiet, close time with Ezra is pretty much all I want in life. I so badly want this to work, but there is this small nagging part of me that feels like I'm getting away with murder. The last time we did this was easy, maybe too easy, but I don't want to be a downer or make him more anxious than he already must be, so I say nothing except: "I took one when I first got home, so I'm ready when you are."

"Great," Ezra says. He stands and stretches. I see the muscles on his stomach when his T-shirt lifts up. I turn away. His abs are really good.

Like, *really* good.

I start the mantra in my head. *I'm safe . . . I'm safe . . . I'm. . .*

"Go get your knitting, your iPad, and a copy of Harry Potter—you choose the volume."

I can't help it. My shoulders sag. So far, this is like the romantic life of a ninety-year-old couple or a ten-year-old couple. I don't bother to argue, though. I just go and get what he's requested. When I return I see that there is a pillow on the floor right in front of the bed.

"By the way," Ezra says as he sits on the bed, "I guess you haven't heard anything about me at ARC? No all-points bulletin or anything?"

"Would have led with that," I say.

Ezra motions to the pillow and I sit down on the floor. I lean back against the bed and position myself between his legs.

"Right. Obviously. They always say that no news is good news. Not sure that's the case here. But hey, what are you gonna do? Such is the life of a wanted man."

I turn to look at him and squint. Ezra is the least fugitive-y fugitive ever. He looks down and smiles, and I have to quickly look away. Slow my breathing.

"So," he says, clearly noticing my reaction, "why don't you start knitting and turn on one of the podcasts that you like listening to?" I begin one of the NPR shows that I wrote on my list. I like them well enough personally, but mostly they trigger a strong emotional childhood response. My parents only listen to NPR in the car, and on any long road trip that's all my brother and I heard. I pick up my knitting. I'm making a warm cowl to fit over my uniform for the coming colder months. I thread the needle through the woolen loop, wrap it, and pull it through. There's a rhythm to the knitting itself that is calming, a *click, click, click* that Zens me out. When I add *This American Life* to the mix, the whole experience is positively peaceful. Ezra is wearing another of my dad's sweaters. The whole setup is about as sexual as Sunday school.

"All right, I am going to put my hands on your shoulders and then your hair. Remember to say your mantra and just know that you are totally safe. Everything will be fine. Nothing—"

"Is going to hurt me, I got it. You can start." I say the words softly to myself as I see Ezra's hands move. Ever so slightly, he rests them on my shoulders. Ezra's hands are big and warm. I can feel the heat through my shirt. My breath catches. I grit my teeth. Things don't feel as easy today as they did last time. I'm emotionally drained from the intake session and it's harder to focus. Ezra's fingers sit lightly on my skin. I feel the Blood Lust start to build.

"Shit," I say as I leap up away from him.

"What?" he says with alarm.

I close my eyes. I can't answer him. I try to control my breathing, but it's coming so ragged and quick. I'm close to panting. I slap my hands over my eyes. Logically, I know that I am safe. I really do, but something else is going on inside of me. I get quick visions, flashes of taking those lovely hands of his and bending each finger back until it breaks. I picture punching him again and again.

With the last shred of self-control I have left, I leap up,

knocking Ezra back. I see him wince. I don't know if I've actually hit him or just knocked the wind out of him and right now I don't care. I tear open the bookshelf, practically rip the access hatch off the hinges, and jump down the hole that leads to the second floor, scraping a good portion of my back on the ladder that is folded up like origami.

I run to my room and slam the door so hard the whole house trembles. The Blood Lust has me, but even I can feel its grip is not quite as strong as it was with the vampire at The Rift. I take my hand and clench the doorknob. I want so badly to go back out there and hurt Ezra that I start to shake. I keep telling myself that I am safe, but my blood is screaming so loud I can't hear it over my own thoughts. Instead of opening the door, though, I punch the wall beside it. I keep punching until the plaster breaks and my hand goes through it. Scarlet droplets pool on the wooden floor at my feet from where my knuckles have been sliced open. I pull my bookshelf down and the books hit the floor with a thunderous boom.

"Ryn?" I hear Ezra say from above me.

"Stay away!" I scream back, although I barely recognize my own voice. It's the throaty, desperate roar of a caged animal. I pick up my bed and fling it backward as if it were nothing more than a sheet of paper. I jump up to the ceiling and grab the pendant light fixture, peeling it away from the wires so they crackle and spark before I heave the light against my mirror. The shards of both fly everywhere, including at my face. I feel a dozen pinpricks of pain on my cheeks and forehead. I stare at myself in the cracked reflection, looking every bit the monster that I feel. Somehow, though, seeing myself in this state makes me stop. I stare. I am a living Picasso. I touch my fingers to my lips and taste the salty copper of blood.

My breathing starts to slow. Reason is slowly creeping in. What is happening? No one can swallow back the Blood Lust once it goes full force.

"But I did," I whisper to myself. That night in the Village. I stopped myself from killing Ezra and that was even before I knew about the drugs or the programming. "And I'm doing it right now."

How?

There is so much about this I don't understand. We're smart, Ezra and I, but we aren't psychiatrists. We're fumbling around, clasping the best parts of the research he's read, but we have no real idea what's going on. I hear a soft knock on the door. The Blood Lust has receded, coiled back inside me like a viper. I walk slowly over to the door and let it swing open. Ezra stands just outside the door frame appraising the damage. My room looks like the back end of a coke-fueled rock star's bender. I hear Ezra's heart start to beat faster. This room scares him. As it should.

"You're hurt," he says, though he doesn't come inside. I stare at my hand. I gingerly touch my face. I'm sure my back is bleeding, too.

"Yeah," I admit. "But you're not. And I guess that's something." I am conflicted about the state of my room. I want Ezra to see how dangerous this is, how dangerous I am, but I am also ashamed. The embarrassment twists my stomach.

Ezra still makes no move to come inside and I certainly don't invite him to investigate further. "Come on," he says gently. "You're going to need me to help you with your face." He reaches his hand out toward me and I look at it, eyes wide.

"Are you insane?"

"Are *you* feeling particularly horny right now?"

For some reason the question makes me wince a little. It hits too close. "No."

"Ryn," Ezra says as he glances beyond me into the wreck that is my bedroom. "Step back from this for a minute. Yes, it's crazy in there," Ezra says, eyeing the chaos behind me. "But we can be rational about this. We can work with the facts we know. The most important fact? You're all soldiers. They did this to you to make you better, less distracted. Boone and Violet are a really great litmus test for this. They like each other, right? That's what you told me? But they haven't killed each other. And that is significant. You can't succumb to the Blood Lust unless you're physically touched by someone you find attractive at a time when you don't feel *anything* else but turned on. If you're terrified, angry, sad, or even, uhh . . . murderous, it can't activate because then you wouldn't be effective Citadels." He moved a little closer. "So, how are you feeling right now?"

"Well, to be honest I'm a little embarrassed at what I've done here . . . and I'm in pain. Pretty bad pain," I admit.

"So come on," he says with his hand outstretched once again. I glare at it and turn my head away. I'd really rather just deal with this myself. "Here," he says, holding up a bottle of red pills. "Take some more of these." I don't know if he's offering me the drugs to make me feel safer or to make himself feel safer. Either way I take a pill out of the bottle. "Maybe you should take two. See what happens," Ezra suggests.

I dump another pill into my hand and walk toward the bathroom. I put them in my mouth and wash them down with water from the faucet. I don't even bother to look at myself in the mirror. I just open the medicine cabinet and take out some tweezers and hand them to Ezra. For the next twenty minutes he goes about digging every shard of glass from my skin in silence. Whether or not he's just concentrating or is freaked out by how I look and what he has to do, I can't say. His hand is on my head. His face is just an inch or so from mine . . . but he's right. There isn't anything sexual about this and the Blood Lust isn't anywhere close to surfacing.

When he's sure that all the glass is out, he takes a warm washcloth and gently cleans off my face. This part is far more intimate, but the act itself reminds me of how my mom or dad used to clean me up after a fall. It's nurturing and I embrace that feeling.

"You're done," he says as he backs away to get a look at me. By now the cuts have all stopped bleeding, and most of them, all but the deepest few, have even closed entirely. He shakes his head. He knows I'm different, obviously, but seeing it like this—my healing—might be freaking him out more than the injuries in the first place.

"What do you want to do?" I ask him while chewing on my bottom lip.

"I'm stubborn. I want to try again upstairs." He leans against the door frame and crosses his arms.

"Are you serious? Were you just where I was? Up in the room and then down in my room . . . all the punching and the exploding glass everywhere?"

He sighs and smiles slowly. "You don't know me that well yet, but I will tell you that when I say I'm going to do something, I do it. I'm determined as fuck. This isn't supposed to be easy, but it's the right thing to do. No one should have to live like you do. I want to help you beat this."

"Well, *beat* could be the operative word here. I'm tired and sore. I don't know if that will help this process or make it worse."

"Only one way to find out," he says, and then walks away and back upstairs to his room.

He's leaving the decision up to me, which I have to say is ballsy as hell. Part of me thinks I should just go straight to my room and start putting it back together. Truthfully, though, I don't want to face it right now. The room is one big failure on my part and I'd rather clean it with some kind of victory under my belt. Even if it's just holding hands again.

I walk up the narrow ladder leading to Ezra's tiny space. He's sitting on the bed and I sit down again in the same position I was, with my back against it and between his knees. I pick up my knitting and start a row. He turns another NPR podcast on. He only waits for a minute or so before he touches me. I suppose he figures that he had just been right up in my face, so there is no point in teasing it out. He slowly puts his hands back on my shoulders. I begin to say the mantra in my head. *He won't hurt me. He won't hurt me . . .* Ezra stays here unmoving for a few minutes. Then slowly, his hands move down my shoulders. He brings them up again and his thumbs trace the muscles in my neck. I tense for a moment. Ezra doesn't move at all. He lets his hands remain there and I do relax. I focus on the knitting. I hear the voices from the podcast talking, though I'm not really listening to what they are saying. Rather, I let their voices become a droning lull that is powerfully meditative. Ezra inches his hands up to my head. He runs his long fingers through my hair. It is here where I really begin to realize the difference between sexual and sensual. The moves Ezra is making, they aren't entirely innocent. The feeling of his hands as they comb through my hair and gently massage my skull is provocative. It's not lust I am feeling but want, *of something*. It makes me ache. I am amazed that this whole thing is working.

I know that I am changing. Whatever was done to me is being erased, slowly, inch by inch. Even what I had *just* done, to my room and the pain in my body, the shame of it, the frustration of it, ebbs away. Ezra's hands are erasing the past. I don't ever want to remember what ARC did to me. But if I ever do, I'm going to have to find a way to make peace with it. I have to accept that I was abused. I have to accept it and walk away from it. I have to focus on the future I want. There can only be trust in this room and maybe love, though I don't want to use that word because that scares me, too.

In a good way.

Ezra takes his hands off me and asks for the Harry Potter book. We rearrange the pillows on his small bed. I turn off the podcast. He asks me to lay my head on his lap. I'm not sure I am ready for this. I know this will put me in very close proximity to an area of his body that just days ago I wouldn't have dared to go near. I have to have faith in myself, in Ezra, in us together. I do as he asks. I lie down on his thigh. He starts to read from the book, and as he does, he once again gently touches my hair and my face. I close my eyes. I don't even need to say the mantra anymore. I feel safe. There is such a tenderness in the way he moves his fingers over my skin that it leaves little room for me to feel anything else. He reads to me for almost half an hour. There is a heaviness in my bones. I am weighed down by the nearness of him, with the possibilities of him. I am sure that if I lifted myself up and touched him, kissed him even, we could take this further . . . except that even thinking of that makes my body immediately tense. I am getting better, but the Blood Lust is still lurking, still hiding out in some forgotten corner, tucked away in the back of my mind. It's a sleeping monster. If I try to wake it too quickly, it will pounce.

Though Ezra was right about going slowly, again, how he knows what to do and how to do it is beyond my reckoning. It amazes me how smart he is, just on his own without being screwed with like me. He's a leader. I didn't realize that until just now. He has a quiet strength and self-confidence that is inspiring. For some reason, though, his self-assurance fuels my self-doubt.

How can someone be so *sure*?

I wonder how much he cares about me. It's hard not to. For one thing, he owes me. He's hiding out in my house. I helped him get out of the Village. He could have easily told me what needed to be done and then opted out. That would have made us pretty even. Or he could have told me what I wanted to hear, read my emotions and simply used me to escape, and already be on the other side of the world by now. But neither seemed like options for him. Because he's here now. He *wants* to be the one touching me and getting close. Maybe I am being naive, but I was lying to Edo when I said one of the skills I've always had is being able to read people. I'm not some lovesick kid infatuated with blue eyes and ripped abs. Maybe it's not love—and hell, I'm not even sure I can call what I feel *love*— but I know he truly likes me. And I think that's what has got me worrying so much. Because this is great—whatever *this* is. But I wonder, once we get past this, once these few days are up: Where will we go from here?

I sit up. I don't want to think about that now. Things have turned so quickly. I used to be afraid of him getting anywhere near me. Now I'm afraid of what will happen when he's gone.

Okay—maybe I am a little lovesick.

Ezra announces that we are done for the night, and as glad as I was for our moment together, I'm equally glad to get out of this little room for a bit.

I go downstairs to make dinner. When it's ready, I bring it up.

I admit I'm nervous. About the future. About us. About the Blood Lust and The Rift and my team and the Immigrants and a million different things. But—as if Ezra senses that—we don't talk about any of those things. Instead we talk about normal things. About our lives and our pasts. He talks about his grandparents in Morocco and his holidays with them. He speaks vividly, moving his hands, describing Marrakech in such detail that I can almost hear the call to prayer and smell the jasmine and oranges. I talk about the lying, how exhausting it is all the time. I admit how sad I am that my parents don't really know me. I talk about guilt. I speak about blood and death and the first time I shot someone, how I threw up beside the body and how Vi held me the whole night as I cried, and how I did the same for her a month later when it was her turn.

We probably could have sat there all night sharing stories, but there is an unspoken acknowledgment that time is against us. Ezra has a mountain of work to do and I need to learn another language. We both agree that the Karekins fit somewhere into this puzzle. They know something about how The Rift works, and whatever it is, they are willing to die to shut it and ARC down. When the smoke clears after a Karekin attack, there is never a single one left alive, ever. But each time they come through they get a little farther past our defenses. I need to try to corner one and ask what they know.

I leave Ezra's room, even though it's the last thing either of us wants. Ezra is a soldier now, too. He understands that our individual needs can't outweigh the mission. I go down to my bedroom. The progress we made in the attic fills me with a new determination. I clean my room up quickly. I don't dwell on what I did to it. After a short while, it's done, and after a quick snack, I start to learn the difficult, nuanced language of the Karekins. The most bizarre thing about it is that there is something familiar, not in the words necessarily, but in the cadence and the lack of certain common linguistic features. It's right there, but I can't place it; no matter how hard I try to nudge the answer, it eludes me. Ezra continues his own work, focusing less on the algorithms and more on breaking a cipher-coded file that he thinks might hold some answers.

It isn't until I've been reading and speaking to myself for four hours that I wonder, if we've never captured a Karekin prisoner, who has?

And how in the hell did ARC get them to talk enough to get an entire lexicon out of them?

CHAPTER 19

I try to hide just how distracted I am at work the following day. I think I do a pretty good job, or at the very least, my team instinctively knows that I need some space and is giving it to me without asking me a bunch of questions or—in Boone's case—making smart-ass remarks. We are in the reserve unit, way back from the deep action of The Rift. It's a good place to be if I want to go all stealth commando, but nothing threatening comes through. I never thought in a million years I would actually want a Karekin invasion, but somehow I need to find a way to get close enough to one of them. Today is not the day.

Before I can make it into the training gym, I am told by a blank-faced soldier that I have to report to Applebaum's office. Violet, Henry, and Boone look at me with concern. They must be nervous about our time at the intake session. I wish. That's the least of my concerns. I tell them not to worry and act like it's all no big deal. Inside, though, I am spooked. I don't think Applebaum knows that Ezra is at my house, or they would have already gotten him. How much *does* he know, though? That's the question. Edo, Audrey, Levi, Kendrick—any one of them could have said something that would get me into trouble regardless of who's hiding out in my attic. Applebaum's office door is open, but I knock swiftly on the door anyway and wait for him to tell me to come in.

"Close it," Applebaum says sternly.

I do as he says and stand at attention.

"At ease, Ryn." I relax my posture but remain standing, vigilant. In just two or three strides I could be over at his desk to snap his neck. I can't help these dark images that bloom inside my head. I know that he didn't come up with the idea of brainwashing us into killer sex machines, but he enforced it. How many consecutive life sentences would he serve if our cases were prosecutable? Child molestation, child endangerment, assault, kidnapping (in a way)—he would get thrown in jail until the end of time. Instead, he's the one in charge here. That's not justice. If one thing is clear, though, it's that ARC couldn't care less about justice. The rules are simply different for them. I know they would execute me if I killed Applebaum. They would have no trouble concocting a lie to sell to my parents. It would be a lie so convincing and with so much evidence that my parents wouldn't even question it. Of course, they'd have to hunt me down on foot—no handy kill switch to throw—but I have no doubt they haven't planned for that contingency.

I can't think of anything more dangerous in the world than a rogue Citadel. I'm sure ARC can't, either.

"I'm going to cut to the chase here, Ryn—we know you've been in the Village."

My face muscles do not move. I already knew they were aware. I might have been far away when Ezra broke out, but I still had my implant in both times that I was there. I can't help but think about the chip now, hidden in one of my flak pockets, protected by the leather of my uniform.

I don't say anything. I just look at him. What does he think I'm going to do? Cry? Confess? When I don't speak, he continues, "You think you're the first Citadel to break into the Village before you turn eighteen? Hardly. It happens more than you think. You're teenagers. You're curious. I get it. We always let it slide. Except with you, it wasn't just once, but twice." He keeps waiting for me to say something and I can tell by the way he's biting down on his jaw that my silence is grating. Good. "I'd like an explanation. Now."

"No," I say calmly.

"Excuse me?" I wonder if it's healthy to have your complexion turn purple so quickly.

"Sir, as a Citadel, I believe I have earned the right to go where I want, when I want. After all, I put a lot of people in there."

Applebaum laughs, though it sounds wrong coming out of his throat. It booms awkwardly. At least his face is turning a normal shade again.

"Oh, so you want me to believe that it's compassion that made you go there? Like you need to make sure all those poor souls are okay? We both know you don't give a shit. Violet— I might believe something like that coming from her, but you? No way. You don't have it in you. In fact, I would question your humanity at all if it weren't for the fact that you were there to see a boy." He looks so smug sitting there. It's taking everything I have not to leap over there and beat him down. How dare he question my humanity? If I'm fucked up, it's because of him and ARC in the first place. What an asshole.

However I feel, I betray nothing. My body remains unmoving. I don't blink. I don't swallow. "If you have all the answers, then why am I in this office?" I'm not going to give him the satisfaction of seeing any part of the real me. He doesn't deserve a single emotion of mine, not even anger.

"Well, the funny thing is, that boy is now missing." He waits for me to react. I'm sure they brought up and tracked exactly where I was during the time frame that Ezra escaped. I was nowhere near the Village. Because I know this, I smile at him coldly.

"Good," I tell him honestly.

"So you're not going to cooperate at all, are you?" Applebaum has stopped laughing. Oh my God, did he actually think I would help him? Seriously?

"I *did* see Ezra in the Village. I *was* curious about what happened to the Immigrants there. I found him to be charming and smart. I don't think he felt the same way about me. I think he was fascinated by me, and curious. I mean, he *is* a scientist. But mostly, he was scared of me. He didn't trust me, probably because I basically put him in that place." I am such a good liar, sometimes I surprise even myself.

"So what did you talk about?" Applebaum pushed. "What was your exact conversation?"

"Nothing that he didn't already know or wasn't able to figure out by himself. He's human. He's smart and he disappeared. So what? What do you think he's going to do? Tell the world? No one would believe him. He'd get locked up in a psych ward before anyone would take him seriously. Let him go and live his life. I doubt you'll hear from him again." Now that I am able to actually say these things to Applebaum, I'm glad he called me in here. Maybe I can convince him to let it go. Let Ezra go.

And maybe they'll shut down The Rift, reverse my conditioning, and let me leave with a million dollars.

"It doesn't work that way. Immigrants cannot live outside the Village. Period. They are too much of a security risk. Eventually, we're going to catch up to him," Applebaum promises.

"I don't know," I counter. "The guy is pretty much a genius. If he gets access to a computer, I don't think you have a chance in hell of finding him." Again, Applebaum laughs. This time, it's even more unsettling.

"What do you think this is? *The Bourne Identity*? You think we're Homeland Security and we have to rely on facial recognition software and CCTV cameras? You think we have to trace a call? We don't need that stuff. We have . . . other ways. So now, is there *anything* you'd like to tell me?"

Shit. What is he talking about? And for the record, I think this is a little too much like *The Bourne Identity*, actually, but I can't say that to him.

"No," I reply stonily.

"Fine. You can go. Just one more thing . . ."

I look at him and I see something cross his face. It's not exactly concern, but something close. I narrow my eyes without even thinking about it.

"If you think that I can protect you from Christopher Seelye, or any of the bigwigs at ARC, I'm telling you that I can't. You don't want to get on the wrong side of them, Ryn. I see you as an asset. They see you as a number."

I gulp, but hopefully not loud enough for him to hear me. None of it matters now. There's no going back. I don't expect protection from anyone but my own team. "All right, sir. Thanks." I turn on my heel and stalk out of his office.

For the rest of the day I train with Beta Team. I am fiercer than I have been in a long while. My punches and kicks in the gym land with both accuracy and brutal force. When we get out into the forest, I am pleased. I haul out, full steam. The team has to work to keep up with me. I am worried. I am anxious and this manifests in my body. I leap higher, somersault cleaner, and balance on branches without making them move even a fraction. I let the power of my body take control because I know that *it is my body*. Technology is not allowing me to have this strength—it is all my own and knowing that makes me feel stronger.

It's an amazing feeling.

I tell Violet, Henry, and Boone that Applebaum got me in his office and asked if there was something going on with me. I don't give them specifics, but they assume it was the intake and I let them believe this. I tell them not to worry, that I can handle Applebaum. I lie as good as I fight, but my close friends aren't going to buy what I'm selling them for much longer. They are too smart. As I head home I begin to form a new plan. I race up the stairs and into the attic. When I get into the room Ezra looks at me and for the first time I see that he has fear in his eyes.

I rush toward him. "What? What is it?"

"Remember all this time that I've been saying that there's a lot more going on here than we thought? Yeah. I was right. Like, horribly, terribly, right. And I don't know that I can do much more on my own."

There are papers scattered everywhere. Furiously written formulas are on the whiteboard and crossed through with black ink. Clearly, Ezra has spent the day getting increasingly frustrated.

There's no point telling him my news without hearing his first. "Explain," I say softly.

"These formulas they had us look at and the algorithms

they wanted us to write? It's not a map. I cracked the cipher on the file I stole. If I had just concentrated on that in the first place, I could have been much further along. I was so sure . . ." Ezra sighs heavily and then rubs his eyes with his thumb and forefinger.

I don't move to sit on the bed or the floor. I remain standing so that he knows I am serious. "It doesn't matter—just tell me what you figured out. I can't help you unless I know what's going on."

"Okay, I know it's not a map because that didn't make sense anyway when I really thought about it. Why map out trillions upon trillions times infinity of Earths that could be of little to no value? It's not logical. There isn't enough time, there aren't enough people to go to each one to survey it. That's not smart—and the people in charge here? They are very smart."

I shrug my shoulders and roll my eyes.

"No, Ryn," Ezra says, his voice rising, "I mean it. I'm a quantum cryptologist and even I feel like a preschooler trying to read Shakespeare. Do you get that? You can't underestimate these people."

"All right, I won't. *I don't.*" I say gently, "Go on."

"It's not a map. The algorithms are a trail. A trail of bread crumbs, and each bread crumb is a key."

I look down to the floor and narrow my eyes as I take in what Ezra has said. "A key to what?" I ask finally.

"A Rift. The equations are passkeys, skeleton keys. With the right equipment they can open a Rift *anywhere.*"

"So let me get this straight—it's a way through a Rift from here *into* the Multiverse so that you can get to *another* version of Earth?"

"Yes, but it's not as simple as that. You see, *you're* the one leaving a trail. Well, maybe not specifically you, but it's a quantum signature leaving it. Every different Earth in the Multiverse has its own unique quantum signature. They *haven't* found a way to lock on to a version of Earth and get there right away. All they can do is follow that quantum signature, but it's not a straight shot. Their technology will continue to open Rifts that have similar signatures until they find the exact right one."

I sigh. I'm getting frustrated. I don't get it. "I'm sorry, Ezra. I haven't done the calculations. Break it down for me like I'm a total civilian?" I ask, trying hard to keep my voice calm. Even still, I begin to pace.

"All right. Imagine that each version of Earth is a musical note. ARC is looking for an Earth, just the same way a musician would look to tune a string on their guitar pitch-perfect. Most people don't have perfect pitch. They need help to make sure the note is one hundred percent in tune, so they use a tuner. You pluck a string and then you turn the machine head, the silver knobs at the top of the guitar, until you get to the right note. That's basically what this system ARC is using does. If each unique quantum signature is a note, their technology basically wobbles with the pitch—or the signature—until it gets close enough to open a Rift. If it's looking for a B-flat, it can eliminate all the other Earths that don't resonate to a B-flat. Then it begins to eliminate the Earths that aren't a *perfect* B-flat.

"Now, in order to really get this concept, you have to imagine that there aren't just twelve notes but an infinite number of notes—each one distinct—and you're trying to tune the thing in a room full of other music. That's why they can't get exactly to the Earth they want to go. There is too much noise. They have to narrow it down. Each little tweak of the machine head would be a jump into another Rift. They have to go through multiple Rifts to get where they are going. Maybe it's ten, maybe it's one hundred—I don't know."

I take a minute to consider what he's saying and then I give an outward groan. "Oh. My. God. You're a musical prodigy. On top of everything else. *Of course* you are. Is there anything you can't do?"

Ezra shrugs a little, but he doesn't confirm or deny the allegation. "Well, I'm not so good with the punching and the kicking and the stabbing people," he offers. No, he's not a fighter the way I am, but he's still a fighter nonetheless. It makes me think about what he'd be like as a Citadel. He's already probably smarter than any of us, without the genetic modifications, but if he could kick ass the way we could? Man, he'd be unstoppable.

"Okay, so is that why you're using a music metaphor? Because I've gotta tell you, unlike *some* people in this room, I did not join the philharmonic when I was in diapers. Maybe you should stick with the math."

"No." He gives his head a vigorous shake. "I'm not using music to dumb it down. I'm using music because I think, I mean, I'm fairly sure, that's what they're using. Sound. To open a Rift, to navigate one."

"Whoa," I say, trying to keep the sarcasm from my voice— and most likely failing. "If that were true, then somebody through history would have stumbled on this magical note and opened a Rift already." I shake my head. "This is crazy. Impossible."

"Oh, really? Well, why don't you flip on over and balance on your pinkie finger and then we can have a conversation about what's impossible?" He says it just a little too smugly for my liking.

"Fine," I concede as I lift my head up to stare at the ceiling.

"It just seems like, I don't know. Magic. Don't get me wrong; I love magic. Magic's the best, but it isn't real."

"What was it Arthur C. Clarke said? 'Any sufficiently advanced technology is indistinguishable from *magic.*'"

"Ahh yes, Clarke. Wonderful chap. Anything else, professor?" I ask in an over-the-top British accent.

He shrugs my sarcasm off. "So maybe this is exactly that kind of situation. Consider this: Sound waves are invisible vibrations. If you couple them with this kind of advanced technology it may seem magical, but so does a cell phone or solar power or breathing. You don't *see* how these things work, but they do, right? I've looked at the specs on this machine. I've looked at the formulas and I've also found what I can only extrapolate to be some kind of weird chart music. This is how they do it."

I don't say anything for a moment. I think about Ezra's discovery, and maybe because I know it has to do with sound, I drum my fingers on my thigh. "Okay, so if we follow what you've figured out through to its logical conclusion and we continue to use the guitar metaphor *and* we assume that the device they've created is the guitar, then—what's the tuner?"

Ezra raises his eyebrows and waits for me to catch on. When I don't chime in right away he throws me a bone. "What's the one thing that every Citadel has?"

"Oh," I say, mentally chiding myself for missing it. "*Come on.* How many things can this fucking chip do? It's like the world's most complicated Swiss Army knife. Look!" I yell with over-the-top infomercial enthusiasm while pointing to the back of my head. "It can change your DNA, locate you anywhere in the world, sometimes kill you, and now . . . at no added cost, it can open a poooorrrtalllll to the Multiverse!"

"Funny," Ezra tells me. "But not that funny, obviously. And

look, the information I decoded about how the implant works in conjunction with the device is sketchy. I think it's some kind of a booster signal. Like, it amplifies the sound or maybe it directs it better? I don't know for sure."

"*Clearly* you're not on your game today, then," I joke, but Ezra's face remains solemn. "Fuck," I sigh as I cover my face with my hands. Like all earth-shattering news, this is hard to process. My mind scrambles as I go over the hundreds of lies that turned me into this person, that led me right into this room. I'm supposed to be superhuman, but it was Ezra with some stolen files and my dad's computer who has finally figured out the truth. The same computer that makes up fliers for Literary Leftovers, our local bookstore, has also uncovered a way to navigate the Multiverse. How does that even make sense? I'm supposed to keep fighting now and Ezra is going to have to leave. He'll never see his family again. He'll always be on the run and I have to figure out what to do with this information. My confusion builds to frustration, which quickly turns to anger. There is one other person who could have told me the truth, who's known it all along.

"That bitch!" I practically yell. Ezra narrows his eyes at me. "I *knew* Edo wasn't telling me everything. I thought it was all about the kill switch. I should have known with her, *with them*, that there would be way more to it. God. Why didn't she just tell me?" I am fuming mad. I almost feel like going back to the base to kill her.

"Ryn, just calm down a minute." Nothing infuriates me more than someone telling me to calm down. I give Ezra a death stare, and I'm both impressed he doesn't flinch and a little pissed my death stare isn't working. He ignores all that and says, "Maybe she didn't tell you because she was trying to keep you safe. Maybe just having this information is enough cause for ARC to terminate you. Maybe Edo was, in her own way, trying to protect you."

I throw my hands up in the air. Every time I think I have something figured out, I uncover something bigger, more horrible. I don't care what Ezra says. Edo should have told me. This changes everything. "Don't you get that the Roones have had this technology all along? If it's in our implants that means they've been able to do this from the very beginning. The only question is, what are they waiting on?"

"If I had to guess, I'd say, numbers." Ezra gives me a look that I can't quite translate.

"Like more math? A better machine, a more accurate tuner? To filter out more of the noise?"

"Yes, that could be true. They could still be tweaking that, which is why everyone at the Village is working on the algorithms. But that's not what I meant. I'm thinking bigger picture. A much worse picture. I mean *numbers* as in more *of you*. More Citadels. Look, I don't know what the plan is. The Roones? They probably want to just go home. But different versions of Earth are dangerous places. They need an escort. ARC? They want to exploit the technology. Maybe. But I'm not even sure they can do this yet."

"So they don't care about protecting The Rift, but invading it?"

"I don't know. Sure, they might be waiting for more of you to do just that. Or they might be waiting because they don't have it totally figured out yet. At this point, the why isn't what I'm worried about. What's really bothering me is that I give off a different quantum energy signature than you do, because this is not my version of Earth. I hate to use the same music metaphor again, but I would pitch to a different note than you, using their machine."

I put both my hands together, almost like I'm praying. I put my hands up to my lips, thinking about what Applebaum said today. Something clicks.

"Today the colonel at ARC, Applebaum, asked me about you. He told me that they have ways of finding you, ways that other government officials didn't have. I thought he was talking about the tracking chip, but now I'm thinking he was talking about your signature. We probably aren't safe here anymore."

"We don't know that for sure. We don't know anything for sure except that they have the technology. But I never saw any data indicating that it's even been tested. I don't know how far away they are from a practical application. It could be days, it could be years. Applebaum could have just been trying to scare you. I think we should stay put. At least for the next twenty-four hours."

I walk toward him at the desk. I reach my hand out, and Ezra takes it and presses it against his cheek.

"You're right, we can't panic," I say to him gently, "because when you panic you make mistakes. But we need another plan and we need to move things along a little quicker." Ezra is still holding my hand and when he looks up at me, I can see in his eyes that he's worried.

"The thing is, it's not that I don't think we need to run. It's that I don't *want* to. I . . . don't want to leave you. Isn't that crazy? What we're standing right in the middle of, it's life or death. It could be the end of a thousand worlds, and all I can think about is you. I've never met anyone like you, obviously."

Each word he's saying is working its way inside me, past all of my natural defenses, past all the lies and the hurt. He makes me better, not happier, but whole. I suddenly realize that I need him, too. He can't leave. The thought is almost enough to take my breath away. I grab his hand tighter, and he smiles.

"Whatever is coming," I say, "we're in it together. If you go, I'm going with you. I don't want to be alone anymore. I don't want to be alive if nobody knows who I am. That's not a life. It's a burden and now that I know you, I'm not strong enough to carry it anymore." I look into his eyes—those glorious blue eyes. I bite my bottom lip. Quietly, almost a whisper, I say, "Put some music on."

"Shouldn't you maybe take a pill first?" he asks tentatively. For the first time it dawns on me that he's dedicated his whole life to school. He went to MIT when he was fifteen. He might not be the most experienced guy when it comes to sex, either. Somehow, that helps relax me.

"I already did, in the car on my way here."

Ezra turns to the computer and hits a button. Damien Rice. He's on my list. I smile as Ezra stands. He is right in front of me. First, he takes my other hand. We hold fast, clenching our fists together. Our foreheads touch. My heart is hammering so hard I think it might break free of my chest. I'm not afraid, though; I'm excited. And I don't bother with the mantra this time, because my head is clear. There's nothing lingering there, because at this moment there's nothing but Ezra and me. No conditioning. No ARC. Just us.

We both look up at the same time. Slowly Ezra moves his mouth to mine. Our lips touch. The kiss unhinges me. I feel like I'm falling, but Ezra's hands are there, to steady me. He takes one of them and cups my face. I've only been kissed once—by that vampire—but that was about lust, if anything. With Ezra, it's so different. It feels like the first time, but it also feels like we've kissed a thousand times and I don't even know how to begin to understand how that makes sense. I wrap one arm around his waist and take my other hand and grip his head—his hair—and pull him closer. I break away from him for a moment just to look at him. Can this really be happening? Am I really able to be this close to him? I'm not me anymore. This part of the Battle Ground lie isn't one I have to believe anymore. He is so beautiful it hurts.

"Is this how it's supposed to be?" I ask, close to tears.

"I guess with us, when it's real, that's exactly how it's supposed to be."

"Is this love, then? Is this how it feels?" I take a step back, unfolding myself from his body. "I know that sounds cheesy, but I really don't know. I don't have anything to compare it to."

"That question is not exclusive to who you are or how you're built, you know. Love isn't a theory you can prove. You can't measure it or weigh it, it doesn't stay in one place, and you can never really be sure of it. But I would say that it's the only word that feels right when I look at you."

Even when he's talking about love he's so nerdy. It's adorable.

"So you trust me? Just like I trust you."

Ezra looks at me doubtfully. "That sounds ominous. But yes, I trust you."

I smile as I pull out my cell phone from the back pocket of my jeans. "Good, because I'm calling my friends."

"Whoa, there, Sparky." Ezra looks at me wide-eyed. "Are you sure that's the best idea? Don't get me wrong—your friends sound great, and I know you trust them with your life, but can you trust them with mine? And even if you can, you're putting them right in the direct line of fire—endangering them."

I put one hand on my hip and cock my head. "We *literally* had, like, a whole soul-mate conversation five seconds ago. Now you're calling me 'Sparky,' which I'm pretty sure is a dog name, *and* you're second-guessing me in a way that makes me feel like you wonder about my judgment."

Ezra sighs and looks straight at me. "That's not it. I'm just—

kind of—nervous because I don't know these people and they don't know what we know. You can't blame me for that."

I smile and put my arms around him. "We can't do this alone. If something happens to me, you're going to need help getting out of here. If something happens to you, I'm going to need help, period. Besides, we have to get the implants out of their heads. ARC could hit the kill switch on them just for being part of my team. They deserve to know. You would want to know."

Ezra sighs and nods. I'm tucked into him, everything seems to melt into everything else, and it's wonderful. I would love to stay like this. I'd love to stay in this bubble, too, this secret little world where it's just the two of us, but we don't have the time. I pull myself away reluctantly, then hit Vi's number on my phone.

CHAPTER 20

"Hey, you." Violet picks up right away and answers brightly. I can't remember a time when that wasn't the case.

I am acutely aware that ARC could be monitoring the call, so I keep my language vague. "Hey, I'm bored. And I'm also over the whole needing-my-space thing. Sorry for acting like an over-the-top emo chick. Please come over, and bring the boys."

"You sure you want the smelly boys around? We could just have a girls' night."

I have to play this right. I can't sound like I want them here too badly, but I have to convince Violet that it's worth the hassle of having the boys around when we haven't had much alone time together lately.

"Let's have mercy on them, save them from an evening of Halo and pull-ups. We can always douse them with perfume.

We could even water board them if the smell is unbearable or Boone gets particularly annoying." Ezra shoots me a look. I'm guessing interrogation humor might only work with the military crowd, but at least Violet is laughing. The fact is I generally never push for all of us to be together. Rather, it always just kind of ends up that way, so it's good she's playing it loose. Violet isn't stupid, and now she knows from this conversation that something is up. The fact that I'm not saying whatever it is out loud is a tip-off, too.

"Well, okay, then, I'll let them know and see you soon."

My nerves are close to exploding as I hit the End button on my cell. I'm not worried at all that my team will rat me out. What I am concerned with is how they will take the news I am about to share with them. They didn't exactly take my visit to the Village in stride. It's going to hit them *hard*. I sigh. Nothing to do but wait.

IN LESS THAN AN HOUR, I hear the front door. Vi could have walked over, but I suppose she was waiting for Boone and Henry to give her a ride. I open the door and welcome them in. I had drawn all the shades and curtains in the house before their arrival, just in case anyone is watching. I don't see any suspicious-looking cars on the street, but still, I feel safer knowing that no one can see into the house. We all say hi and Violet stands there staring at me with one eyebrow raised. Oh, yeah, she for sure knows something is up. Before anyone can say anything else, I raise my phone and power it down. I point to it and to them so they can follow my lead. After Boone's eyes roll so far up and back that he looks like the little girl from *The Exorcist*, he finally turns his phone off along with Henry and Vi. I usher them back past the kitchen and into the family room, which has far fewer windows.

"Okay, Jane Bond. What the hell?" Boone asks.

"I don't want to sound like a total drama queen, but you're going to want to sit down." I motion to the couch.

"Oh my God, you are killing me," Boone says in a huff, but he sits down anyway. After everyone is settled, I remain standing. My stomach drops. I so don't want to have to do this.

"First of all, I am going to show you two things because if I try to explain anything before I do, I'm not sure you'll believe me. Before I start, I want you guys to promise not to freak out. I mean, you can freak out, just wait until we've explained everything. Then you can feel free to lose your minds. Only for tonight, though—by tomorrow you have to be normal again." I bite my lip and tap a jittery finger on my thigh.

"Who is *we*?" Violet asks. I breathe out hard. No going back now. Ezra has been waiting on the stairs, listening. He knows this is his cue. When he makes his way down the steps, Violet looks around. "Who's here?" She can hear him, and so do the others. When Ezra appears before us, the three of them look at me and then each other, mouths gaping.

"You broke him out of the Village? Are you insane?" Henry asks in that tone he has, which makes him sound particularly terrifying.

"I did not. He got himself out. But he's hiding here. He was working in the Village. Ezra is a computer genius hacker guy. He found some stuff out, stuff that affects us all, and it's really serious and . . . bad."

Bad? Stubbing your toe is bad. Sending out a nude selfie by accident is bad. What is going on here is so much more than bad I wonder how I'm going to explain it.

Well, at least I can let them know part of what we figured

out without having to use any actual words. I hold my hands out, palms up, beckoning Ezra straight to me.

"Ryn! What are you doing?" Vi screams at me.

"Stop!" Boone says right after.

We ignore them. First Ezra takes my hands, then he pulls me inside of his arms. I hear my friends gasp. Henry jolts up. I look over Ezra's shoulder and tell my very tall and very large team member to sit the hell down. Ezra runs his thumb over my lips and I smile slowly. He keeps his hand in my hair as we kiss. We kiss hard and long and deep. We put on quite a show for my dumbstruck friends, who are just staring at us like we might burst into flames.

I won't lie—I couldn't care less about them at this moment.

"Holy shit. You guys figured out a way to have sex!" Boone announces with a fist pump.

"Really, Boone?" Violet says, exasperated. "I get it. You're horny. The entire town, if not the entire planet, understands how horny you are. But don't you think there's a bigger-picture thing going on here that we might want to ask Ryn about?" she demands with a mixture of awe and annoyance.

Ezra and I sit down on the large ottoman in front of the couch and we lay out everything we know.

"OKAY, TWO QUESTIONS," BOONE CHIMES in the second we are done talking. "Can I get some red pills off you right now, like immediately? And also, what are we going to do?"

"Shut up, Boone," Violet says. "But . . . yeah, I'd like some red pills, too," she says sheepishly.

"There are enough red pills to go around. But honestly, you two are going to have to take it super slow. I mean it. You're both Citadels, so that means double the danger. This is not a game. And this is not about getting laid. This is about feeling both vulnerable and safe at the same time. Not so easy," I warn.

"Not that I don't want to engage in sex as much as the next guy," Henry chimes in, "but isn't the bigger deal here that the implant inside of our head could explode at any moment? *Killing* us?"

"No—it's about getting laid," Boone says.

"Boone—come on," Violet says. "Henry is right. That has to be our priority. I know it's been hard—"

"I *wish* it's been hard!" he says, gesturing to his lap.

"Jesus," I mutter, but I realize this is just Boone being Boone. If anything, it means he's focused.

And so is Henry. "This is serious. There's a chip in our head that can end us, and crazily, that's not actually the biggest issue."

"What is?" Violet asks.

"The biggest issue is what if this theory of Ezra's is right? That ARC has a way to jump from Earth to Earth? That would mean that not only every iteration of this planet in the Multiverse would be at ARC's mercy, but every iteration of us, too—talk about being able to play us off each other."

I look at Ezra and I can't believe that I have not considered this liability. If they have to go to ground, all ARC would have to do is abduct a version of Vi, or Ezra, or her parents, or even herself to use as leverage. No one that I know or care about would ever be safe, *anywhere.*

Ezra shrugs, his eyes wide, and it's apparent this is a new thought for him, too. Which means he hasn't thought of a solution to it.

Great.

I turn back to my team. "Look, let's just focus on what we

can do. We can solve the intimacy problem, which *is* a pretty big deal. I can remove the implants myself. I just need Violet's help." I lean forward as I try to read them all. I think ARC's betrayal will eventually hit them. For now, like the soldiers they are, my team is focusing on the logistics. I guess I should have known that they would be reluctant to show any weakness in front of Ezra, who is not only a stranger, but an outsider. Still, I am worried about how they will process this information and I hope they won't internalize it all. That once the shock wears off they will remember that we're a team and that they don't have to grapple with this alone.

"You want me to assist?" Vi offers.

"I want you to sneak into your father's office and get the drugs and supplies we need," I tell her. Even though I hate this idea, I see no other choice.

"My dad is a vet," Violet says flatly.

"Well, vets use scalpels and local anesthetic. I know it sucks, but there isn't another way. I won't ask Edo to take your implants out, because I don't want her knowing that I've told you all—not yet. I don't care one way or the other about lying to *her*, I just want you to all be as safe as possible. I'm well aware that she helped me, but she has an agenda. Maybe." I run my fingers through my hair and sigh. "Maybe I'm just pissed off at her and all the Roones for what they did to us and it's messing with my ability to see things clearly. Maybe she's as innocent in all this as we are."

"No," Henry says right away. "We don't trust anyone from ARC, not anymore. Edo may well be a victim, but there wouldn't be an ARC without the Roones, not an effective one, anyway. We need far more information before we start choosing who to trust."

"Agreed. And to that end, Vi, you know you're going to have to get this stuff during your dad's office hours," I tell her.

"Wait, what? No, I can't. It'll be way easier to grab them tonight when everyone's asleep." Vi sits up on the couch a little straighter while I sigh and let my shoulders drop.

"Ezra? Can I be super rude and ask you to go back upstairs for a while? I just want to talk to these guys alone for a few."

Ezra stands and kisses the top of my head. I can tell by the body language of my friends that they are unsettled by this affection. They want it themselves, but it scares them.

"Sure, It was nice to meet you all. I'm sorry, obviously, that the circumstances weren't better." Ezra walks away and the four of us sit in silence for more than a few seconds. They are waiting for me, but they aren't going to like what I'm about to say.

I pull my legs up and fold them beneath me, crisscross style. "Violet, it worries me that you would even suggest going to the clinic tonight. You're smarter than that."

"Ryn . . ." Boone warns.

"Shut it down, Boone. We don't have time to dick around, and Violet doesn't need you to play the hero. She is totally capable of defending herself. I don't blame her or any of you for not fully comprehending the situation yet, but we can't afford to be reckless. Every move we make from here on out has to be precise," I explain. Boone grits his teeth. They are all used to taking my orders on the field, but out in the world they are used to a certain level of autonomy. I've just stripped that away with a single conversation. No one, including me, is really in control, but I have to take charge. "Violet, ARC is monitoring us. You don't think it will be suspicious if they check where you are tonight at three A.M. and see you in your dad's office? I pushed things with the intake and Kendrick, but that was before I knew that them finding Ezra was even a possibility. If I had known then what I know now, I never would have gone in that room," I admit.

"But you *did* go in that room," Henry jumps in aggressively. "You went to the Village. You're harboring the world's biggest fugitive in your attic. You've made a lot of impulsive decisions and now you've just made us all your accomplices. I'm not saying that I wish I didn't know, but . . . well, maybe I am saying that. I wasn't exactly the happiest guy in the world, but at least I thought I knew where I stood. I had a job to do and I did it. Now I don't know what the fuck is going on."

"Are you serious right now? Your *job*? You don't even know what your job is! You're cool with basically being a slave?" I snap.

"Don't get all high and mighty with me, Ryn," Henry growls. "You didn't go looking for answers because you sensed that we were in danger or your conscience was suddenly bothering you. You did all of this for a guy. You were following your snatch, not your morals." Now it's my turn to growl. I get up off the ottoman and stare at them all.

"It doesn't matter how we got here. It doesn't make a damn bit of difference how I figured this out—and in the future, Henry? We're going to leave my vagina out of this, thanks."

"Don't even try that shit, Ryn! Are you kidding me? We've known about this for two seconds and you've known about it for days—for weeks, for all we know. You're going to sit there and dare to judge what *I* say or do? Fuck you." He gets up, and for a moment I think he's going to leave and I realize that would be a disaster. I also realize that he's right. I'm being self-righteous and sanctimonious, and I definitely didn't begin this with anything like the high-minded ideals

I'm spouting now. I think, perhaps, that I'm shocked by Henry's language and anger.

The problem is, though, there's no time for that. No time for his anger, or *my* anger, or any of it. Shit is real *now*, and it's clear they haven't yet accepted my command on this particular mission.

That needs to end.

"Sit down, Henry."

"Go to hell, Ryn."

"Henry. Sit. *Down!*"

There is no mistaking my tone. This is how a team leader sounds. I don't yell it, but every part of me, from my voice to my eyes to the set of my legs, indicates there is no arguing anymore. Henry doesn't hesitate—he sits down, even as Vi and Boone sit up a little straighter.

"Listen to me. It doesn't matter how we found out about this, because the *now* of it isn't as pertinent as the *then*, ten years ago, when they stuck this shit inside us. But they did do something that will help us: They made us great soldiers. And that means knowing when to follow the chain of command. This is not a committee. *I* am in charge here. If you don't like that, you should have asked for a transfer a long time ago." I stand perfectly still, but my eyes soften just a bit. "The fact is, you've trusted me with your lives countless times, and there is no duty I take more seriously than that. There is nothing I wouldn't do for you three, do you get that? All I care about is keeping us safe. If that meant going into the kitchen and grabbing a butcher knife to dig that thing out of your skulls, I would do it right now. This is going to get messy. This is going to get ugly—it's going to hurt. But you all need to understand that unless we stop this, or expose it, or—I don't know what the plan is yet—but unless we do something, *we* are the bad guys. We are the axis of evil, the Empire, the Legion of Super-Villains, and literally the Frightful Four. Maybe you think I have morality issues, Henry—and maybe you're right," I concede, throwing him the tiniest of bones, "but I don't want to be *that*, I promise you. I'd rather put a gun in my mouth than be their weapon."

"It won't ever come to that, Ryn," Violet assures me.

I sit down in front of Henry, on my knees. I grab his hands, which are clenched together on his lap. "I hope not. I want to live. I want to do good in this world. They made us different and I want to make a difference. Henry, do you really believe that knowing the truth has made things worse? Really?"

"I don't think we know the truth," he says as he takes hold of my fingers. "I think we only know part of the truth, which means we are flying blind. We don't have the tactical advantage, no matter how high you believe our moral ground is, and that's a dangerous place to be." Henry's look softens. "I know you mean well, Ryn, but we might not survive this." He untangles one of his large hands and tenderly runs one of them down the length of my hair.

"No," I admit. "But if we die, we die for our cause, not theirs. We can take something back now that they stole from us. I like those terms a hell of a lot better, even if it means we're flying blind."

"And we can have sex," Boone adds, and the rest of us collectively release heavy sighs. "I mean, yeah, yeah, saving the world or worlds, plural. I'm in. But I was pretty much down for anything once you told me about the red pills."

"Hey, it's Mr. Romance!" I exclaim with tween enthusiasm, and get up off the floor.

"Go, freedom fighters," he cheerleads. "And sex. Go, having sex."

"We're with you, Ryn. All the way," Violet says earnestly.

I nod and smile, happy they've decided to follow me. Happy my team is still with me. But Henry is right.

We have no idea what we are in for.

CHAPTER 21

I spend what's left of the night up in the attic. Ezra and I use the small bed like a lifeboat, clinging to one another, each of us adrift on a sea of variables and theories. We have no real answers. We only have uncharted maps of skin: arms and legs and torsos. We trace the lines of muscles and sinew. We wrap our limbs together and find our way in the semidarkness.

I know that Boone is keen to have sex. I am not ready yet to go to that place, and Ezra does not push me. I know my body. I know how it can bend to fight and kick and hit, but I have never felt it arch like it does when one of Ezra's hands is on the small of my back and the other is on my thigh. I know how to hurt, but I don't know how to caress or touch with feather strokes, or grab and claw to elicit moans instead of blood. We don't have a lot of time, but I am not willing to give up the excitement of this process to expediency. The inevitable might be racing toward us, but here, in this bed, I want to be slow and deliberate. I want to stretch out each new discovery I make. This will never be new for me again. I don't know anything about sex, but I do know that the first time only happens once, and I am young. I think I love him, but I am overwhelmed. Could any boy make me feel this way? Or is it just him? I feel like the first time you should know, for sure.

LATER ON IN THE MORNING, I have to leave for work. I know I have to go, but that doesn't make it any easier. I reluctantly kiss Ezra deeply and close the front door. I have been distracted these past few days, but that distraction is over. I feel singular in purpose: Find out what ARC plans to do with the Citadels and find out if they have discovered where Ezra is. I drive to Battle Ground High. I ignore the other students completely, get quickly through the school to the ARC section and hop on the train, all the while putting Ezra and my feelings for him in a lockbox that I mentally kick to the back of my brain. Right now, I have to be a soldier, not a girlfriend. Which is actually pretty easy, considering I've been one most of my life, and the other—if I'm even that—for like three minutes. Once we arrive, I walk with renewed determination to the changing rooms. Let them try to stop me, I think. I am in a mood for violence.

I see Violet dressing once I enter. Her lip is split and she has a light bruise on her cheek. I sigh.

"So much for taking things slow, huh?" I whisper once I get close enough.

"We did, at first. We held hands for an hour while Boone made me hold some rare edition of an *X-men* comic."

I can't help but laugh at that. "What did he have to endure, I wonder?"

"Oh, I'm sure he'll be more than happy to relay that I made

him turn on Josh Groban. God, by the way he bitched about it you'd think I made us listen to *Rent* or *The Little Mermaid*." I peel off my clothes and start to shimmy my way into the field uniform.

"Is *The Little Mermaid really* not on your list, Vi? How about *Aladdin*?" I zip up the zipper and Violet puts a hand on her hip.

"Oh, right, sorry, I forgot you're the coolest girl on Earth. So, *Star Trek: The Next Generation* wasn't on mute last night when you and Ezra were doing your thing?"

I wince a little because I had actually thought about putting it on until I realized that Imogen Heap would give us a sufficient emotional buffer. The list is all well and good, but it's kind of hard to set the mood with aliens and eighties hair. I love *Star Trek* because it's always been my dad's favorite show and we could watch it together without talking. Then I started to like it. Actually, after a careful examination of the list, I have had to accept that I'm a pretty big dork, and cringingly, most of my choices are things that my parents liked first. Damien Rice is my mom's absolute favorite and he's become one of my favorites, too. Our taste in music is one of the few things we have in common. Ezra, true to his word, has not judged me, but why would he? *He's a computer geek*. We might look a certain way, but we're both nerds on the inside, which suits me just fine. Besides, my list is not all sci-fi fantasy stuff. *Downton Abbey* is on the list, and so is *Gilmore Girls* and *The Great British Bake Off*, or as I like to call it, visual Xanax. Wow. I watch *a lot* of TV.

When I'm done dressing, Violet and I walk to the transport bay. No one has noticed Vi's face. Injury is common among Citadels. It's almost more unusual for us *not* to have some kind of visible bruise. Boone and Henry meet us there. I notice that Boone looks far worse. His eye is black and his jaw is swollen.

"I thought you said you just held hands," I say very softly so no one else can hear besides us four.

"I said we did that for an hour, then we tried kissing. But I dropped the comic book and then we were kind of making so much noise I couldn't hear the music and yeah, it got a little violent. But just a little."

"I—"

I cut Boone off at the pass. "Don't say it, Boone. None of the terrifying shit we've figured out is going to matter if you two kill each other before we can make a plan. Seriously," I say just before the jeep rolls up, "you've been waiting for, like, a hundred years just to touch each other. Do you have to turn into porn stars overnight?"

"Speaking of that," Boone says conspiratorially, "Vi wanted to put porn on the list."

We are in the vehicle now, and the regular army troops look back at us from the front seat. I give Vi and Boone a dirty look, warning them to watch what they say.

"*The Notebook* is not porn," Violet argues.

"I was being ironic, Violet," Boone deadpans. Then he mouths the words so that only we four can possibly hear or understand him. "Every movie she has on that damn list ensures that I will never, *ever* get an erection."

"You guys need to shut up now," Henry says without much emotion. It must be so hard for him. He knows I have Ezra. Boone and Vi have always had each other, but Henry doesn't have anyone. There are a few other openly gay Citadels at ARC, but none are as cool or handsome as Henry. Besides, we don't even know how or when we are going to tell the others about our discovery. Henry isn't any better off than he was before, and I get a rush of shame that everything has changed in my life, but as of right now, nothing has changed for him.

He can't touch anyone or be touched and we are going off to work, just like we always do.

We take our positions in Foxhole Six today. If there is serious action, we will be a part of it. Omega Team is taking point. I haven't seen Audrey (thank God), and I'm not sure if Levi is working today. That makes me think: Should I tell Levi? He could have sold me out to ARC about getting into the Village, but my money is that Audrey's cooperation in return for shift work at The Rift site is how Applebaum found out. Levi is an asshole, straight up, but he is an excellent Citadel. He's a brilliant tactician and a natural leader, not to mention that no other Citadel can beat him in a fight, except for maybe Henry. I'm just not certain we can trust him. Considering what he did to his ex-girlfriend, he would likely be on our side, so there is that.

Still, he has that whole total-jerk thing going on.

We had all agreed that talking about what Ezra and I have uncovered would not be smart with so many ears around. Instead, we sit silently in the foxhole. The trench is uncomfortable and cold. When it starts to rain, each of us pushes our backs farther into the mud, trying to get some cover from the small ledge above our heads. I close my eyes. This is another part of my job I hate. The superhuman strength is great and all. I love healing fast, and by the end of the day Boone and Violet will appreciate it, too, probably when the marks on their faces are gone. But this? This mundane waiting outside in the pouring rain? I'd be happy to walk away from this.

Suddenly, I feel the air change around us. It crackles and hums. I already have goose bumps from the cold, but I feel the hairs on the back of my neck stiffen. I get that same sense, that pulling ache in my belly. The Rift is about to open. Omega Team confirms my instincts just a few short seconds later. We wait until it reaches Stage 4, but we don't have to wait long. Instantly, I hear a great booming crash and the trees about two hundred feet behind us explode. Bark and dirt rain down on us in the hole.

It's the Karekins.

My teammates and I look at one another. We had talked about this last night, and it's as if the gods heard us. I need to get to a Karekin and question him alive, and I need my three teammates to help me—and now we have a chance.

We leap out of the foxhole. Right away I know that something is different. Thirty Karekins flank what looks to be a tank, and even more Karekins follow behind it. This species has always been deadly, with sophisticated weapons and armor, but the fact that they manage to drive a vehicle through The Rift tells me that something has changed on their part. The tank starts firing, and a fiery red laser pulse cuts down the Citadels that have jumped from the Nests.

Damn. They are going to need all four of us in this fight. But there's something much bigger going on than this battle, and the Karekins' tank is definitely part of that. My team is holding back, probably thinking the same thing. I nod to let them know our plan is still on. We might be putting some of our fellow Citadels' lives at risk by stepping away from the combat, but we could be saving everybody's life if I can corner a Karekin and get some information.

Through the smoke and chaos I see Levi. He's cutting down the Karekins as if they were nothing more than sheets strung up on a laundry line. I watch as he shoots one squarely between the eyes and then kicks another so hard into a tree that the trunk actually snaps with the force of it. There is such precision in his combat that he makes it look effortless. Then, as if he knows somehow that I'm watching, he turns his head and looks at me. He looks puzzled: Why aren't I fighting?

Shit.

The four of us pick the enemy soldier who is closest to the edge of the forest. He is by no means on his own, but there are at least ten feet between him and another Karekin. The tank continues to blast and our troops start firing back. There are turrets in the Nests for this very reason and despite the misery of a foxhole, I'm beyond grateful we weren't assigned to one today. Vi might be the best shot with a rifle, but for some reason, I'm the most accurate with the heavier artillery. I would have had to stay behind.

We all lunge for the single Karekin. He goes to pull out his weapon, but we are close enough that Boone can shoot him in the hand so that his gun drops. Henry and I get behind the Karekin. I give him a running kick to the kidney, which pushes him forward a foot or two. Boone and Vi are the bait. He doesn't have his gun, but he's pissed that Boone shot him. He starts to pursue them, his giant strides covering more ground than ours can, but it doesn't matter because we are way faster. I pray that Levi doesn't follow us. I manage a quick look and I don't see him.

Thank God.

So far, this is working. Henry and I are right behind him so he can't run back, not that he wants to by the look of fury on his face as he chases Boone and Violet. The Karekin's blood, a red so deep it almost looks purple, spills out on the needles and brush below. I don't let the amount of it fool me. This species is tough: A gunshot wound is barely more than a scrape to them unless it's to a vital organ.

The Karekin reaches out for Boone and swats him deftly

in the head. Boone goes down for just a moment, rolling on the ground and then bouncing up again. We are farther away from the action now, but not far enough. Henry races forward, running at full speed, and pushes the giant forward with all his strength. The Karekin goes flying past Boone and Violet, at least ten feet. He gets up again quickly, but not fast enough, and Vi lands another swift kick to his back. He staggers forward. We have to keep him thinking that we want to fight. He won't follow us if he thinks we are just herding him away from the rest of his unit. Does he know anything about us? Because if he truly knows what we are capable of, he can't possibly think that he can best all four of us together. It could be that he does know, but his temper and his emotions are stopping him from thinking clearly. Maybe none of it matters at all. Maybe he knew he was going to die anyway and figured he'd just take as many of us with him as he could.

The Karekin is on his knees with only Boone in front of him now. He lunges forward and grabs Boone's ankle. It would be easy for Boone to simply kick out with his other leg and land one good one to the Karekin's face. Instead, Boone lets the soldier pull him down, feigning weakness, allowing the Karekin to believe there's a chance. The Karekin pulls out a knife from his utility belt and leaps on top of Boone. Violet jumps forward and yanks the enemy's hand back. Then she takes her knee and plants it squarely on the Karekin's elbow between her own two hands. The Karekin is on his knees and forced to drop his knife. She may have broken his arm. Boone takes off running again and the Karekin, enraged, throws off Violet, gets up, and follows. Finally, I think we are far enough away. I signal to the rest of my team to hold up and disable the mics.

When we all stop, he screams. It is a primal, throaty roar. He must realize that he's surrounded, that he's been stupid and let his anger get the best of him. I hold my hands out and make my posture less rigid.

"We don't want to hurt you," I say in his own language. "We just want to talk."

The huge being narrows his amber eyes at me. "Get my words out of your mouth." His accent is a lot different than the one I heard in the MP3 files. The nuances are hard to catch.

"I don't mean to offend you. I apologize. I learned your language, but I had to steal it from the people in charge here. They don't want us to communicate. Why do you think that is?"

The Karekin remains unmoving. He says nothing and he keeps his body taut.

"We fight your kind. We kill your kind, but we aren't the enemy. We were taken as children and the ones in command changed us; they turned us into soldiers. I want to stop this. I want to close the . . . big green thing."

There is no Karekin word for Rift. I don't know if anything I am saying is getting through to him. Still, I am closer to him than I have ever been to another one of his race that I'm not in the process of killing. Usually everything happens so fast on the field and when you're fighting for your life, it's difficult to observe all the little things. For the first time I notice a small black device in his ear. He sees that I've seen it and immediately reaches for his head. He's fast, but I'm faster. I grab his hand and the others grab the rest of him. He goes down. Henry grabs one arm, Violet grabs the other. Boone restrains his legs, but he is flailing wildly, trying to get us off. I quickly reach into his ear and pull out the tech he's got in there. It's definitely a communication device. I hold it up to my own ear, and hear a faint buzz and possibly a voice, though it sounds distorted and like it's underwater. It's too faint to make out what anyone is saying.

"What is this?" I ask, holding it up. "I'm telling you the truth. I don't think you want to die, so tell me something useful! Can you talk to your army through this?"

Suddenly, the Karekin stops moving. His mouth transforms into a maniacal smile. He begins to laugh. "I am a loyal servant. *I am loyal.* You will learn obedience in time."

I blanch, distracted, which in turn distracts Violet. The Karekin sees his opening. He breaks his good arm free in a flash and grabs the knife strapped to my thigh. Before I can make another move, he drags the knife swiftly across his throat. Deep crimson blood arcs in the air. The Karekin has severed his artery; he will bleed out in a matter of moments. His violent suicide has stunned us all and we stand there watching as his life drains away.

"What did he say, Ryn?" Boone asks as he crouches down to get a better look at the Karekin.

"He said he was a loyal servant. He told me that we would all learn to be obedient and loyal." I take the knife from the Karekin's hands and wipe it off on the hard ground below.

"Oh, good," Boone says dramatically. "I thought he was going to say something scary. Fuuuck." He swears in a long whisper that ends in a flourish of annoyance.

"Loyal to who?" Vi asks solemnly, looking squarely at the Karekin's mutilated body.

I shake my head and back away. "I don't know. But whoever it is, they're scarier than slicing your own throat open, so yeah, no answers, only more questions." I begin to walk away. I hope the other Citadels have contained the Karekins near The Rift.

I don't feel like fighting anymore.

CHAPTER 22

I am staring out the window from my kitchen sink. I have washed my hands twice already and the air is thick with the scent of lemons and bleach from scouring the table. It's almost dark. In this weather, the sun doesn't so much fade as slam shut like a door. One minute it's light, and the next the light is gone, erased from the sky, a blanket smothering the heavens. I wish we could have timed this better. I'd have liked to do this in the day, but lately time is becoming more and more aggressive, turning against our little band with hundreds of counter moves. Pretty soon it will be the enemy outright. I can't stop it. I can't even slow it down. I don't stand a chance against it.

It won't be long until the rest of the team arrives. Boone and Henry are on their way from home, and Violet has gone to rob her father. That's how she said it, anyhow; she's clearly still not comfortable with what she needs to do. At this point, though, comfort isn't really our priority. God knows I would have loved to get some more alone time in with Ezra, but I know that from here on out, there is safety in numbers. I go upstairs and tell Ezra what happened with the Karekin. He doesn't have any more insight than I do. I give him the earpiece that I managed to retrieve. Right away he notices a small button down toward the bottom. When I suggest he push it, he immediately says no.

"This is an advanced race. I doubt they need to use something as basic as an On/Off button to turn this thing on. By the sounds of it, he was willing to die brutally rather than talk. I wouldn't be surprised if the earpiece had a self-destruct option that kills not only the signal but also the person wearing it. I'll try to take it apart while you guys do . . . your own thing."

I lean down and kiss Ezra on the mouth. He tastes like peanut butter. I don't think I will ever get tired of kissing this boy. "Cool, well, yeah, you mess around with the potentially highly explosive device up here and I'll go and perform some brain surgery downstairs on my friends."

"Have fun, hope you win," Ezra says with a little click of his tongue while pointing his thumb and forefinger in the shape of a gun.

I walk back downstairs to wait. I go to the sink to wash my hands yet again. I feel the skin tighten around my knuckles when I pat them on a paper towel. I tell myself that I can't touch anything else because I don't want to scrub them a fourth time. Dry skin I can handle; cracked skin will distract me from doing what needs to be done. I hear the doorbell. Immediately I know something is off. The team would have just knocked or let themselves in. No one rings the bell. I know my parents aren't expecting a package. They have already given me the flimsiest of excuses to check in way more often than they need to (like making sure the sprinklers have really been disabled for the season and did Mom return that shirt to Nordstrom or is it still on her closet shelf?). A delivery would have been big news.

I cautiously walk to the door. There's no time to call up to Ezra and tell him to stay put without whoever's outside hearing me yell—I can only assume he understands that a doorbell is not a good time to come downstairs. I push down on the latch and the door swings open.

Christopher Seelye is standing there.

The breath is knocked out of my lungs as if someone has punched me in the stomach. *What is he doing here?* Seelye is one of the most, if not *the* most, powerful people on this Earth and he's standing at my door, casual as anything with a grin that is impossible to read.

This is very, very bad.

Our eyes lock, and in those brief seconds I imagine pulling him inside, grabbing hold of him, and twisting his head the wrong way round till his neck breaks. I consider hitting him on the most vulnerable part of his skull with the fireplace poker. I think about slicing his throat with a kitchen knife. I know physically I am capable of doing any and all of these things, but I also know that while I may be a killer, I am not a murderer. I may think I'm a monster sometimes, but I am not.

Unless Seelye tries something stupid—and then all bets are off. I have no qualms about defending myself.

"Hi, Ryn," he says in a tone slick enough to be an oil spill.

"Hello," I respond, but I do not budge. I don't open the door any wider. He may be smiling, but I'm not.

"Can I come in?" Seelye asks, with just the barest hint of sarcasm. As if I'm not being polite, as if somehow I'm the one intruding and he's indulging my teenage rudeness by not being more welcoming. Of course, I don't want him anywhere near here. I don't want to look at him. I don't even want him in the same state. But if I slam that door shut, I will no longer be playing the game. I reconcile myself to the fact that I am an expert liar and Seelye doesn't stand a chance no matter how clever he thinks he is.

"All right," I concede, and once the door is open, he waltzes inside with the kind of smug sense of entitlement I would usually associate with royalty. He's tall and slender, with the sort of frame that makes me think he has to work to put on weight. Seelye makes himself right at home and sits on one of the chairs in our living room while unzipping what looks to be a very expensive jacket. He's wearing jeans and a navy sweater that looks soft enough to be cashmere. Seelye is not unattractive in the face, but he's still fairly repulsive.

I reluctantly take a seat across from him. I cross my legs and lean back, forcing my muscles to relax, to pull away from my bones. I don't say anything; I am waiting to hear whatever bullshit reason he has for being here. Seelye doesn't say anything, either; he just looks at me with narrowed hazel eyes. I work hard to keep my breathing even. Ezra is upstairs and the boys are due any minute.

Finally, he crooks his head to one side and says, "You're not going to ask why I'm here?"

I fight the urge to look at the white grandfather clock against the wall that really did belong to my grandfather in Sweden. I don't have time for this, but it's imperative that Seelye believe I have all the time in the world.

"No," I say as if bored.

"Aren't much of a conversationalist, are you?"

I shrug my shoulders. "I must have missed that day in basic training."

Seelye lets out a loud, arrogant-sounding laugh. I don't crack a smile. I just continue to stare at him. His laughter stops abruptly, unnaturally. "Where are your parents, Ryn?" It should be a question, but the way he's asked it sounds more like a statement, like he knows exactly where they are.

"Not here," I answer back, careful not to answer too quickly. I steal a glance at the clock. Any minute now Boone and Henry are going to walk through that door and God only knows how they are going to react to Seelye's presence here.

"Well, I can wait for them." Now it's his turn to lean all the way back in the chair.

I clear my throat. I don't like having to disclose this. "They're out of town."

"So you're alone," Seelye responds slowly.

"Why do you care where my parents are? What do you want them for?" I sit up a little straighter now.

"Well, I did tell you that I was going to be taking a more active role, nurturing that raw talent of yours. I wanted to tell them how special I think you are, how well you're doing. And to give them the heads-up that we might be putting you in charge of some special projects and that you might be away from home for extended periods of time. It's the burden of leadership, Ryn. Sacrifice. For them and you." Seelye looks relaxed, but there is something undeniably predatory about the man. Did he really come here to explain to my parents that I might be gone for a while? Or is he just warning me that ARC can take me away whenever they want? Both, probably, the former as justification for the latter.

A lot of Citadels love Seelye. I've seen them watch him doe-eyed and breathless—even the guys—during Seelye's speeches. He's never fooled me, though. I've always suspected that he has Hollywood screenwriters on the company payroll.

His words never ring completely true or heartfelt, no matter how hard he tries to sell them. He's like those slimy Evangelical preachers on TV who go on and on about Jesus but then make millions of dollars off little old ladies who live on cat food. I need to remember that now. He's just a man—a powerful one, to be sure—but a man all the same.

I'm the one with the superpowers.

"Cool," I say without expression.

Seelye gives a menacing chuckle. "I like you, Ryn." He folds his arms, one over the other. "There's something about you. I can't quite put my finger on it—it's not like you're the friendliest person. I think it's the fact that you're an original . . . and a bit of a rebel. Maybe you remind me a little of myself."

I grit my teeth. I fight to stay calm.

I am nothing like you.

If the boys walk in right now this could be the end of everything. They are not yet unchipped, and Seelye, more than anyone, has complete access to the kill switch. For all I know he could have a remote in his gajillion-dollar jacket pocket right now. I wouldn't put it past him to push that button just to prove a point. He might have a weird affinity for me, but as Applebaum said, the rest of my teammates are nothing more than a designation.

From the floor above, the ceiling gives a tiny groan. And then, we both hear Ezra's footsteps. The hanging light overhead vibrates with the noise. I grit my teeth.

"I thought you said you were alone."

"I never said that," I tell him as calmly as possible. *Please, please don't come down here, Ezra.* The footsteps walk across the ceiling. I hear the bathroom door shut. I let out a breath I hope Seelye hasn't seen me holding.

"Well, if your parents are out of town, that must be your brother. Abel, right?"

There are thousands of Citadels all over the world. The fact that Seelye is sitting here in this room and knows my brother's name means that he also knows a lot more about me. The implications of that are too awful for me to even think about right now. Boone and Henry are supposed to be here already. If Ezra comes down and the boys walk in, this will turn into a fight. Seelye might not walk away from it, but we'll be hunted down by every Citadel and ARC associate in the world. There won't be a single place on Earth where we'd be safe.

"I'd like to meet him. Why don't you go get him, bring him down?"

"No," I say sternly, standing up. I have got to get him out of here. Seelye looks momentarily befuddled. He's not used to hearing that word. He's backed me into a corner. Playing it cool isn't working, and I realize I've got to come out swinging. "Look, I will work for you. I will show up on time for my shifts and put on my uniform and follow orders. But my private life? My family? Off limits. You stay away from them. Got it?"

"Or what?" Seelye counters unfazed. The fact that he has chosen to remain seated while I'm standing tells me that he's not threatened in the least. Why not?

"Please . . . give me permission to show you what that scenario looks like," I practically whisper.

The plumbing in the walls slushes and flows. The door upstairs creaks open. I can hear it, but Seelye probably can't. I stare at him in a way that makes it obvious that he's not welcome here. Finally he stands. He looks me square in the eyes. "Oh, I know you can fight. But do you think you can win? Really?"

"Keep talking and I might be willing to give it a try," I tell him with a sly smile. Upstairs, Ezra's footsteps stop at the stairs. *Stay there!* I wish, not for the first time, that mind reading was one of my abilities. I look at the door, hoping that Seelye will use it, praying my friends won't walk through.

"You don't want to make an enemy of me, Ryn. You *really* don't."

Finally. An actual threat. His double talk was just pissing me off. I can use this. I hear the tiniest creak on the landing from upstairs. I hope to God Ezra is listening to this conversation. He'll stay put. Or shit, maybe he won't. He's thoroughly pissed off at ARC; I hope he can keep it together. He's probably the most rational person I know, besides Vi, maybe. But reason and logic can go out the window when you're having to listen to the douche bag who would have imprisoned you for the rest of your life threatening your girlfriend. I mentally will Ezra to stay where he is. I hope he knows that I can handle this for both of us.

"Why don't you tell me, then, what exactly it would take to become your enemy? Would it take implanting a chip inside your head without your permission? Would it involve a constant terror every time you go to work that you might die? Being forced to kill people? How about never having a normal life? Never being able to have sex? Would that make me your enemy?"

Seelye sighs audibly and gives me such a condescending look of mock sympathy that it takes everything I have not to pick him up by the balls and throw him against the wall. "Oh, the melodrama . . . ," Seelye wails as he clutches at his chest like a southern belle about to faint. "It's good to know that all teenagers are the same, regardless of any kind of *special talents* they may have. You all think the world is against you. I remember that phase."

That's it. I've had enough. He could be Mother Teresa right now (which he *so* isn't), but this man has got to fucking go.

"Yeah, okay," I say, refusing his last bait. "Like I said—when I'm at work, I belong to you. I will carry out any and all duties asked of me. I will even go along with whatever weird special project you probably have in store for me. Just give me my private life and leave my family out of it. I don't want them tainted with this shit any more than they already are. I think you owe me that much at least."

He stares at me and the floor above creaks again. Seelye's eyes look sideways.

"I'm going to go," Seelye says almost kindly, as if I've actually asked him to stay and he can't. What a dick. I don't bother to respond. I also realize that he hasn't agreed to my terms, so I just go to the door and open it.

"Good-bye, Ryn," he says with fake sincerity. He zips up his jacket and walks outside. "Don't do anything crazy, now."

"What?" I ask with a grimace.

"You know, because your parents are out of town and everything. Don't do anything stupid."

I don't bother to answer him. I cross my arms and watch as he gets into a black SUV that's been waiting for him. I watch it drive off, wait fifteen seconds, and race up the stairs. When I turn the corner of the landing I see Ezra leaning against the wall.

"What was that?" he asks, his words a mix of fear and anger.

"Trouble."

"What do you think he knows?" Ezra peels his head off the plaster of the wall to look at me head-on.

"I don't know. Nothing. Everything. I mean, obviously he's

zeroed in on me for some reason, but I have no idea. Applebaum is a prick, but I don't think he'd willingly offer up any information to Seelye about me, or you, unless he absolutely had to. As far as he's concerned, he's the colonel, the boss. He doesn't like answering to ARC and I think there's a part of him that doesn't think he should have to. I think he walks a very fine line, like we all do."

Ezra tucks a piece of my hair behind my ears. "This is getting more dangerous by the minute. You know that, right?"

I take his hand and gently press my lips into his palm. "I know. And I also know that I have to get those things out of my friends' heads as soon as possible. After that, I'll just have to be insanely careful. There's nothing else we can do. Not yet, anyway."

"You're right. But it's also okay to be super freaked out that your James Bond villain of a boss was here to 'check up on you' or play King of the Douche Bags or whatever." Ezra says, trying to make me laugh, which is not at all the same as making light of the situation. Because he's right: I am a touch unnerved by this unprecedented visit. But if Seelye is King of the Douche Bags (which, all in all, sounds about right), then I'm the Queen of Lies.

"I'm fine. You should go back upstairs just in case he shows up again. Also, I don't think you want to be around when I have to tell the team about Seelye's visit. It could get ugly," I joke. Well, I'm only half joking really, but Ezra's had enough excitement for one day. I walk down the stairs and sit on the steps. I glare at the door.

Five minutes later the boys walk in. "Hi," I say solemnly. I never thought, as their team leader, I'd be so happy they were running late.

"What is it?" Henry asks, dropping his knapsack right

down in the middle of the hallway. Jesus. Maybe I'm slipping. Maybe I'm not the liar I thought I was. *Or* maybe, probably, the encounter with the president of ARC has left me more rattled than I thought. I care about Ezra, but it's different with my team. The trauma we've gone through together has bonded us in a way that Ezra and I will never be able to. Which is for the best, really—I don't want him knowing all the gory details of everything I've beaten and killed . . . or when I've been beaten and nearly killed. Henry can read things in my body language and my face that I hope Ezra will never have to.

"Just come in. I'll explain everything once Violet gets here," I tell him, because it's a laborious story and I don't want to have to do it twice. I make myself busy by prepping the dining room table. I lay out clean sheets and position rolled-up towels so the team can be on their stomachs with their necks straight. Boone and Henry eye my preparations warily.

A little while later, Violet rushes in. She has her backpack clutched to her chest and she begins talking the moment she closes the door. "Oh my God, that was terrible. I had to sneak into the surgery room while my dad was in the exam office just down the hall. I'm so glad he makes me help sometimes in the office or else I wouldn't have known what the hell to get, but then I started feeling guilty because I'm always so annoyed that he makes me go in there with all his lectures about responsibility, when I would just rather be dancing when I'm not on duty. But then, you know, I thought about it and I was like, 'Why am I even thinking about dancing? I'm never going to be a dancer! I'm a crazy soldier with a weird bomb in my brain that could go off any second,' and of all the things I imagined I would be doing, having my best friend cut into my head was not one of them." Vi is frantic, rambling as she unloads the supplies in her bag onto the kitchen counter.

Boone gets up and puts his arm around her. It's such a small thing, but it's also huge. For one thing, it means that Ezra and I aren't a fluke. For another, it means that we can finally have the chance to be platonically intimate with someone we're sexually attracted to.

"I know you're feeling guilty, Vi, and afraid," I tell her as I begin to examine the supplies that she has brought. "All I can say is that I know I can do this and we don't have a choice. These things have to come out. If your dad knew all the facts, I'm positive he would understand."

"Oh, please," Violet says as she takes off her jacket, "let's not even go there. I hate the What Would Our Parents Do game. It sucks."

"Great. Violet has arrived, with her *mouth*, that won't stop *moving*. Are you going to tell us all what's going on now?" Henry asks impatiently as Violet gives him the finger in the form of scratching her eyebrow. Part of me really liked it better when it was just Ezra and me worrying about this shit. It's hard to give people answers when you don't really have any. It's hard to watch the team become paranoid, and feel increasingly unsafe outside of The Rift. But I know, if we're going to make it out of this, we're going to have to do it together. As a team.

"What? Did my dad call?" Vi asks in a panic. There it is, paranoia. Check.

"No," I assure her. "Okay. Well . . ." I hold my arms up and scrunch my shoulders, as if I'm about to tell them a funny story. We can't afford a total freak-out right now. "Christopher Seelye came over right before you guys got here." The three of them look at me stonily. A silence that is beyond awkward ensues.

"Way to bury the lede, Ryn," Boone says finally.

"Tell us everything, and I mean *everything*," Henry commands in a voice as hard as the scalpel Violet just swiped. So, I begin with the doorbell. I give them every detail of the entire encounter. I include every word and every gesture, implied or otherwise. When I am done, I am rewarded with more silence.

"So basically what you're saying is that he knows," Henry throws out.

"She's not saying that. She never said that," Violet jumps in, trying to defuse the tension.

"Right now, in this moment, it doesn't matter." I lean back on the dining room table. I want them to see what's behind me. I want them to realize where the real emergency is. "The most important thing is that we get these things out of your heads. Right now. Beyond that, I'm not sure. It could be that he knows a lot of Citadels and he knows how they usually act and I'm not acting 'normal.' I think it was some sort of an assessment, a test."

Henry rakes his long fingers through his short hair. "Well, if that's the case, then it's a test you failed. You were belligerent. You *threatened* him."

I straighten my spine and dig my fingers into the underside of the wooden table. "He doesn't *know* me, but he knows that I'm not a kiss-ass. If I had started bowing and scraping, it would have been far more suspect. If anything—and I know it's weird to say—I think he kind of respects me more now."

Henry snorts and looks away. Violet and Boone give each other a knowing glance. "What?" I blurt out, throwing my hands up in frustration. "What do you want me to do? I can't go back. It's done. I'm sorry. We have the chance to stop something potentially catastrophic, and maybe we take that chance next month or next year, but we're gonna take it because I don't think any one of us wants to be on the other side of this wishing we could have done something. Okay? Enough."

I close my eyes for a moment and take a deep breath. "Now it's time for me to cut your heads open. Who's first?"

"Me. I'll go," Henry volunteers. I know this is as much about his bravery as it is his having my back. I smile at him gratefully right before he lifts up his shirt and throws it at Boone. Good Lord, Henry has a body. His muscles are so toned and defined they almost don't look real. He lies facedown on the table. I position the towels so that one is under his forehead and the other is under his shoulders.

"Boone, I'm going to need your help making sure his head stays still. Vi, you're going pass me the things I need. Ready?" I pull the floor lamp closer to me so that I have enough light and a clear view.

"Don't fuck this up," Henry mumbles.

"You'll be fine," I assure him, even though really my heart is hammering a thousand times a minute. "Vi, fill up the syringe with the anesthetic."

Violet takes a hypodermic needle from a plastic pouch, opens it, and then plunges it into one of the bottles—just another important skill learned as a Citadel: emergency triage. As she is doing that, I shave a small patch of hair just above Henry's neckline. I'm not sure how we are going to hide this. We do heal quickly, but a big bald patch of skin might be obvious. Well, there's a chance someone could notice and there's a chance someone could flip a switch and kill us. I like the removal odds better. I swab his entire neck with peroxide.

I begin to stick the needle in Henry's neck. I numb the entire area and wait for a few seconds. When he says he can't feel my finger, I ask for the scalpel. I make an incision about an inch below his occipital lobe. Violet gives me tiny clamps so that I can pull the skin apart. I can't directly access the skull without drilling into it, so I must go just under it, from the bottom. I see the implant immediately, but this next part is trickier. I freeze the surrounding area inside the wound and grab some tweezers. Gently, I pick up the device and cut the almost invisible thread of an electrode on the right. I do the same on all the other three sides. I do this in the exact same order that Edo had done it in my head. When I am done I give a little tug. The implant is free. I take the tweezers and with a flashlight look for the residual threads that connected the implant. When I pull them out, each one is at least a foot long. Vi shudders and makes a gagging face. I put the implant in a cup and take the clamps out. Instead of stitches, I use medical adhesive, basically Krazy Glue, to close the incision. The scar won't remain for long, but if anyone does see it, at least they'll think it's a gash or a cut. Stitches would be far too obvious.

"Okay! You're done and you probably don't have brain damage. Who's next?"

Violet volunteers to go; Boone reluctantly hops on the table last. Everyone is a little sore—including me, because it's amazing how tense your muscles can get while performing brain surgery on your friends—but fine. About this, at least, I feel good. I have given my friends a fighting chance at a normal life. If they want to leave ARC, disappear, start new lives, they can do that now. If they want to stay and do what I fear needs to be done, they can do so without worrying that someone can simply kill them by pushing a button on a computer.

Before Henry walks out the door, he pulls me aside. Clearly, he's been thinking of the implications of removing this along with Seelye's visit. "You understand that eventually every Citadel all over the world will need to get this device removed." He says this quietly while Boone and Vi are preoccupied, giggling at some private joke between them.

"I'm well aware, Henry," I answer bluntly.

"And so you're also aware that will require a total change in the regime at ARC."

I raise a single eyebrow at him. "I understand the implications. I also understand that even though we are young, we are patient. They trained us well. It could take years to infiltrate the entire system. We can't let Seelye's showing up here push us into a hasty decision based on fear." I put a hand on Henry's arm and squeeze. "But eventually, it has to be done. We can't leave ARC in charge, not of The Rift and most especially not of us. If for some reason the time line needs to be moved up, we'll adapt, because we're good at that, too. I've already got some ideas, but you should start thinking of a plan as well. In the next couple of weeks, between the four of us, we should have at least a basic working strategy that we can start implementing."

Henry sighs and looks down. His short, black hair isn't long enough to fall into his eyes, but his body language suggests that it should be. He doesn't look like a soldier in that moment. Instead, he looks like a kid caught up in something he knows he's not quite emotionally equipped to deal with. He needs my help. As his team leader and his friend, I know he hates feeling vulnerable, but he's going to have to accept it. "Remember that first day all of us were together in Beta Team?"

Henry looks up at me and nods ever so slightly.

"We were expecting the worst, Karekins or some other predator type of monster, but then it was just a bunch of people."

"I remember that day vividly," Henry responds.

"At first we were so relieved, because it was just people, and we could send them along to intake and we wouldn't have to fight anyone." At this point, Boone and Vi have stopped gushing at one another and are listening to me. "They weren't normal people, though. They were from some fucked-up Mad

Max Earth without society. They were crazy and rabid with blood on their faces and scalps sewn onto their arms so they looked almost like wings when they stretched them out. You guys remember that, right?"

Vi nodded as she grabbed Boone's hand. "They smelled so bad. Oh my God. I wanted to barf as soon as the wind hit them."

"We didn't fully understand until that day, that humans could be monsters. We had been told, but we didn't get it." I stop for a minute, reliving those horrible first few moments. I put my index finger on my lower lip and trace it back and forth. "I don't think any of us were ready to actually kill another person. That was the day we really became Citadels—because of *you*, Henry. I fought, but I was mostly just defending myself. I couldn't even take my gun out of the holster, let alone use it. One of them pinned Violet and, Henry, you stepped up." We all look at Henry, who is now standing a little taller. "You put five slugs in that guy. You didn't hesitate. You didn't even think. Violet was on the ground and you did what you had to, to keep her safe."

Henry blows out a breath. It makes a whooshing sound. He puts both hands on his hips. "It was the first time I killed anything. I was fourteen years old."

None of us need to say what is obvious, that fourteen is too young to even see something that awful, let alone actively participate in it. "ARC doesn't look or, to Vi's point, smell, like those guys, but they are just as barbaric. We'll take them down because they've got all of us on our knees already. No one should have that kind of power, and when we take it we're going to have to make sure that we don't turn into monsters ourselves. That needs to be part of the strategy, too."

I stop talking. I let my three friends consider what I am

saying. No one is incorruptible. Not completely. Because the Rifts are so lethal, we can't vote on what to do every time one of them opens. How are we going to create a situation under martial law that's democratic and fair?

As if reading my mind, Henry bends down and plants a swift kiss on my head, possibly more affection than I've gotten from him ever. "We'll find a way," he tells me. I grab his arm again, this time tighter.

"We have to, because if we can't come up with a solution to keep ourselves in check, I'm afraid we'll end up being worse than ARC ever was."

CHAPTER 23

I send my friends home. I make Boone and Vi promise not to try and hump each other, at least not tonight after the procedures. Henry offers to keep Boone with him, which is a good idea. Violet could stay over—maybe she should—but I am getting greedy now and want to have Ezra all to myself. I take a shower once they leave and change into my pajamas. Ezra is passed out asleep on the small bed by the time I get up to the attic. He must be so tired. I climb into bed beside him. I fold my body into his, knees against knees, feet on feet. I feel him stir and we both turn over so that now my back is up against his chest. He kisses my shoulder and the back of my neck and then mumbles something, but I'm pretty sure he's actually asleep. I thought guys were always trying to have sex no matter what. I guess my guy is different. Well, that and the whole traveling through the Multiverse, breaking out of prison, hiding in an attic, working out complex quantum equations for twelve hours a day thing he has going on. He needs to rest. I, on the other hand, am fine for a few more hours.

I roll over to let him get on his back, then lie against him, tucked in his arm tightly. I bury my face in his hair. I trace a line from his shoulder down to the tip of his finger. I make myself as small as I can against him because this life I am living feels so incredibly big. When I find myself in that place between sleeping and awake, suddenly out of nowhere the Blood Lust overtakes me. Even as I feel the fury build I am confused, because I actually thought that when we kissed it had gone away for good. Now it is back, roaring with rage.

I jolt up. The panting begins. I hold the sheets in my hands, fistfuls of cotton, as if they can somehow keep me back. Noiselessly, I jump to a crouch. I look down at Ezra's beautiful face; his long black lashes curl slightly on his cheek. I want to kiss that cheek and then I can feel all my reasoning and logic slip away as I get the overwhelming urge to pull the skin away with my bare hands so I can see his skeleton beneath. I try to block out the violent images, but it doesn't help. I leap out of the bed, pick up Ezra like a rag doll, and throw him against the one solid wall in the room. His body hits the plaster with a dull thud and his eyes fly open. I am going to kill him. I know it. This is it. This is the end. How will I live with myself when the Blood Lust recedes and Ezra is gone? In this moment, I don't care. I practically fly over to him and pin him back against the wall with my forearm at his throat. He grabs my elbow, eyes pleading. I rear back and punch him in the face. I expect him to struggle, but he remains, unmoving.

I think for a moment it's because my punch was hard enough to kill him. I begin to relax at that thought.

The fact is, I can't see much. The room would be pitch-black, but there is a big, swollen full moon and the light is pouring through the tiny window. Up against the wall, we're in the shadows, but it's enough. Ezra manages to use his hands to pry my arm away from his throat.

"Ryn, stop."

I want to stop. I am desperate to stop, but I also want to kill him even more, especially now that I know he's still alive. It's like an affront to me. I give him another swift, hard punch to the face.

"I'm not going to fight back, Ryn," Ezra manages to say, though he doesn't sound so great. I'm guessing his nose is broken. "I told you I would never hurt you and I meant it. You're always going to be safe with me." He somehow relaxes his posture. He has turned off his fight-or-flight response, which takes an amazing amount of self-control. His nose begins to bleed, and as the moonlight hits the crimson it becomes silver. It's as if everything around me loses color. We are both black and white. I let him go. I step back.

"You're safe. You're safe. You're safe . . ."

He keeps saying it over and over, to the point where it's all I can think in my own head. An endless loop of him telling me "You're safe." I continue to study his face. Slowly, the colors begin to seep back into his skin and eyes. The blood is red again. Something has turned. Something has switched off. He told me he wasn't going to hurt me and in this moment, for the first time, I guess, I truly believe him. He actually would have died rather than fight back, rather than risk hurting me. I feel different. The Blood Lust is nowhere to be found. It's not lurking or hiding. It is gone. But at what cost?

"Oh my God," I whimper, bringing my hands up to my face. I am so ashamed. I don't know that I've ever truly felt shame before. I know what guilt is. I have felt guilt. Guilt is how you feel when you've done something bad. Shame is what you feel when you know that *you* are bad. The Blood Lust may be gone, but it doesn't change the fact that I almost killed him. Ezra is such a good human being. Maybe if I was born good like him, like Violet, the deprogramming would have stuck after we kissed. I think there must be something fundamentally bad about me. "I am so sorry. Are you okay?"

"Are you?" he says without the least bit of sarcasm in his voice. He is worried *about me*.

"I am. I think that it's finally over, but I wish we never started this. We never should have risked your life like this. It wasn't worth it. *Sex*. People can *live* without sex. I should have kept my distance. If I was a really decent person, I would have."

Ezra doesn't hesitate. He just comes straight over to me and holds me. I tell him it's over and he believes me just like that? How is that possible? At first I can't imagine being so trusting, but when I think about it, I know that I would believe anything he told me now. I didn't know what real honesty looked like before Ezra. Before Ezra, I existed in a world built entirely on lies, so how would I know how to trust? Now I do. He's given me another gift, and all I've done is hurt him.

And that doesn't seem to bother him at all. "You are decent and you are good," he says. "I didn't think I was going to get out of this without being hurt. I knew the risks. But it's worth it, Ryn. It's not just about sex. It's not even just about being with you, though that's becoming more and more important to me. No, it's about fixing something that is morally wrong. It's about a small victory in what is likely to be a massive war, but it's a victory we need." He pulls me away from him and looks at me. I see that his jaw is swelling, along with his nose. "You deserve to be normal. You deserve to be touched and loved on and wanted. If a busted nose is the price I have to pay for you to get that, then it's a small one. If you needed to go all Blood Lusty so that you could see that no matter what, you were safe, I'd say we got off lucky."

I touch his face and shake my head. "I don't think you understand. I really could have killed you. You gambled with your life. You had a theory and you bet on it."

"Yeah, but what you don't get is that together, you and me? We're the House, and the House always wins. Let it go. If it's over, then let it be over. Don't let tonight ruin us."

I sigh loudly. Could it be this simple? I fuck up and he just forgives me? I mean, I know it wasn't technically my fault, but I still did it. Isn't he afraid that it's not over? Aren't I? I rifle through my brain. I scurry through every thought. I'm looking for even the smallest shadow of the Blood Lust. I've lived with it so long, I know exactly how it feels, especially when it's dormant, but it's gone. If he can forgive me, then I can forgive myself. Yes, I could have killed him, but I didn't. I was able to let go and listen. That has to count for something. "Tonight's not going to ruin us. It's going to make us stronger," I promise him. He hugs me again and I don't feel anything but grateful. He leads me over to the bed and we lie down. I turn over and he holds me. He doesn't let go until morning.

I don't think I'll let go, ever.

CHAPTER 24

Eventually I untangle myself from Ezra and go downstairs. I spend some time in the bathroom and then I put on a robe instead of getting dressed right away. The nightmare of last night feels like exactly that, a nightmare, a bad dream. He has forgiven me and I have forgiven myself. I should have known that it wasn't going to be as easy as watching a few TV shows and reading Harry Potter. The kind of trauma I suffered runs deep. It gets in the marrow. It infects with thousands of invisible threads that have sewn me together out of pieces that were cut too jagged and small. I believe the Blood Lust has gone for good, though. Or as gone as something like that can possibly be. It is no longer a wound, but the scar remains and always will. I have to accept that once upon a time I was a little girl who was a victim. I couldn't save that girl, but I can save the woman she'll become by acknowledging that abuse and then putting it far away from my heart where it can no longer hurt me.

I sigh when I look in the bathroom mirror. These last few days are taking a toll. I feel like I look years older. I suppose, given the magnitude of what's happening, I shouldn't expect anything else. I've always known this job was stealing my youth. It's just happening at a faster pace. Even though it's the last thing I want to friggin' do, I'll have to go into work eventually this morning, but I have some time. If I put my clothes on now, part of me will be thinking of the day ahead. Right now, I just want to be here in the house with Ezra. I need to start making some decisions, but our time alone here is precious. I walk downstairs and into the kitchen. I start to collect the things from the pantry and fridge that I need to make waffles. I lift the waffle maker out of the bottom cupboard and plug it in. As I am whisking the ingredients in a big orange bowl, Ezra walks into the room. His hair is wet and he is wearing nothing but a pair of shorts.

"Hey, I was going to surprise you with a big manly breakfast," I tell him with a wide smile even though I gulp hard. I have to turn away for a moment. I scratch a nonexistent itch on my shoulder by running my chin along it. Underneath his eyes are two crescent moon–shaped bruises. His nose is swollen but not misshapen. I don't think it's broken, but I jacked it up for sure. I hate that I did this to him. I know logically this is not my fault, but on an existential level, it is. It's a good thing I'm not a philosopher because I have to shake off this guilt. It won't do either of us any good and he clearly doesn't seem to care. I smile even wider and look back at him. He's still as gorgeous as ever.

"How very fifties housewife of you," he acknowledges as he walks toward me. I back up a little until I'm up against the counter.

I sigh loudly. I love us being here together—me in my robe, Ezra clean and wet from the shower. This is what normal couples do. They sleep in the same bed and then get ready for work and talk over breakfast. We are not a normal couple, though. "You should probably go upstairs. I'll bring this to you and we can eat together in the attic." Disappointment colors my voice.

"Nah. Let's risk it. You'll be gone all day and I don't want to be away from you for any longer than I absolutely have to. Besides, I am starting to go a little stir-crazy in there."

I put down the mixing bowl and fold my arms. "Well, if that's what you really want," I say provocatively.

Ezra raises an eyebrow. "Here's what I *really* want."

It only takes two steps for him to get to me, and when he does, his mouth is electric. We have always gone so slow, he's been so gentle, but this morning, there is an urgency there that we both feel. I moan inside his mouth, against his tongue. He lifts me right up off the floor, spins us both around, and then sets me down so that I am on the open island of the counter. I wrap my legs around his hips. Ezra keeps one hand in my hair, pulling my face into his own as he continues to let his tongue massage mine. With his other hand, he unties the belt on my robe so that the fabric slips off my shoulders and down to my waist.

He begins to kiss my neck as I lean back. He continues down my collarbone until he gets to one of my breasts. I arch my back and squeeze my legs tighter around him, pulling him in aggressively against me. He licks a single nipple and I feel like I am about to explode.

I actually *hear* an explosion, and my eyes shoot open to see the back door destroyed in a shower of splinters.

I whip my head around to look and I am horrified to see

Levi. He's breathing heavy and I can tell that the Blood Lust has taken over. What is he doing here? Before I can even wrap my head around how much he must have seen, Levi races into the house, leaps over the counter, and tackles Ezra to the ground. I scramble to wrap my robe around me. If I'm going to fight Levi, being half-naked is only going to make the situation worse. Levi reaches his arm back, his hand balled into a fist to land a punch. I manage to grab it and wrench it back before he can execute it.

"Ezra, run!" I yell, but Ezra backs up and away, giving him just enough distance to use his elbow to jab it hard and quick into Levi's throat. Levi's eyes widen. We do have superhuman strength, but not even Citadels are impervious to a hit to our windpipes. I use the distraction to pull Levi up by his shirt. I cross my forearm into his already damaged throat and throw all of my weight against him so now he and I are backed up against the counter.

"Stop, Levi," I say with as much calm as I can. I lean in close, though he's thrashing and struggling to breathe and get away from me. "No one is going to hurt you. You're safe." He gives me an odd look. He doesn't understand. He's confused, turned on, scared, and furious. I whisper into his ear. "They've been lying to us this whole time. It's all a lie." Before I can get out another word I hear boots on the ground. Regular troops, not Citadels, burst into the house with guns drawn. I hear a rifle shot and see the tranq dart lodge itself into the back of Levi's shoulder. Before they can get me, I duck down and watch the dart shoot into a cupboard behind me. Levi slumps and falls to the ground. He's out. Great.

"Now you really have to run!" I shout at Ezra, who is standing now. He just shakes his head: *Where am I going to run to?* I realize he's right: We are surrounded. I'm so annoyed that I have to fight in a slinky robe that I want to scream. No choice—I'm about to become a cliché in almost every action movie where a chick has to fight. I use Levi's thigh to jump off for more height. I fly over the counter and tackle two soldiers. When they fall, I continue to move through. There are at least eight soldiers in the kitchen now. I'd like the odds a lot better if I was in my uniform and they didn't have weapons. But I still like my odds.

I hear the gun go off again. It's Ezra this time. The dart lodges itself in his leg. I rush the soldier that just fired, grab his gun, and hit him squarely in the face with it. I don't want to have to kill anyone, but if it's us or them, I'm going to have to make the selfish choice. With the rifle in my hands I use the butt end of it to hit another soldier in the jaw and then again quickly on the temple. I block the punch of yet another soldier and take the end of the gun again to hit him in the ribs. I kick out behind, knowing another is coming at me, and they keep coming through the blasted kitchen door. I'm hitting, punching, blocking, and all the while dodging the bright red blooms on the end of the tranq guns.

When I feel a sharp sting in my calf I know that I have lost. There were just too many of them, at least twenty now by my count, and no place to fight with any kind of tactical advantage. The room begins to spin and my eyes feel like they have twenty-pound weights attached to them. I stumble, reaching out for one of the kitchen chairs to brace myself. I miss the chair by inches and fall to the ground. My last coherent thought is about Ezra. Have they taken him already? Is he okay? And did he remember to slide the ladder back up into the linen closet before he came down? If he did, we may just be able to hide what we know for a little while longer.

CHAPTER 25

The first thing I hear is voices. They cut in and out as if I am listening to them on a cell phone with bad reception. I try to focus, though it's difficult because the sedatives are still fighting with my instincts and my senses. If I make a move to shake my head or open my eyes, whoever is talking will stop talking. That can't happen. I just need to concentrate without giving any clues away about me being conscious again. I zero in on the voices themselves, their tone and timbre. A male and female. Once I figure that out, I realize it's Edo and Applebaum. Are they really that dumb? Are they really going to have a conversation about me while I'm lying right here? I guess they are. The fact that they would be so incredibly short-sighted is something I can use to my advantage. They under-estimate us Citadels, which seems impossible. They created us; they should know our limitations and where our strengths lie, but I suppose they just look at us as weapons instead of people. How stupid. A gun doesn't change, but a teenager? That's all we do.

"So your theory is that the conditioning failed? Can that happen to all of them? Or is it just her?" I hear Applebaum say.

"It worked for years, Colonel. Every human has a unique body chemistry. I believe her tolerance for the medication simply became higher. Her case is an anomaly," Edo says with confidence. I bet she doesn't like this line of questioning any more than I do. I hear Applebaum sigh and walk closer to me.

"Edo, your people swore up and down you could make the conditioning stick. You never thought to mention that anomalies could occur?" There is a faint tapping. Edo must be typing on her tablet. I kind of love the fact that she is not giving Applebaum her full attention.

"The statistical probability was so minute that no, we never thought it needed to be addressed. I'm as surprised by this as you. Think of all the thousands of working Citadels there are all over your Earth. This is the first time it's happened," Edo argues. I seriously cannot believe they are having this conversation right here beside me, unless, of course, one of them *wants* me to hear it.

"So she doesn't know anything? This was a fluke?" I hear him ask with that same lick of condescension in his voice that never fails to set me on edge.

"I would not say that she knows nothing. Both Immigrant Ezra and Citadel Ryn are technically geniuses." There was more *tap, tapping* on her tablet. "You are the one who put Ezra in front of a computer. You allowed him access to the data set we have been working on to solve our problems navigating The Rift. I can't say how much he gleaned from the information you gave him."

It's kind of amazing how Edo is totally relieving herself of any responsibility. She is putting the entire thing squarely on Applebaum. She is a good liar. No, a great liar. I can't ever forget that.

"A bullet in his brain will solve that problem."

It takes everything I have not to reach up and rip Applebaum's esophagus out of his throat when he says that. He wants to kill Ezra? I had always assumed he would just stick him back in the Village. Maybe they would rough him up a bit, let him spend some time in the brig, or both, just to intimidate him into being quiet. I never really imagined that Applebaum was a straight-up murderer. I force myself to remain calm. As bad as I want to protect Ezra, I have to play it cool. If I kill Applebaum now, well, I suppose that would make me a murderer, too. Is that what I am? I allow myself to linger on this moral dilemma for a moment. Ezra is innocent. Applebaum is not. Is it okay to kill someone who is guilty of terrible things? I'm sure Applebaum believes that he, too, is protecting innocent lives by taking out Ezra, so how guilty is he? And where is the line? I've killed people before, but only ones who were actively trying to hurt me. Now I have to question that, too. If we had been trained differently, if we spoke nonhuman Immigrant languages, how many lives could have been spared?

I wonder now if ARC could have turned adults into Citadels all along but chose not to because as children, we would be more likely to follow their insane orders without question.

Shit—I think we've been Ender's Game*d.*

There have been so many lies. I think back to that very first day when I found out what we were. Everyone just sat there as Seelye explained the new order of things. I know they drugged us with one of their brainwashing serums. I resisted even then. My body went along, but I didn't like it. I fought it. I also know that my case is not an anomaly. Applebaum said that others had broken into the Village. We are not supposed to do that. The drugs are supposed to suppress that curiosity. It only makes sense, then, that I'm not the only one who has this freaky genetic quirk that gives me a higher tolerance. Clearly I'm not completely immune, otherwise I would not have been able to get physical with Ezra easily, but I had enough resistance to ignore orders.

I wonder how long it would have taken me to wake up to the truth without Ezra's intervention. My tolerance would have built up, obviously, but would I have been brave enough to question ARC's authority on my own? I want to think I would have been, but I also know that Ezra's feelings for me and the risks he's taken for me have given me a moral clarity I never had. The others like me haven't rocked the boat. So I have to believe it's Ezra. It's love that's made the difference. It sounds so cheesy in my own head, but it must be true. Love is more powerful than ARC, than their fucked-up brainwashing that allowed teenagers to keep such a huge secret from our parents. It's more powerful than all the Roone technology that's meant to keep us in line. It isn't my tolerance that makes me different. It's the fact that I may well be the only Citadel on Earth who's allowed herself to fall in love and be loved in return.

Wow.

"So what do we do?" Applebaum asks, and I know by the way his voice has carried that he is now looking directly at me.

"I assure you that we can erase any memory she has of this experience and recondition her to be more compliant, but it might take an extended time period. After that, we simply increase the dosage of the drug each day in the protein shake," Edo says flatly as I try not to wince. "The only problem we have now is explaining Ryn's absence to her family and friends. Of course, that is out of my purview," Edo says deferentially.

"That won't be a problem. Just get started as soon as you can." I can hear as Applebaum begins to walk away.

"And the boy? We could try something similar with him. He does have a valuable mind. It would be unfortunate to waste such an asset."

Thank you, Edo! Applebaum doesn't answer right away.

"No. We'll interrogate him, find out if he managed to use that genius brain of his to figure anything out that might be of use, then we'll eliminate him. It would be too dangerous to let him live."

"Whatever you think is best, then," Edo tells him passively. At least she tried. She has to get points for that. When I hear the door open, then shut, I keep up the knocked-out routine, thinking about what my next move should be.

"I know you are awake, Citadel Ryn. The moment they wheeled you in here I gave you a shot to counter the effect of the tranquilizer."

I open my eyes and sit up quickly. Maybe a little too quickly—my head spins and I have to exhale loudly to get my bearings. I look down. I am wearing a hospital gown, but at least I have my underwear on still. I hate the idea of being totally naked and vulnerable to any member of the ARC staff.

Edo takes out a penlight and grabs hold of my head in her small hands, shining the light into my pupils. "You have a problem, a serious problem, and I am going to offer you a solution, though you will not like it."

I move my head away and swing my legs over the bed. "Is the problem the fact that I know you lied to me the day I confronted you? That I thought you might have been the *one* person in this whole friggin' place who I could trust, and now

I don't think I can trust anyone here? *Jesus*. Why in the hell didn't you tell me?"

"I was going to. Eventually. You didn't need to hear that information all at once. The fact that you and the Immigrant boy have figured something out that no other Citadel knows is significant. My instincts about you were right. You're the one we've been waiting for. You may not trust me, but I trust you," Edo says with as much sincerity as I think she is capable of.

"Oh my God. Really? I'm 'the one'? Ha!" I say with as much sarcasm as I can muster through the fog of the sedatives I'm fighting off. "Don't put that shit on me. We both know that's not true. I'm one of many, even if Applebutt hasn't figured it out. None of this would have happened without Ezra. Maybe *he's* 'the One.' "

Edo gives me a considered look. I don't break eye contact. If anything, I stare at her harder. "All right," she concedes. "I apologize if I sounded overly dramatic. You are not *the* one, but you are the first, which makes you important. I don't know how to adequately express how vital that is."

I hold up my left hand to Edo's face and then snap my fingers back on my palm in a dismissive gesture. "I don't know what you're talking about. I don't care. You operate on this fucked-up level of, like, reverse transparency that I cannot deal with. I have to get Ezra before he's murdered, okay? I don't have time for whatever crazy you're selling today."

I hear Edo sigh, a winded whirring that sounds like a broken machine. "I understand that. However, it is entirely too risky for one of your dramatic fighting escapades. There is only one truly safe way out of here. And it starts with knowing you have more time than you think. Ezra will not be executed immediately. You must be smart now, as smart as I believe you to be. You must be methodical and put your emotions away."

"You don't need to tell me how to be a soldier. I know how to do that," I snap at her. I swing my legs around and try to put my weight on them. It feels good to stand. Even with bare feet, I feel stronger.

"But you don't know *why* you need to be a soldier."

I fight the urge to scream. The only things keeping me from bursting through that door and finding Ezra are her assurance that he's okay for now, the fact that I can't really burst out of anything, and the dawning reality that she might be right. I can't trust her, but I also can't afford not to at least hear what she has to say. If I was right in telling my team that something big was about to happen, clearly ARC's reasons behind this whole situation could be key. I grit my teeth, but eventually say, "Go on."

"The thing is, I think you already know part of it," Edo says. "I know what information Ezra stole. I know what he read and I'm fairly certain that, between the two of you, you figured out that we have a device capable of navigating the Rifts."

"Yes—we put that together. And I'm pretty sure I know why the Roones would want to navigate the Rifts—because it's a way home. What I don't get, what I can't imagine, is why ARC wants to be able to go into the Rifts. What are they going to do? Colonize other Earths? Steal technology from them? What exactly is the plan? I mean, if it was noble, if they meant to return all the Immigrants back to their own homes, then we would have known." The dizziness has passed and my eyes can focus fully.

"I assume *all* of those things will be happening. Immigrants will be returned home and, knowing ARC, different versions of Earth will be infiltrated."

"And you're allowing that to happen. No—you're *facilitating* it." I sigh and shake my head. "So getting home is worth any price? I get that ARC doesn't seem to have a conscience, but the question is, do you?"

Edo places her tablet on a table beside the bed. She stands before me with her tiny frame, looking so much smaller than she ever has before. "When we first arrived here, we couldn't have known where our work would lead us. You have to understand—and I must be blunt, so I apologize in advance—but to us, humans are little more than barbarians. You are a violent race grasping for power. Some of your own grandparents were born during a time of a terrible war where millions died horribly, simply for choosing to worship one of your Gods in a way that their persecutors felt made them inferior. That's a living memory for your most elderly, not the distant past." Edo walks over to the cabinet beside the bed and opens it.

I close my eyes and grind my teeth in frustration. "Edo, the Holocaust was a terrible thing, but I'd like to think we've learned from that as a species, grown from it." I do not want to talk about history. I want answers about the here and now.

"But you haven't. Genocide continues to this day among your people. Those being murdered are poor and hail from less developed nations, and for some reason that matters less, which I find even more disturbing. Even as we are speaking right now, there are any number of groups that would love nothing more than to destroy this country and everyone in it based on religious differences. There has been some progress, but it is marginal compared to what you are capable of." Edo opens the door of the cabinet and hands me a field uniform. "All we ever wanted was to go home. But we are only a few, while humans number in the billions. We have had to work inside a very flawed system. The Citadels were created to be peacekeepers, but even the vision of what you could be was corrupted by people like Applebaum and Christopher Seelye. We are prisoners. We have no power here."

I take the uniform and slide it up over my body. I feel a hundred times better once I have it on, more like myself, more capable of doing what needs to be done. I check my flak pocket. The implant is still there as I expected. Edo would never willingly offer that information up to Applebaum, considering she's the one who removed it. "But you really don't care how barbaric we are if it helps you to get home. In fact, it kind of looks like you're using our weaknesses against us. That doesn't sound very enlightened or noble to me. You talk a big talk, but really what you are saying is that the end justifies the means. Maybe we aren't so different after all."

Edo takes two large knapsacks out of the bottom of the cabinet and struggles with the weight before depositing them on the bed in front of me. "I am an imperfect creature," she admits. "I have made mistakes, but I believe the Citadels can outsmart ARC and travel through the Rifts, being the ambassadors we created you to be."

I furiously grab the side of the bed and lean forward. Edo jumps with my sudden movement. "Let me just get something straight with you: You did not *create* me; my mom and dad did. You experimented on me, you brainwashed me, you abused me, you turned me into a killer. If you had wanted us to be ambassadors, I'm fairly certain we skipped that part of the training."

Edo does not look away. It's hard to stay mad at someone who is clearly trying to help me and who also looks like a cute cartoon character.

I stay a little mad anyway, because she also has been a part of the program that kept me a monster.

"Like I said, we had much different intentions with the Citadel program, but it was taken out of our hands."

"Yeah—like *you* said."

"I do not understand your logic," Edo says while giving an almost imperceptible shake of her head. "You say you do not trust me, and yet you want answers you will not take as truth. You tell me that you must save Ezra Massad, but you stand here debating philosophy and diplomacy. What will it be, Citadel? We can continue this discussion or I can tell you my plan—you decide."

I fight the overwhelming urge to kick something. I hate having to put any kind of faith in Edo, but as it stands, I see no other choice.

"Okay, let's hear this plan of yours," I say.

"You and Ezra, you have to leave. You have to go through The Rift. These packs are full of supplies. Inside are provisions—hazmat suits, gas masks, medical supplies, clothing for both hot and cold climates, tents, and a computer that contains all the information we have on how to open a Rift and how to follow Ezra's quantum signature through each one until you get to his version of Earth. I've also included a detailed schematic of the device you'll be using with very straightforward instructions on how to operate it." Edo's smooth and shiny rocklike face is devoid of emotion. This sounds reasonable to her. It sounds like something very different to me.

It sounds like the beginning of an old Fantastic Four comic.

However, for all her sound logic and calm reasoning, she's left out one key explanation. "And what are you getting out of this, Edo? It seems like if I leave and ARC figures out where I've gone, you're screwed. They'll kill you."

Edo does not look frightened at this notion. She doesn't seem scared by this idea at all, which I find interesting—and troubling. "I am getting proof. I expect that you will escort Ezra to his Earth and then return here to this one with the data. I think that is a fair trade for my help."

I don't say anything about her motives. She's proven time and time again that she operates within the gray areas of honesty. She'll help me, but only as far as it will help her. For all I know, she put together these packs the moment I confronted her about the implants. There's no point in asking her more questions about it. I'm never going to get the whole truth from her. I open up one of the bags and look inside. Even if she is lying about other things, the system they built *does* work and the Rifts are navigable. I don't need to take her word for it. This morning—with them finding Ezra, and our earlier fight with the Karekin—is proof enough.

The things she listed seem to be there. We may be well prepared, but there's no way that she could prepare us for everything we could potentially encounter. "Is this laptop the only place you have these signatures stored?"

Edo cocks her head to one side. She wasn't prepared for me to ask this question.

"No," she answers reluctantly.

"So, technically, anyone could find us. That seems like a flaw in the plan. And besides, if we make it through, why would I ever risk coming back here? I would be shot on sight. Just like Ezra, I would be too dangerous to keep alive." I laugh a little as I pick up one of the packs.

"Please do not attempt to convince me you are someone other than who you are. You would never leave your family or your team behind. You are honorable; you will return to them and you will return my favor today by letting us know that the QOINS function in the way we believe they will. Besides, you don't need to use an existing Rift to travel back to this Earth. You can open one anywhere, somewhere less conspicuous." I grab the other pack and heft it onto my free shoulder.

"The coins?" I ask.

"Yes, the Quantum Operating Interdimensional Navigating System. We felt the acronym was appropriate given that it needs two parts—the Head and the Tail. I don't think I need to clarify where the heads are located."

"That's cute, yeah. Great, I got it. But what I don't think *you* get is that ARC might not know where I've gone, but they are going to know that *you* let me escape."

Edo shakes her head. "Let me worry about ARC and Colonel Applebaum. I will tell them exactly what they need to hear." I scrunch up my eyebrows. I can only assume she will lie on my behalf, but what if she's been working with them the whole time? The further into this I get, the more complicated it becomes. "After you leave here, you must retrieve a Tail—the other part of the QOINS—from the storage facility room 81B. It will be heavily guarded. Then you must go to the intake area of the bunker to rescue Ezra Massad, who will also be under heightened security protocols."

I give Edo a burning look. "Oh, cool, is that all? I thought this was going to be hard. So first I have to go beat down some soldiers before they call for backup. Then I have to pull a *Mission: Impossible* thing with some piece of technology I've never even seen. Then I have to drag all this stuff and my sedated and possibly tortured boyfriend out to The Rift site. No problem at all." I roll my eyes. I don't see how in the hell I can do any of that alone. "Where is my team?"

"Foxhole two. I'm sure they will assist once you get to The Rift. And I do suggest you use the existing Rift here instead of the QOINS right now. We know this Rift is viable and you can enter it quickly. Until you get a better understanding of the technology, I believe that would be the more prudent option."

It had never occurred to me to try to open a Rift on my own. The idea that I can seems crazy. I consider, for a moment, my options. Something is beginning to take shape in my head, something inescapable. Something awful. I can't leave without telling my story to as many Citadels as I can. The truth has to come *from me*, firsthand. That part is imperative. I also can't leave without making sure that after my story is told, the Citadels who hear it will be safe. The other obvious advantage to leaving is that I not only save Ezra's life but most likely my own as well. Applebaum will be watching me like a hawk, making sure the fake reprogramming has stuck. If I'm going to dismantle ARC, how can I do that if every decision I make and everywhere I go is monitored and picked apart?

If I go.

If I choose to leave, my options have narrowed down to one inevitable, terrifying truth. I told Henry that the time line for this might have to change and that we would adapt, because we were good at that. I'm about to put that theory to the test. I'm going to need Edo's full cooperation in order for the ultimate end game here and at HQ in Livermore to work. I might not get another chance to land the Roones squarely on my side. It would be careless of me to leave, though, without some kind of tangible proof that I can trust her.

"I'll go. I'll go and test your device for you," I offer, "on one condition."

Edo's eyes widen just a fraction, as if she would be raising her eyebrows if she had any. "You have very little bargaining power, Ryn. Choose your words carefully."

I don't believe that. She doesn't want just any Citadel to be the first to Rift out. She wants *me*. That's leverage enough.

"I want your laptop. I want your personal files. I want to know what you don't want ARC to know."

For a long moment Edo says nothing. The onyx of her skin reflects brightly in the harsh fluorescent light. It almost hurts my eyes to look directly at her small, smooth head. "It's entirely in Roonish," she finally says.

"You can provide a flash drive with the whole lexicon," I counter.

"It's in code," Edo says right away.

"Ezra can break it."

Edo looks away, considering. If she wants me to trust her, here is her test.

"I could just take it," I say with bravado. "I could just march into your office and take the damn thing. You couldn't stop me, not physically. You can't call security, because I have these two packs here that prove we are working together."

Edo sighs slowly. I've got her and she knows it. Then she surprises me by letting out a short laugh that sounds like a pickax striking granite. "The laptop will provide you with answers, Citadel, but that doesn't mean you'll necessarily understand the truth."

I shrug. "Not *necessarily*, no. But it's better than being in the dark about all these lies."

"Fine. I will give you my laptop and my language, and then you will go off and begin your great quest. But you must really leave now, Ryn. If my laptop is the price I must pay for your obedience in this matter, then I will comply."

Edo turns on her heel and walks briskly out of the room. When she returns five minutes later she has her computer and a flash drive in her hand. I take them from her and shove them into one of the packs.

"Just so we are absolutely clear—because I don't want any

backpedaling later on, you understand that, by agreeing to do this, it means that we're in this together? We're on the same side, Citadels and Roones." I pick up the other pack.

"I understand that it is part of your training to attempt to get such a guarantee, but I do not believe it is necessary."

"That's not an answer." I deliberately remain where I am so that Edo sees I am not going to move unless I get one.

"Fine. I will do everything I can to make sure you are safe, and to keep ARC in the dark about your whereabouts. I cannot guarantee anything beyond that. I cannot speak for every Roone, just as you cannot speak for every Citadel."

I may not be able to speak for every Citadel, but I know that not one of them would want the implant left where it is. That truth is compelling enough for me to do what I know I have to do next. If I explain this to Edo she will try to stop me. She may even decide that her assistance is no longer a fair trade. Her desire to get home has led us to this moment every bit as much as the moment I decided to break into the Village. Like I've said before, every future is made up of a series of past choices. "That sounds fair," I say as I back up. "I'll see you when I get back."

"Be safe, Citadel Ryn," she says with as much warmth as her scratchy voice will allow. "And be smart."

I nod and smile, but all I can think is that it's already far too late for that.

CHAPTER 26

I keep my head down as I walk quickly toward the elevators. I am frustrated that I have to carry these two huge bags with me. It's unusual for a Citadel to carry anything other than a weapon, and I know if I don't double-time through the hallways someone is going to notice.

I catch the elevator down to the lowest level. When the door opens, I am met with an armed soldier standing in front of a caged metal gate.

"What are you doing here?" he demands. "You aren't authorized to be here."

"Yeah, sorry about that," I say even as I throw one of the packs at him, which he catches. It gives me enough time to drop the other pack and leap onto the cage behind him. I hold on backward to metal holes in the gate and then quickly wrap my legs around his neck. I squeeze my thighs and apply pressure. I am not going to kill him, just choke him long enough for him to lose consciousness. The pack drops from his hands. He struggles and reaches for his sidearm, which I kick away swiftly with one of my legs. He holds on to a thigh, digging his fingers in, trying to get me to let go. The suit absorbs most of his futile efforts. Poor guy; he doesn't have a chance. After a few seconds, he falls to the floor. He's out. I prop him up and open one of his eyes long enough so that the scanner can read his iris. The gate opens. I put him in the entryway to stop it from closing—and momentarily feel bad for using a living person as a doorstop. I get over it, though. Then I go and retrieve the packs. Once they are on my back, I step over the soldier to get inside the long narrow hallway of the storage area.

I drag the man to the first door. I crouch down and reach for his swipe card that's hanging from his neck. I swish it through the machine and the door opens. It's not the room where the Tail is being kept, but I have to stash this guy some-where. I drag him inside and take his com system. I break the door handle so he'll be locked in with no way to call for help. I decide to leave my packs just outside the door. Speed is the key to success here, and those bags are making this ten times harder than it needs to be.

As soon as I step out, I see another guard. He looks at me and narrows his eyes. I watch as his hand goes toward his ear so that he can call for backup. *Sorry, pal—not going to happen.* I run at him full speed and knock him to the ground. I stand over him and take his head in my hands. He's putting up a fairly good fight, his leg kicking up, trying to get me.

It's cute.

I bang the back of his head on the cement floor twice. He's out, too. I take his com unit and destroy it under my boot heel. I open the door closest to me, pick him up, and throw him into it, breaking another door handle so that he can't escape. I have to move quickly. I have no idea how often these troops have to check in. I run past doors, checking each one for the number I need.

Once I reach it, I open the door. I suppose I was expecting a small room, one the size of a supply closet or something, because it's supposed to be storing a Tail, which is supposedly only about four by four inches. That's not what I see. The room is large and fifty feet long, maybe longer. The built-in shelves on either side make the narrow room seem even skinnier. I go to the closest shelf and open a box—it's filled with Tails. My stomach drops. I look at the room, and see the shelves are filled with identical boxes.

My God . . .

There isn't just one Tail. Every shelf, from top to bottom, holds *hundreds*. And there are so many shelves . . .

They really do mean to send all of us through The Rift. I stop for a moment and think about the numbers. I was the fifth crop of Citadels. There were five hundred of us when I began. There are now another three hundred, with another seven hundred implanted and waiting to come of age. If I add the number of Citadels from the other Rifts using the same math, that's more than twenty thousand soldiers. Next year, the number gets bigger. I don't know what it would take to stop that many of us. Nuclear bombs, maybe?

I could destroy all the Tails, but ARC would only build more. Besides, there are thirteen other Rift sites. I have no doubt they have storage facilities just like this one. Something needs to change, but getting rid of the QOINS is not going to do it. I quickly grab three of the Tails and run back the way I came. I go into the room where the packs are and find the soldier is still passed out. That's good, at least. I shove two of the Tails into one of the packs and then the single one into another. I heft the packs back onto my shoulders and run for the elevator. So far, this part of what I need to do was easy. I doubt the next part will be the same.

I exit the elevator and walk quickly in the direction of the intake area. I stand in front of the retinal scan to get into the section. Adrenaline starts to pump through me. Applebaum could have already locked me out of the system, I have no idea. The scanner reads my eye and I hold my breath until the machine beeps and lights up green. I'm in. They haven't taken away my clearance. I briskly take myself down the hall. No one seems to be paying much attention to me, which is kind of weird. I am a Citadel in uniform with two large knapsacks. Maybe they are afraid to stare at Citadels—afraid it will annoy us and we'll go off. They probably think we are monsters.

They're probably not far off.

I assume that one of the intake rooms serves as an inter-rogation room. It's got the two-way mirror so that everything can be observed, and the equipment so that everything can be recorded—although I know that Applebaum won't be recording *everything* he plans on doing with Ezra. I go to the door that Greta took me to, the one where I saw the Maribeh intake. I actually don't want to be on this side of the room, but I am not sure where the other door—the one I watched the Maribehs walk in from—is in this maze. I'll start here and think of something.

Before I can reach the handle, I feel a hand on my shoulder.

"Ryn, hey, what's with all the stuff?" It's Kendrick and he's looking at the two packs with interest. What do I do? Can I trust him? I don't trust anyone in here really, but I don't think he's the enemy. He may be self-serving and have an agenda, but I don't think he would be down with murdering an Immigrant just because he escaped from the Village.

I take his shirt in my fist and pull him down lower so he can hear me. It has the added benefit of showing him just how strong I am, in case he needed a reminder. I angle my head behind him so that no one can see what I am saying. "I need to get into that room. You're about to question a hostile, correct?"

Kendrick pulls away from me and scans my face intently with his deep brown eyes. "What's going on?" he asks in a tone more serious than I've ever heard from him. "Ezra Massad is in there, and the brass say he murdered a guard in the Village. Is that true?"

"No, of course not. He did escape, but that has nothing to do with why he's in that room."

Kendrick tries to pull away from me but finds he really can't budge me. That surprises him, but I don't want him alarmed, so I let him go. Just by reading his face I can tell he isn't going to help me unless I give him more. "You know he's a computer genius, right? Well, his job in the Village was to look over data and decode algorithms. He found something. He figured out something that ARC doesn't want him sharing. Once you're finished with him, Applebaum is going to have Ezra killed. I heard Applebaum say it when he thought I was tranqued."

Kendrick is looking at me like I've sprouted two heads. He doesn't believe me. I clench my jaw and I feel my back teeth grind together. I might as well go all in now, or else Kendrick will force my hand—literally.

"ARC has a way to navigate the Rifts. The implants in our heads aren't implants; they're tracking devices and part of a locating system. They're going to use us, the Citadels, to conquer, or colonize, or . . . I don't fucking know, okay? But everything ARC has told us about who we are and what we're doing here is a lie. If I don't get Ezra away from here, he is going to die. Are you going to help me?" I notice that others are looking at us now. I don't need this kind of attention.

Kendrick takes a good long look at me. This time his face is unreadable. "You realize you sound totally delusional, right? Like you need a psych eval."

I grab his shirt again, even harder this time. He jerks forward. Kendrick's eyes widen.

"Don't be an idiot. You've seen Ezra. You think he's capable of murdering someone? What makes more sense: Ezra being a coldhearted killer? Or ARC—who has kept this whole thing secret, and by the way, *did* this to me without anyone's consent—lying?"

Kendrick places his hands over my own and I look down at them, and then up at him. I raise my eyebrow, as if asking, "What do you think you're going to do here?"

He pulls his hands back, holding them up like he's surrendering, so I let him go. He backs up. "Fine, I'll help you. But let's get one thing clear: You don't ever touch me again, and you protect me if this goes sideways."

"Agreed," I say. I don't even smile at the thought of him threatening me.

"I'll get him out of the room. Just wait here and try not to look like you're about to snap someone's neck. Be cool."

I open my mouth to warn him not to tell me what to do, but he's already gone. Minutes tick by. People pass and I lean against the wall, with the two packs at my feet, trying to look casual. The people walking by don't look at me. I am not sure whether or not this is because I am succeeding with my act that it's just a normal day at the office, or because I am a Citadel and the other personnel in the base instinctively avoid us.

Kendrick is remarkably fast. He emerges from the intake room with Ezra, who is wearing military sweats with the ARC logo. At least they had provided him something to wear other than the boxers he was captured in. He, too, must have been given something to counteract the tranquilizer. His eyes are sharp and focused, but there is a thin sheen of sweat on his brow. He is scared but keeping it together.

"I told the other intake officers that I was taking him to medical. You don't have much time before they figure out he's not there. I hope you have a plan," Kendrick says warily.

"I do. Just keep your head down, and whatever happens, try to stay out of the way. I'll make sure to tell my team that you helped me today. They'll look out for you."

Kendrick watches with obvious curiosity as I heave a pack over my shoulder and give the other one to Ezra. Kendrick must have questions, but he is smart enough not to ask them, smart enough to know that I probably wouldn't tell him the entire truth—if any version of the truth at all—so there is no point in demanding answers.

"You're a good Citadel, Ryn," Kendrick says kindly, "but you're a better person. If you say there is something going on that isn't on the level, then I believe you. I care about the Immigrants. It's my life's work. I need you to know that. When they brought Ezra in, I knew they were being cagey about it. I'm happy to help get him out of here."

It's nice to know that not every adult in ARC is a jerk. It's nice to know that there is at least one person, just an ordinary flesh-and-blood person without superhuman abilities, who's willing to put it all on the line to do what's right. "Thank you, Kendrick. I really mean that."

I begin to walk down the hall, leaving Kendrick behind. Ezra is beside me, matching my steps. He turns to say something to me, but I silence him with a look. I want to touch him. I want to hug him, kiss his mouth, feel with my own body that he is okay. But more than that, I want to get out of here.

We wind around several corridors and then take the elevator up to the floor where the transport bay is located. Adjacent to the double doors that lead to the outside is a smaller, unassuming one. I crack it open and pull Ezra into the room. It's one of the armory rooms, but of course, it isn't empty. There is a counter running the length of the room and a large bulletproof Plexiglas wall. A soldier sits at a desk on the other side of it.

"I'll take the Glock 19 with three clips and a set of zip ties."

He looks familiar, though he's not posted here on a regular basis. He has a burliness to him that makes me think he must be a Marine, but it's hard to tell. After a while, the troops all started to look the same to me. I don't know whether that's because there's a certain type of soldier ARC chooses to work here, or because I stopped really looking. The soldier glares at Ezra and then me. I do not break eye contact. I cannot reveal that there is anything out of the ordinary going on.

The young man goes to one of the many large black metal sets of drawers. He unlocks the top shelf and retrieves the gun, and then from another set of drawers, the clips I had asked for. Finally he gets the zip ties. He passes the items through a window that he unlocks from his end and slides them onto the long counter between us. I take the clips and put them in various flak pockets. When I get the gun, I look it over and then cock it back. "I'm feeling a little resistance. When was the last time it was cleaned?"

The soldier looks at me sideways. I hate this look I get from newer ARC military, like, "What the hell would a little girl know about a gun?"

"Yesterday," he says with a slightly irritated tone. "Did it myself."

"Well, maybe I'm imagining it. Why don't you come out here and have a feel for yourself?" I keep my tone neutral.

He sighs loudly and exits through a metal door.

I have kept the gun out, ready for him to take, but as soon as he's close enough I hit him with it square in the nose. Blood immediately starts pouring out of his face. Rather than reeling back, as I assumed he would, he lunges for me. I manage to spin us around just before my head hits the concrete of the far wall behind us. I quickly maneuver my feet to the side so I can run them up the wall. I scramble up high enough to flip in the air and land behind him. I take the Glock and hit him in the back of the head. The soldier staggers. I hit him again and he goes down, unconscious.

"Ezra, grab his keys; they'll be in one of his pockets."

Ezra drops his pack and immediately begins to search. I use the zip ties to bind the Marine's hands and feet. When Ezra finds the set in his pants, I ask him to unlock the door behind the Plexiglas. After he does, I drag the soldier back into the room and stash him under the desk. If anyone walks in, no one will be able to see him. With that done, I leave the sectioned-off room and join Ezra in front of the counter, putting my gun in the holster on my belt.

"Please tell me there was a good reason for doing that," Ezra says with a judgmental tone that instantly makes me clench my molars.

"We needed the room," I say as I put the pack at my feet.

Ezra looks at the pack and then back at me. "'We needed the

room'? We couldn't have just talked somewhere? Jesus, Ryn." He runs a hand slowly through his hair.

"When we get to wherever it is that we are going, we are going to have a serious discussion about Intelligence."

Ezra narrows his eyes and crosses his arms—a harmless gesture, but one that seems aggressively directed at me.

"Not that kind of Intelligence. Spy stuff. How to signal someone, how to make a drop, how to disguise yourself, sweep a room, create code words, that kind of thing. But the first rule of spy stuff, Ezra? Don't stand in a corner and whisper. It's suspicious."

Ezra keeps glaring.

"Why are you looking at me as if I've just killed him? I knocked him on the head. They took us and now we're escaping. What the hell did you imagine was going to happen? That we were going to skip out of here, holding hands, singing 'Follow the Yellow Brick Road'?"

That was too harsh. I drop my shoulders and relax just a fraction. "Come on," I say as I pull him toward me into a hug. He holds me tight. We cling to one another. I'm scared, too, but I'm used to fear. I'm used to acknowledging it and then pushing it back someplace deep enough so that it won't affect my decision making or my fighting. I am literally built this way. Ezra is not a coward, not by a long shot, but he isn't used to this.

We put our foreheads against each other and then we kiss. We kiss surrounded by guns and ammo and tear gas canisters. The room smells like oil and copper pennies. I want to keep kissing him, but there is no time. "We have to go," I say finally, breaking away from his mouth but keeping my arms around him.

"I know, but where?"

"I made a deal with Edo," I begin. Ezra pushes me back just a fraction to get a better look at my face. "I told her that in exchange for her help to escape the base and for her personal laptop, we would go through The Rift."

"I want to say yes because I really want to get out of here, but I also want to say no. No. No. Please, God, no. Can I say that and not sound like a pussy?"

I put my hand on his face and smile. "That is a totally valid response and not pussy-like in the least. Just hear me out. The Roones' navigation system works. That's how they found you at my house. All the things you theorized were right. You need to leave this Earth. The safest way for you to do that would be with a Citadel. The Roones need data as to how many Rift jumps it takes for their system to lock on to a quantum energy signature, so they need a Citadel for that, too. And finally, we need to decode Edo's laptop together and try to find out if we can get a clear picture as to how much power the Roones really have. It sounds drastic. It sounds crazy, but honestly, I think it's the smartest move."

Ezra folds his arms and sighs. "I don't know, Ryn. It's awfully risky. How do we even know for sure the technology will work on another Earth?"

"We don't. But staying here is not an option. I need Edo and the Roones on our side. The Roones will do anything to get home. They aren't the hippie Vulcans they want us to believe they are. They need us. For something. We need to figure out what that is, away from their reach. Edo handed over her laptop under the assumption that we wouldn't be able to understand the information stored on it. The more they underestimate us the better. If we stay on this Earth, we lose the advantage on several fronts."

"I agree with you. We have to go. But . . ." Ezra says as he massages one of his temples with a couple of his fingers. "You have to tell the rest of the Citadels about the implants, about what we learned. It's not that your team isn't great, but they aren't you . . ." I can tell he's reaching for the right words, trying not to offend me or my friends. "You're a leader, Ryn. You're *the* leader and this is your story to tell. If it's not explained in the right way, it could go very, very badly."

"I know. That's why I am going to tell everyone the truth and *then* we are going to leave."

"Okay." I can see Ezra putting it together. "I don't . . . how are we going to . . ."

He keeps interrupting himself because what I'm proposing makes little sense, at least to him: How can we escape on the sly but still make sure the Citadels we leave behind are safe?

I can't help but grimace. Ezra is not going to like this part of my plan any more than I like having to execute it. "You're right—there won't be any Rifting out with the kill switch still in play." There is dead silence, and I watch Ezra's eyes change as he starts to put together what I mean.

"What are you going to do?" he asks.

"I'm going to take over the Command Center," I say with more confidence than I feel.

"You mean *you're going to start a war.* Right now? You're going to Pearl Harbor all over this sweet little clandestine operation? Alone?"

I cock my head to the right and look to the ceiling. "It actually sounds a lot scarier and more aggressive than it will probably be?" I don't mean to put this in a form of a question, but it just kind of comes out that way. "I can neutralize everyone in Command by myself. And there's a good chance I won't have to kill anyone."

"Seriously, Rambo? Call your friends. Why would you do that by yourself?"

I'm getting a little frustrated now. I realize we're partners, but he doesn't understand much about guerrilla warfare and I don't have the time to explain it. "I need the element of surprise, and pulling my team away from The Rift will set off alarm bells at Command. You've really got to trust me. It sucks, but I have to do it. I have to tell the others the truth and I have to make sure they're safe when I do it."

Ezra shakes his head in annoyance. "There's no way I can talk you out of this, I know it. I'm not even going to try. So let's go before that guy wakes up and ruins whatever crazy plan you've got. Just know, for the record, I think this is fucked up—you doing this alone. But if you say you can do it, I suppose I have to trust you."

I reach up and kiss him on the cheek. "Thank you," I tell him, and I mean it. His faith in me is astounding. Standing beside him, I feel like I can do anything. I feel like I can make everything right because I am on the *right side*. He makes me feel like a hero. "You're going to go ahead," I tell him. "I want you away from this base right now. I'm sure your instincts are telling you to wait for me, maybe even to help me. But honestly, Ezra, the most helpful thing you can do is get away from here so that I don't have to worry about you while I do what I have to do next. Are you okay with that?"

Ezra rolls his eyes. "Uh, no. I'm not okay with it. I hate the idea of my girlfriend going off to save the day while I hide up in a tree or some shit . . . but I will. I'm not going to let my ego put you in even more danger."

I squeeze his hand and smile. It was the perfect thing to say.

We pick up our packs. I open the one that has all the specs and instructions about the QOINS, pull out the spiraled papers and hand them over to Ezra. "Here," I say as he takes them. "This will give you something to do. Memorize it and keep it safe."

Ezra skims through the papers. Once he understands what they are, he doesn't say a word. He just hugs the packet close to his chest while adjusting the pack on his back with his one free hand. We walk out of the armory and after a few short feet, push open the double doors that take us out to the transport bay. The wind is biting and cold. The sky is flat. I walk over to a soldier. There are always at least four posted here, not just as sentries but drivers as well.

"I'm going to need you to drive this guy to the intake rendezvous point. He's doing some consulting work for us."

"That's fine," the soldier says, and walks toward one of the jeeps. He offers to help with the packs, but I wave him away. He goes and sits in the driver's seat while Ezra and I walk around the back to dump our packs in.

I secure the bags in the jeep and turn to Ezra. I wish I could hug him. I can't. He does lean in, though, and I catch the briefest hint of his smell, that spicy oak, which makes me sigh.

"Be careful, Ryn, *please*." He doesn't wait for me to respond. He has already walked ahead, around the vehicle to climb into the passenger seat. I signal the driver with a thumbs-up sign that he sees in his rearview mirror. The two of them drive off and I exhale slowly. Once I do this, there is no going back. I am about to start a war and I'm doing so without backup, without input from my friends, and without the approval of my new Roonish ally, who is going to be pissed.

God, I hope I'm doing the right thing.

CHAPTER 27

I go back inside and take the elevator down to the Command level. There is a soldier posted outside the door of the Command Center. He nods.

"Open the door," I demand.

He gives me an odd look but does as I ask. As soon as we step inside, I reach down and relieve him of the weapon in his holster and give him a kick that's hard enough to send him flying into the air before he lands on the floor headfirst in the middle of the room. I step over his unconscious body. The entire room stops and looks at me. There are about fifteen people in all. Ten are seated in front of computers and there are two armed soldiers. Applebaum is standing in front of the dozens of monitors that show The Rift site from various positions, and finally, Levi and Audrey are there, too.

Well . . . *shit.*

I definitely wasn't counting on that. My mind scrambles, one thought tumbling over the next. Why would they be in this room? Levi had been tranqued, but he must have gotten the drug to counter its effects because he looks alert and ready to take me down. I wonder what Applebaum has told him. The way the colonel is looking at me, though, it's clear he anticipated my arrival—Audrey's presence is testament to that. *Well, I suppose she makes the perfect pet if you can keep the leash tight enough.*

I look over to Applebaum to try to get a read on him. He seems unfazed. More than that, he has the barest hint of a lopsided grin. "Oh, Ryn," Applebaum says in mock sympathy. "I'm so sorry it's come to this. Sergeant Rossi? Enact the Midnight Protocol on designation 473, authorization Applebaum, Thomas. Charlie Hotel three three seven one Foxtrot Bravo." Before I can even swing my head around to look at who he is talking to, I hear a keyboard furiously click away. Applebaum has a shit-eating grin on his face. And then . . . nothing. Applebaum's brow furrows. "Rossi! Do it!"

"I did, sir."

I walk over to the man who just tried to kill me. I wonder if he has a family, if he's married, if he has children. I try to humanize him. It isn't easy humanizing a man who would so casually murder a seventeen-year-old girl just because he's been given an order. He didn't even hesitate. I take his head and quickly pound it hard against the keyboard. Blood spurts from his nose. I smash his head down again. The armed soldiers in the room aim their rifles at me. I don't want to have to do this. I hate having to do this, but I don't have time to tell them that they are on the wrong side. Two lives for every other Citadel on the base. It's not fair, but nothing about this situation is fair. I point the gun I have just taken from the officer posted outside and fire off two quick rounds to the other soldiers' abdomens. They won't die right away. Stomach wounds take a long time to bleed out; they might have a chance to live if I can finish here quickly enough. Audrey begins to giggle. I'd like to shoot her next, but first things first.

"Everybody stand up, move away from your computers, and get against the wall," I demand. Chairs scrape and I hear them scrambling to do as I say. "Oh, come on, Tom," I say, looking right at Applebaum. "You gave us all this superior intelligence. You can't honestly be surprised I figured that one out. Then again, honesty isn't exactly in your wheelhouse."

"Ryn, what are you doing?" Levi asks with stony intensity.

"Well, not dying, for a start, which probably bums out a lot of people in this room. Sorry."

Applebaum hasn't moved, but his hands are up, at least. And that lopsided grin is nowhere to be found on his dumb face.

"Now, Ryn, let's talk about this. I'm sorry I had to do that, but you've lost it. You're a danger to everyone in this room. Do you really want to kill these people? I don't think you do. I think you want answers, and I can provide them to you. Just let everyone go, then you and I can sit down and I'll tell you everything you want to know."

I sigh and cock my head. "Maybe later, 'kay? You know us Citadels—we always play hard to get."

Levi begins to walk slowly toward me. "What's going on?" he demands.

I turn and aim the gun directly at him. "Don't take another step, Levi. Seriously. I don't know what he told you about me, but I promise you that whatever it is, it is a lie. The implants? They have a kill switch in them. Applebaum just tried to activate it, but I had mine removed. And yet I still have all of my abilities. How can that be? Well, there's a complicated explanation for that, but the easy answer is that you all"—I swing my gun around a little bit—"are a bunch of evil fucks."

Levi looks baffled and Applebaum is starting to sweat. Levi looks over at the colonel and, Levi being Levi, sees everything he needs to know written all over Applebaum's face. It's not just that he's angry—because obviously, being the egomaniac the colonel is, any Citadel challenging his authority would piss him off—it's that he's scared. Terrified, actually, and just a little bit guilty. Levi sees this. He's piecing it all together. *He knows* I'm right. I have to be quick now. If something comes through The Rift, the Citadels on the ground will be expecting to hear from Command.

"Audrey," I say, focusing my attention on her, "I know you're crazy. It's cool, I get it. But I am not your enemy. ARC is the enemy. The whole 'hurting people we want to get with'? That was brainwashing. And not just normal run-of-the-mill mind control, either. I mean seriously messed-up stuff where they exposed us to sex and beat us."

Audrey shrugs her shoulders and makes a little sound like she couldn't care less. "I'm not so concerned with how they did this or why they did this. I like what I am and if ARC is responsible, then my loyalty is to them. We are not on the same side." Audrey changes her stance. Her body goes rigid—she is ready to pounce.

I can't say I'm surprised about where she stands. I turn to face the other Citadel in the room, and even though I'm fairly certain he's on my side—I'd probably be dead already if he wasn't—it doesn't hurt to reinforce it. "Levi, you know me. I would never do anything this drastic unless I had a very good reason. I know I promised you I would never touch Ezra, and I broke that promise *because I actually could.* I figured out what they did to us and it's awful, but we fixed it. You don't have to live like this. We're on the same side—I swear to you we are. Even if you kind of hate me or whatever, I need you. I am not crazy. I am not a danger to anyone besides the people who did this to us."

Levi's breathing becomes heavier. It looks like he's ready for a fight, too. He walks up to me and looks me straight in the eye without giving anything away. Because of ARC, he nearly killed his girlfriend, but maybe he feels he's in too deep already. Maybe he doesn't want any part of the truth. Maybe he just wants to follow orders and not do any soul searching about what his place in all of this is. The truth here is ugly. It would be so much easier for him if he just believed that I had gone rogue. He puts his hand on my gun.

"How could you ever think in a million years that I hate you, Ryn? I don't know what the hell is going on, but I'm with you. I've got you."

I smile at him gratefully. "Thank you for trusting me. I know how difficult that is for you, for all of us. But I'm worthy of it, I promise. Once you hear the whole story, you're going to think differently of me. You're not going to think I'm a little kid anymore," I say with a kind of half laugh.

"I said sometimes you *act* like a kid. But let's get something straight: I don't see you as a child, Ryn."

He's giving me a super-intense look. I absolutely have no idea what to say to that. "Ohhhkayyy" is the best I can come up with. I think it's best we skip over the implications of his statement and get on with this, so I give him an order. "You handle Applebaum. But don't kill him—not yet. We do need more answers. I'll handle loony tunes over there."

Levi takes the gun from me and pushes it right into Applebaum's forehead. He doesn't bother to speak, but if I was Applebaum, I'd be very afraid. Levi's eyes are colder and more intense than I have ever seen them.

I turn around. There are about ten feet between Frenchy and me. She is smiling a particularly disturbing smile. "Okay, Aud—" but before I can even finish saying her name, she runs and leaps forward, kicking me squarely in the chest. I am thrown a few feet backward, into one of the desks. My shoulder blade hits a computer, smashing it to pieces. I'm now lying on the desk, but before I can get up, Audrey is on top of me and her hands are around my throat, squeezing. I grab her wrists and whip my head up so that my forehead connects violently with her nose. Audrey still won't let go, even though from the blood and immediate swelling, it's clear I have broken it. To be fair, as hard as it must be for her to breathe, it's a bit harder for me, what with the choking and all.

I still have her wrists in my hands, though, and the head-butt must have distracted her a bit, because finally I am able to pull them apart and off my neck. I keep them locked in my own hands and jump up into a crouch. I leap off the desk into a somersault and land behind her. Her arms are pulled the wrong way now, and it won't take much effort to dislocate her shoulders. What Audrey lacks in strength, though, she makes up for in speed. Using her legs to get leverage, she scrambles up the side of the desk and pushes back so that we both land on the floor. In a flash, she leaps up and kicks me again in the side. There is enough power in that kick to send me flying into the wall. I land on the floor with a thud.

I spring forward using my hands and whip back up to standing. I'm a good fighter, but I don't revel in it the way Audrey does. She isn't just skilled, she *loves* it. And yet for all this zeal, I can't help think: *But . . . she's* French.

Audrey runs at me, her hand balled up into a fist, and manages a swift punch to my jaw. Before she can land another, I block her hand with my own. She tries another kick, but

I leap out of the way. As we get into a rhythm, it's obvious that Audrey truly is crazy, and that her manic style—while unpredictable—is also undisciplined.

That's when I know I'm going to kick her psychotic ass.

I dodge another attack and punch her again in the nose. She staggers. I use that lapse to my advantage, jumping up and using all of my body strength to hit her in the face once more. Audrey falters; she is covered in blood. Her nose—or what is left of it—is making a sound like a twenty-year-old Nissan trying to get up a steep hill. I take the back of her head and then slam her face into my rising knee three times in rapid succession. I can feel the crack of her jaw and hear at least one of her teeth being dislodged from her mouth.

I'm sure she's done, but then she surprises me by jumping on my leg and flipping out backward, away from me. She gets in a solid kick that uppercuts my chin, and I taste blood in my mouth from where I've bitten down on my tongue. This is getting ridiculous. I should have just shot her, not killed her or anything, but disabled her. The problem is that she's wearing a uniform and the only place I could have shot her would be the head, putting her down permanently. And as batshit as she is, I don't necessarily want her dead.

Audrey tries another kick, but this time I'm ready for it. I grab her leg with both hands, scramble around to the other side of her, jump back a bit, and then kick her hard in the shin. I kick her so hard that her tibia breaks and pops through her suit. She must be in agony, but she is still smiling. I've had enough. I pick her up and throw her with all the force I have against the wall. Her head thuds sickeningly against it. Maybe she's dead, maybe she's just out. At this point, my tongue is killing me, and I don't care—the clock is ticking.

The colonel has not moved. He doesn't seem worried, and this worries me. There's a protocol for everything in ARC. How long is it until what's happening in this room is noticed by everyone else?

"Who else has access to the kill switch?" I demand.

Applebaum says nothing. He won't even look at me, but instead is looking over my head to the door.

"You're not going to tell me? Fine, we don't have time for an interrogation." I move Levi's hand away and punch the major swiftly in the throat. Applebaum starts to wheeze. His eyes bulge, which is perfect. I take the knife from the holster on Levi's belt. Without hesitating. I push him easily to the ground. I get on top of him, my knees astride his body. I lean down and quickly push the tip of my blade into the outside corner of his eye socket. Applebaum screams, which is no mean feat with a partially collapsed windpipe. I hold his head steady and push the knife deeper in and then scoop up. His eyeball pops out. I grab it and cut it away from his head. It's a fairly radical thing to do, but I figure that having access to Applebaum's iris can only be a good thing.

A few of the others in the room start to scream. There isn't a single part of me that feels bad for what I have done. Applebaum deserves this and a lot worse. "Everyone shut up!" Levi hollers. "The next one of you who makes a sound gets a bullet." If Levi is disgusted by the act of torture I've just committed he isn't showing it.

I lean down closer to Applebaum, who is whimpering. "Tell me who else has access to the kill switch. You have five seconds before I take your other eye." I wait for two, then raise my knife again.

"Okay, okay," he pleads between sobs. "The Roones on the

base can enact the Midnight Protocol, but besides them, only I have the authority. ARC HQ in Livermore can do it remotely, of course."

I force myself to stop and think for a moment. I have been working on adrenaline and instinct all day. I need to stop thinking like a fugitive and start acting like a true leader. I look around. There is blood on the walls and pools of it underneath the fallen soldiers, who are turning white with shock. Audrey is laid out like a busted mannequin. The rest of the staff are keeping themselves small. Heads down between knees, arms wrapped around legs, hoping I won't see them, praying that they are invisible. This room stinks of fear and sweat and shit. I have turned it into a living nightmare.

Now they have an idea of what my life has been like since I discovered their demented secrets.

I'm almost certain the Roones are not going to kill us, not now that Edo and I have our deal. Levi and Beta Team have to fully take over the Battle Ground Rift without anyone in Livermore knowing what they've done. Just the idea of it makes me sweat, but I'm sure they can do it, especially with Edo's help. She won't like it, but she won't have a choice, not if she wants my data once I return.

I turn to Levi. I stand straighter, ignoring the pain in my hands and my throat from the fight with Audrey. He may not think I'm a child, but he doesn't think I'm much of a leader, either. I have to change that perception right now. I cannot show weakness or indecision. Yesterday, I would have been happy with him seeing us as equals; now I have to prove that I am more, that I am capable of leading the charge. "Stay here," I say with authority. "Secure the room. Shoot anyone who tries to come in, *except* for Edo. Give me a few minutes down at The Rift and then call her. Tell her to come here alone with her medical kit. You can trust her, sort of. She's going to be pissed that I did this, but she'll work with you. She won't sell you out."

"So you're just going to go down there and tell everybody? That's your plan?"

I narrow my eyes at him. "Just to be clear, that wasn't a request." I feel around my flak pockets, checking my ammo. I pull my old chip from its secure front pocket. The circuits are fried. It's useless now. I'll need to take one from Beta Team before I leave. I know Levi would be furious if he knew my end game today and I have to admit, I'm a little scared to tell him. Then I realize I don't actually have to. I have a weakness when it comes to Levi. He intimidates me and I have to get over it. Generals aren't vulnerable. They are fair, but not kind. They certainly don't offer up vital information in a room that's not totally secure. I walk out the door without giving him another word.

CHAPTER 28

I leave the bunker from one of the original exits, more hatch than door, a big metal contraption that groans when I push it open. It's better that I get to the intake rendezvous on foot rather than draw more attention at the transport bay. I race toward Ezra. The late-November trees with their bone-like branches blur around me as I run. It doesn't take me more than a few minutes to get to him. He is sitting off the gravel road, reading the instructions for the QOINS with the packs at his feet. He has managed to get the soldier to drop him off and not wait for me. I'm not sure how he managed this, but I am grateful he did.

He hadn't heard me, but when he sees me, he quickly shoves the papers back into his pack and stands. I practically jump into his arms. We stand there, holding each other without speaking. His heart is beating faster than normal.

"You're hurt," Ezra says with pain in his voice. He pulls away and looks me up and down. I don't know what my fight with Audrey has done to the way I look. It's not like I checked myself out in the mirror before I ran here. I guess I have a few bruises. I don't want to tell him it could have been much worse.

"I'm fine. Really. Applebaum isn't dead, but he's not in command anymore. Levi is."

Ezra looks at me sideways. "The same Levi who broke into the house this morning?"

"That wasn't his fault, and there is no one besides my team that I'd trust more right now. I did what I needed to, now all I have to do is tell the Citadels, which might not be as easy as I thought." I look up to the sky and let my shoulders sag. "This is so screwed up. I wish I had more than my instincts to go on right now. I wish I had more time," I admit.

Ezra draws me back into his arms. "Your instincts have done more for your people . . . Huh, that's not right . . . your *kind*? Is that racist? You know what I mean. Your instincts have taken the Citadels out of the dark, and the light isn't always pretty. Things almost universally look better in the shadows. So yeah, it might be harsh and ugly out here in the sun, but you can't doubt yourself now. You've got to stop this before it gets worse."

"You're right, thank you," I say as I pull away from him, though I would love nothing more than to stay there. Levi is alone in the Command room. I have to get on with this. Ezra and I begin to walk toward The Rift. We walk until we are about a hundred feet from the line of Citadel reserves. I know they've heard us already; I've been practically stomping in my boots. Trying to sneak through would give them the wrong idea. The reserve line doesn't bother to hide. They are usually only needed when the Karekins come through. They are the last line of defense between Camp Bonneville and The Rift. The teams generally double up so that there are eight Citadels grouped together under one call sign instead of four. I know that there are dozens and dozens of them between us and where we need to go. Then of course there are the other Citadels who are hiding in the Foxholes and Nests. At any given time there are well over one hundred Citadels on active duty. At least three of them are Beta, which is a relief.

I see the first team soon enough, and thankfully I'm on pretty friendly terms with the team leader. "Hey, Meghan," I say casually.

Unsurprisingly, she looks hesitant. "Hi, Ryn. Didn't think you were coming in today. They pulled someone from Rho Team back here in reserves to sit in the Foxhole with Beta." She is eying Ezra with obvious scrutiny. "Who's this?"

"My . . . boyfriend," I say, because I guess he is and today is not a day for lies.

"You have a boyfriend? And you brought him to The Rift?" Her puzzlement is gone. Now she looks angry.

"Yes I did," I answer defiantly. "Hey, everyone!" I shout, because I know they can all hear me, even from this far away. "I need to speak to you all. Leave your positions and meet me in the clearing." I can hear most of the reserve team leaders calling back to Command. You just don't walk to The Rift. You especially don't bring a civilian, and you never, ever leave your post unless given orders to do so. I know that Levi is on the other end of the com, though. He's telling them to do as I say. All the Citadels, even the older ones, respect Levi because he is one of the best. They respect me, too, but I'm not as lethal as he is. Levi is such an excellent fighter that he makes some of the other Citadels look like normal people when he spars with them, and that's saying something.

Ezra and I walk into the trees. I can hear the reserves following behind us. We aren't being stopped or questioned yet, which means that things are going our way so far. I feel The Rift, as I so often do, before I see it. Today the pull is especially strong, almost as if it knows, as if it's waiting for me to jump inside of it. We get to the clearing and most of the Citadels are out there already. We stop in the middle, just in time to see the remaining soldiers jump down from their Nests like high divers and land quietly in the soft muddy ground around us.

Immediately I look for my team. They've already spotted me, though, and are walking toward Ezra and me rigidly. The three of them have no idea what's going on, but they must know something is very wrong for me to be here with him. I want badly to believe that all the Citadels will listen calmly to what I have to say and then join the cause without much questioning. But after Audrey, and as I look around at everyone's faces, I know that this will not be the case. They are looking at me as if I'm contaminated. I feel like they have already judged me and made their decision without even bothering to hear what I have to say. I understand in this moment that leadership is more than positioning troops and choosing artillery. It's about persuasion and charisma. I need to talk these soldiers over to my side. I might have doubted that I could do such a thing if I wasn't so passionate about the cause. The Citadels must be told the truth. I take off my knapsack and give it to Ezra. I make him strap it on front facing. I figure that if things go sideways, the packs might serve as an extra layer of protection.

I start at the very beginning, that first day when I arrived at Camp Bonneville and received what they called a "tetanus" shot, but which in reality activated our dormant, altered DNA. I talked about Ezra, how I met him, breaking into the Village, and the wrongness of what goes on there. I relayed

Edo's truth, even though I was sure it wasn't the whole truth. I showed them my fried chip, then I asked for Henry's, which he handed over easily enough, but he looked obviously alarmed when I shoved it into the pack strapped to Ezra's chest. I told them about the abuse and the drug cocktail. I held Ezra's hand, brought it up to my mouth, kissed his fingertips, and I heard the Citadels murmur and gasp. I told them all of it, all the truths I knew and the theories I could guess at. I explained that ARC planned to send us through the Rifts to pillage and murder, and how the threat of that, combined with the kill switch in the implant, had forced my hand with Applebaum. Finally, I told them about my deal with Edo and how I was going to go through The Rift first. It was time to take back control of our lives and it had to start with this first jump into the unknown. I look at my team. They don't like this last bit of information. Henry is giving me a death stare. I cannot quietly confer with them. The Citadels need to see that we are all equals and that this is not a popularity contest.

Now that I am finished there is only silence and a palpable tension as thick as a brick wall. Was someone going to say something? Crows caw above us, and the green glow of The Rift casts a menacing light instead of the shimmering ethereal emerald I am used to. Finally a boy steps forward. I know this kid, but I've never liked him. He's a bully. I've seen him be cruel to helpless Immigrants. I don't think I'm going to like what he's about to say.

"We may not like the methods. I'm sure we can all agree with that," he begins without emotion, "but so what? Our job is to keep the world safe, at whatever cost. So far, it's worked. You can't argue with results. You've really fucked things up, Ryn. You've put this entire system at risk because, what? You don't like following orders? You're horny?"

I go to say something, but Violet jumps forward. Her face is red. I've rarely seen her angry. Sad, yes, frustrated, of course, but this mad? Never. "Shut up, Duncan!" Violet sputters and shakes her head. "You're like that blond telegram boy from *The Sound of Music*."

"What are you talking about?" he asks.

I'm kind of wondering the same thing. Count on Violet to reference a musical from the last century during a confrontation.

"Don't front like you haven't seen *The Sound of Music*. *Everyone* has seen *The Sound of Music*, and you're the Nazi boy," Vi hisses. This is Violet's version of mean. In her mind I know she believes she's opened a can of verbal whoop-ass on Duncan. In reality, her equating our situation to a musical is not doing much for our cause. Even I have to struggle not to just shrug her off.

"Did you just call me a Nazi?" Duncan steps forward and I see in that instant how the group divides itself. It's as if someone has said, "Okay—all those who are on Ryn's side stand over here, and everyone who feels like Duncan—the asshole Aryan bike boy—stand over there."

"If the shoe fits," Boone says.

"What?"

"That's what Nazis do," Boone says with more intensity than I've ever heard in his voice. "They force people from their homes. They steal. They take whatever they want because they believe they're entitled to it. They kill. They torture. They make lampshades out of people's skin and stick little kids in gas chambers because they're following orders. The Nazis didn't believe they were monsters. They believed they were saving the world. It's a fair comparison. I mean, look at us—we are kind of the ultimate Hitler Youth Movement."

I see Duncan's facial features tense, but like any good Citadel, he is keeping his emotions in check. "I'm not a Nazi. I'm a hero and you're"—he spits, looking at me—"a traitor. I'm not some mindless drone. I wouldn't stick a kid in a fucking oven. We're the good guys."

For someone who claims he isn't mindless, I have to wonder at this point if Duncan's IQ was ramped up to our level. Besides the fact that I was talking about Nazis and not Hansel and Gretel, he totally does not get it. I step in front of Boone so that now I'm the one just inches away from Duncan. "But you would," I argue. "You would do anything if you knew that ARC could kill you and your friends by pressing a button. You'd strangle a baby. You'd rape a woman to death if the Blood Lust got you. We are dangerous. We are *too* dangerous. And you're going to stand there like a good little soldier and call yourself a hero because you're too dumb or too afraid to see the truth?"

Duncan nods his head. I see some of his supporters shuffle away from him and on to our side, but not everyone, and my heart sinks. I'm so frustrated I want to shake them all. Then, faster than I can react to, Duncan backhands me. This is a gesture of defiance, a show of strength meant to embarrass, not hurt me. Still, I feel the blood pool in my mouth from where my incisor has cut the inside of my lip. I don't even bother to say anything. With the same speed, I haul back and punch him in the face. I punch him so hard that his body flies up and out at least ten feet.

Discussion time is over after that.

The group explodes. There are far more Citadels on our side, but Duncan's faction has a lot of muscle. It's Vi who launches first, at a beefy girl named Jessica who has at least half a foot and fifty pounds on her. I know this doesn't matter. Violet is so quick and lithe that Jessica doesn't have a chance. Violet leaps, kicking the bigger girl straight in the throat.

Meanwhile, Duncan has gotten his bearings. He flips himself up with his hands and lunges toward me. I know that Henry's and Boone's first reactions are going to be to protect me, but I also know that I have to fight Duncan and win if I want control of his supporters. I step forward, toward his charge, letting Henry and Boone know that I have this. Then, before Duncan can get to me, I spin away and elbow him in the back. I'm sure he doesn't feel this through his uniform, but this is just as much a pissing contest as anything else. I am not going to be so easy to catch. Before he can turn fully around to face me, I catch a glimpse of Ezra. He's no coward, but he knows wisely to stay out of the fray. "Run toward The Rift!" I manage to yell at him, but the break in concentration costs me. Duncan lands a strong uppercut to my jaw. I bite my tongue—for the second time today—and spit blood out on the ground.

I hope I get out of here with it all in one piece.

Out of the corner of my eye I see Ezra race toward the shimmering tower at the edge of the field. I have to bait Duncan toward The Rift now. He tries to land another hit, but I parry. I punch and he blocks me. We dance this way for a good thirty seconds, our fists moving so fast that I feel like I'm fighting on instinct alone. He's trying to get me away from The Rift, but he can't outmatch my speed. If he doesn't want to be hit, then he has to move in the direction my feet are taking us.

I finally manage to catch one of his wrists in a failed attempt at a jab. I squeeze down on the bone as hard as I can and twist it back until I hear a snap. It's broken. Duncan is at a major disadvantage now and he knows it. He screams, not in pain but anger. He kicks me in the stomach and I sail into the air. It knocks the wind out of me more than it hurts. He's also managed to kick me in the wrong direction. I fix this by doing a massive handspring up and over him so that now I'm facing The Rift.

A light rain begins to fall; thousands of delicate slivers of water jump from the clouds. I know that in a few moments those slivers will become an icy sheet. Autumn rain in the Pacific Northwest doesn't fall in big fat drops. Soon the ground will be a muddy slick and my visibility will worsen. I have a second or two before Duncan throws the next punch to take in what's happening. It is eerily silent on the field. Our punches and kicks are muffled by our suits. For the most part we don't scream or grunt as other fighters might. We have been trained to fight like ghosts. Invisible hands reach out and grab throats, our bodies twist and leap with the ease of something carried on the wind. And yet, even though the only thing I hear is the thud of a Citadel thrown against a tree or the splinter of a bone under one of our boots, it is absolute mayhem.

Duncan lunges for me and instead of dodging him, I meet his force. I take a step forward and kick out, nailing him hard in the pelvis. He rallies, returning quickly, and with his good arm tries to get me in a choke hold. I'm guessing, based on his size and weight, his specialty is jujitsu, which is all about getting someone down to the ground. His center of gravity is so low that he can inflict the most damage to his opponent when they are on the floor, like a wrestler. I cannot let him get me there.

I manage to break free of his choke hold and swing around, rolling over his back to deliver another blow to his side. Duncan falls to one knee and I see my opening. I keep kicking in short, powerful bursts to keep him from flying and also so that I know, even through the suit, I'm doing damage. I get a good one off to his face, and his mouth explodes with blood. I go to kick again, but he surprises me by reaching around with his good hand and holding on to my leg. I struggle to break free quickly because in this position, it would be easy enough for him to break my leg. I arch backward and plant my hands on the increasingly muddy ground. I use the one free foot I have to slide under his knee and throw him off balance. He wobbles and falls but doesn't release my leg. I push off with my hands, using a fair bit of strength to throw us both up and back into an awkward cartwheel.

The maneuver works, and Duncan has been thrown clear, but he quickly scrambles to where I have landed in a crouch and manages to get me down on my side. I look over and see another Citadel lying unmoving on the ground five feet away from me. He's one of the younger ones, a year or two even younger than me. I don't really recognize him. I have no idea whether or not he was one of Duncan's or mine.

I hate this.

With his good hand, Duncan tries to throw a punch, and because I'm thrown by the boy in the mud, by the blood on his face and his neck, which is lying at an obviously unnatural angle, Duncan's punch lands squarely in my eye. I kick out and grab Duncan by his bad wrist and his other fist before he can punch me again. I throw his body behind me and flip around to sit on his neck, keeping his legs restrained by leaning back and shoving them into the ground with my hands. He can punch me with his uninjured arm, but through my suit he won't do any damage. I squeeze around his face with my thighs. "Stop this, Duncan!" I yell. "We're going to kill each other."

His face is an atlas of bruises. I've won this fight and I don't see why he can't accept that. "Of course we are," he spits back at me. "What in the fuck did you think was going to happen here?"

I look around, trying to see my friends, my team. They are all deep in combat. Ezra is standing as close as possible to The Rift. Henry has gotten close to him, protecting him as best he can while fighting, literally, for his life. Still, Duncan's question unnerves me. I thought there might be a scuffle. I assumed some Citadels would be more difficult to win over than others. I even allowed that one or two would be fanatical like Audrey, but not this many.

I never thought in a million years it would be so bad. This whole episode out here strikes me as ridiculous and very, *very* wrong. I squeeze harder, keeping Duncan's face between my legs like a vise. His skin is getting purple. "Nobody else has to die—so enough," I scream in his face. "We are smart, we can find a way to work through this." I feel Duncan stop struggling beneath me. There is hatred in his eyes, but he knows that he's been beaten. As I said to him before, with us, it's self-preservation at all costs.

"Okay," he manages to wheeze out, and I release him. I stand over him and offer him my hand to help him up, which he bats away. "Just get away from me."

I open my mouth to say something else, to try to convince him that I'm right, but I stop myself. The truth didn't work. Fighting didn't work. There has to be another way to get these Citadels back on our side.

I step away from him, toward Ezra. I wonder if Edo will know what to do. If everyone was conditioned to believe ARC's propaganda, then I suppose they can be reconditioned to see it for the bullshit it is. I hate the idea of brainwashing my peers again, but I'm running out of options. Now I'm worried about the remaining Citadels who have yet to hear my story. How will my team handle telling them? And how can we trust them once we do? I wonder, and not unreasonably so, if the Roones have some kind of test to verify whether someone is telling the truth, some way of watching our brains light up like a pinball machine if we are lying.

Watching all this chaos around me only strengthens my resolve to go. I may be a hero to some Citadels, but after what just happened with Duncan, I realize that some truly see me as the enemy. It's best that I take a step back for a little while and let the other, less polarizing Citadels push forward.

Perhaps more than that, I'm tired. I'm done fighting. My head hurts. The skin on my knuckles is raw. I cannot take a full breath; one of my ribs is cracked. I look down at Duncan. His hand is covering his face. I can't imagine what he's thinking. Does he realize now that he's been used horribly? Or was it truly hatred I saw in his eyes? How can he think I'm a traitor for not wanting to be a weapon? It's too much. It's time for me to go. Ezra and The Rift are close, maybe thirty feet. He's as near to it as I've ever seen anyone, though he has his back to it. He's been watching me this whole time, probably worried out of his mind, feeling helpless knowing that there was nothing he could do. His mission was to keep the packs and equipment safe. Every time he had to witness Duncan hit me must have killed him. He's smart, though. He knew that if he tried to get involved he would have put both of our lives in danger.

The Citadels are still fighting. I walk briskly to Ezra. I get close enough to read the relief on his face. We're going to get out of here, together. I'm almost there.

And then in an instant, a split second, everything goes to shit. Levi leaps into the air from out of nowhere, like he's been shot out of a cannon. He pushes Ezra hard. He pushes him with such force that Ezra goes flying into The Rift. I don't even have time to register what has truly happened because Levi tackles me to the ground, and that's when I hear the shot go off. I look over my shoulder to see Duncan, still on his back in the mud but with his one good arm extended out, the gun pointed right where I had been standing. Levi rolls me over so that the second shot Duncan takes misses us both. We scramble up to our feet, ready to dodge another bullet, but that's not what happens. Instead, Duncan's arm drops. I look around and watch as the other Citadels in his group fall one by one. I've seen many things over the years in this job, but nothing, I don't think, as disturbing as this is. One minute they are fighting, alive, wondrous even, in their fury.

The next, they are gone without warning, just bodies on the ground.

The faction of Citadels who remain look around, stunned. Before I left Levi at Command, I told him to call Edo. I know in an instant this was her doing. Her choice has taught me a horrific lesson: The Citadels aren't nearly as important to the Roones as I thought they were, and this terrifies me. She must have been watching the whole time, carefully gathering the names of those against us so that she could enact the Midnight Protocol. I have no idea why she did this. Was it Duncan's gun? Was it all the other Citadels on my "side" that she was protecting, or was it just me? Whatever the reasoning, this will never happen again. I will remove every implant, in every Citadel, myself—*today*, if I have to. Ezra and I . . .

I bury my face in my hands. It finally hits me that Ezra is gone. I stare into The Rift. I look at Levi and I just want to kick him, but I can't. Edo's hand could very well still be on the kill switch and I'm not about to lose another Citadel, even one I'm furious with. Beta Team comes running toward me. Maybe they expect some kind of explanation as to why I was going to leave with Ezra. I don't feel like explaining myself to anyone right now. "Henry," I say with gentle authority, "divide the remaining Citadels up. You and Boone need to go back to the base and secure it with one group and then round everyone up, civilians and military, and put them in the training arena. I'll be there in a few to talk to them. Vi, you need to stay here with another group to defend The Rift." The three of them stand there looking at me as if they are waiting for me to say something else. Instead I say, "Go," with more intensity and volume in my voice.

Surprisingly, they hustle to do as I've ordered. When Boone tries to pick up one of the dead Citadels, I stop him. "Don't do that. Put her down," I tell him authoritatively. "The next shift will be arriving at the base soon. I want them to see what ARC can do to us if we don't assume command."

Boone puts the girl down gently; her eyes remain open, staring lifelessly at the opaque sky.

I just stand there among the corpses with Levi as my friends organize the remaining troops. Boone and Henry head toward the base with a large group. Violet reforms teams and places them all back into position. She joins Kappa Team on point behind the rock closest to The Rift. A better, more experienced leader might have gone with Boone and Henry right away to deal with the bunker, but I don't feel entirely connected to my own body. I need a moment to let the enormity of what's just happened sink in. I don't feel responsible for these deaths. That fault lies squarely on ARC's shoulders and, to a lesser degree, on Edo's. But there's no denying that they would all be alive if I hadn't started this. I need to sit with the idea that I am both entirely to blame and not at all to blame for what has happened here.

I wince as I try to take a deep breath. I turn my back on the dead soldiers around me and cross my arms. Once again, I stare into The Rift and ignore the way it's tugging at my gut. I can feel Levi's eyes on me.

"Tell me what you're thinking, Ryn," Levi says softly. I still can't even look at him, let alone share my thoughts. I don't say anything. I hear him sigh loudly. "Don't do this, don't shut me out," he warns. "If you had just been honest with me. If you had come to me from the beginning, then all of this could have been avoided."

I grit my teeth, which hurts. My jaw must be bruised. "Don't go there, Levi. Don't you dare. There was no avoiding this." I finally turn to face him. "All of this," I say, sweeping my arms out, gesturing to the fallen Citadels and the blood on the field, "would have happened eventually. ARC needs to be brought down. That means war."

"But if you had just told me, we could have come up with a plan. Jesus, Ryn." He sighs in frustration. "I know what you think of me, but look at what I've done for you! I let you deal with those thugs who tried to rape my sister. I helped you get into the Village. How much more proof do you need?"

I look at him, truly baffled. "Proof of what?" I ask, my mouth gaping. By way of an answer, Levi just shakes his head and purses his lips as if I should totally get it. I throw up my hands. "I seriously don't know what you're talking about. The only proof I have when it comes to you is that while you are an excellent Citadel, you are as mean as a snake and probably the angriest and most judgmental person I've ever met."

"I'm not this way with everyone, you moron!"

"What are you? Six years old? I can't believe you want to get into this right now, but it's so typical, Levi," I say with as much conviction as I can muster, *"this is war,"* I tell him, desperate to get through.

"But you were just going to leave with him! Is that how you think you're going to win a war? I don't believe *you*. You were going to run away and leave us with this colossal mess to clean up."

I don't know why I feel compelled to justify my choice to Levi, especially when I'm so pissed at him, but for some reason I do. "I made a deal. A deal that would secure an alliance with the Roones, prove that the Rifts are navigable, and which offered up a significant amount of intel about ARC and Roone technology. I got all that by agreeing to Rift off this Earth. I was *not* running away," I assert.

We stand there, eyes blazing at each other. It's clear by the look on Levi's face that he's hearing me but not really listening. "Are you serious right now?" He practically spits at me. "Rifting out shouldn't have even been an option. You must know that *you* are the most valuable asset to this cause, to this lovely new war that *you* began. You send someone else, someone less vital. Even the greenest Citadel knows that much."

I narrow my eyes and take a step closer to him. "You could have grabbed the gun from Duncan. Shit, you could have shot Duncan yourself. You didn't need to throw Ezra in there. You're hateful."

Levi rears back like I've slapped him. "I saved your life. That's all that mattered to me. It was a gut reaction. Besides, he was going through anyway."

I shake my head and look up. The rain has stopped for now, but I am wet and cold and fed up. "We don't put civilians in harm's way. We protect Immigrants. It's our job. It's why we're made the way that we were. God, Levi, he might be dead already." I sigh and press my palms into the back of my neck, then I move them over my eyes and press even harder. I feel tears threatening, but I don't want Levi to see. "He's smarter than us. I know that will come as a shock to you, but he understands computing and physics in a way that we don't. You aren't getting that the deal I made was conditional upon Ezra and I Rifting out *together*."

"Fuck the deal. You can't leave."

"Why not?"

"Because."

It's almost funny that Levi expected me to confide in him, that he thinks I should *magically know* how he feels about me. Especially since I don't even think he really knows and that's been the problem since I discovered the first bits and pieces of the truth about the Citadels. How can I trust someone who is so angry and irrational? He claims that he could never hate me, but he acts like he does. He says he doesn't think I'm a child, but he's reprimanding me like I am one. His emotional landscape is a minefield. If I say the wrong thing, he'll blow up at me. I don't have the time or energy for that. We are standing in a graveyard. It's disrespectful of him to play games. "Are you trying to tell me that between you and Boone and Henry and Violet you can't secure the base? You can't come up with a plan to dismantle ARC?"

"Of course we can—that's not the point," he argues.

I back away from him. He's still conditioned, and until that changes, he'll be guarded. I realize, though, it doesn't matter. There's been too much fighting already, and this argument isn't going to change my mind. "I'm so glad that you know what the point is, Levi. That's great. Because I have no friggin' idea what it is. Is it to save people? Protect people? Is it to keep this ugly green thing a secret from the world?" I ask in a hushed tone. I'm feeling defeated and vulnerable. Levi is just about the last person I want to be around right now, but he's here and I've got to keep it together. "We don't know *anything* except how to take orders and fight," I manage to get out. I cover up my mouth with my hand. I struggle to keep everything inside me, as if my palm can push it all back down.

Levi sees this and steps toward me.

I take my hand off my lips and put it up to stop him. "No," I say, feeling stronger. "I fucked up. Like a thousand other commanding officers before me, I made a bad call today. Despite what you may think, or Edo or whoever else, I'm only human. I'm *not* special. This isn't my *destiny* or whatever. I have a higher tolerance to the drug they brainwash us with and I have, or at least I had, Ezra. That's it. I rattled the lock. But picking it? Let alone breaking down the door and walking through? That's going to take all of us, together. No single person is going to fix this, no *one* person can."

Levi looks confused. His lip curls up. He gets that same superior look on his face that, admittedly, I love to hate. "What are you talking about?" he asks, clearly exasperated.

"It doesn't matter. You'll find out. You don't need me here. But you do need me to go through there," I say, gesturing to The Rift. But Levi doesn't take his eyes off my face. "And not because I'm special, but because I've had a head start. I've had weeks to wrap my head around this and I'm the only one who Ezra really trusts, so I have to go."

Levi's eyes get wide and he reaches out and grabs my wrist.

I yank it back, offended. "Not *now*, you idiot. I have to resupply, and heal a little bit, and get Ezra's signature locked into a QOINS device, and deal with a shit ton of other details like helping to come up with a plan to manage the Citadels who worship at the cult of ARC. But you don't need me to implement it. So, no. I'm not going this minute, but as soon as I can, I'm going to leave. I know it pisses you off that you can't bully me into doing what you want, but you aren't going to get your way. Not on this."

"Fine," he says in a tone so sharp it feels like a slap. "But don't pretend you're doing this for some stupid deal or some altruistic agenda. You're going for him. You're going to save *him*."

"Yes—I am going for him. Is that so wrong? But it's not the only reason, and it never was. Like I said, I've had time to live with this, and let me tell you, it's fucking Hydra on steroids. It's in every choice we've made, every fight, every kill. It's at home with our families, it's even in our food. It doesn't have a blind spot. I don't know anyone who hates or distrusts ARC more than you do, and though it might be hard for you to accept, you *are not* really processing this right now. Look around, Levi. Look at what we've done. If I have the chance to save anybody else, I have to try."

Levi does look around and then he looks right back at me. "What in the hell is Hydra?"

"Seriously?" I shake my head. Now he's just being a dick. "Go away, Levi. Leave me alone." The fight's gone out of me, and in an act of unexpected mercy, Levi must realize this and doesn't push. He slowly turns and walks away toward the base instead. All I can do is exhale gratefully in his direction.

I know I'm not alone. Violet is here, as are dozens of other Citadels, but I feel alone. There are dead soldiers all around me, littering the muddy ground like broken dolls. They aren't really soldiers, though; they are just kids—kids who weren't supposed to be anything special. Kids who were chosen for a lonely, gruesome job by a handful of statisticians and suits who claimed it was our duty but who would never have allowed their own children to be Citadels.

There is a practical side of me—a soldierly side—that understands why the Rifts were kept a secret. Regardless of the security element, the absolute spectacle of them all would have made them damn near impossible to police. But there is another side of me that's more human, perhaps only beginning to emerge, and maybe naive. It's the part of me that keeps the memory of when I first broke into the Village close, right on the surface. It's the first day I spent time alone with Ezra and the first time I ever saw a unicorn. In that creature's luminous eyes, I did not see a liar or a killer or a girl without freedom. I saw instead a thousand bright futures laid out before me. I felt hope—for the world, yes, but also for myself. Like *I* could be better.

And the way ARC has handled us, handled the Rifts—it just doesn't connect with that vision world.

Because each Rift is a scientific marvel. Yet ARC took something miraculous and turned it into something dirty and shameful, something you only talk about in hushed tones and underground rooms. The truth is that every child could be implanted—immune from disease and made smarter, stronger, faster. With a population like that, we could cure every illness, end global warming, and stop fighting each other. I know that without the brainwashing twisting us up inside, we are fundamentally better people. Everyone on this Earth could be a Citadel, so why aren't we? Who decided humanity didn't deserve that? Who's really in charge?

I turn and look into The Rift. It may be amazing, but today, it is the enemy. I blame it for everything terrible that has happened. It doesn't shimmer like an emerald tower. I don't feel like Dorothy standing on the yellow brick road looking off at Oz. It is a sickly green to me. It's the color of mold, of infected skin, of the oozing monster underneath the bed. I hate it today more than ever. As if sensing my strong emotion, The Rift gives a hearty tug at my center. I stare it down and give it my most dangerous smile. "Just wait," I whisper. "You think you want me, but once I climb down your throat, I'm gonna kick the shit out of you the whole way through." I half expect The Rift to scoop me up and grab me, but it doesn't change. It sits there like it always does, a silent, glowing beast. I turn my back to it and walk away.

ACKNOWLEDGMENTS

The idea for Ryn came to me in a rush. One minute, I was knitting, and the next, she was there, plain as day, kicking all sorts of ass. However, getting that germ of an idea into the actual book that you are reading now took a lot of work—and not just on my end. There were so many people involved in the process that had they not helped me, Ryn would have been left on the page, and I think we all know Ryn needs to be where the action is.

My literary touchstone when I was writing *The Rift Uprising* is the insanely talented Judy Blume. The first novel I ever read was by Blume, and as I got older, the characters she created were there every step of the way, guiding me to maturity. Judy Blume wrote young adult books *for* young adults. She didn't shy away from what was considered taboo, so I took my cues from her. I stuck to my guns, and luckily, everyone else in this process supported my vision, which is a book that is most certainly not for young children. And just for the record, that's not the easiest sell these days. So, Ms. Blume, thank you. I don't know that I'd be the person I am today, let alone the writer I am, without your brilliant words.

My second huge massive thanks goes out to my sister from another mister, my literary agent extraordinaire, Yfat Reiss Gendell. You've always believed in me, even when *I* didn't believe in me so much. You sold the shit out of this book and made me feel like a total rock star in the process. The entire team at Foundry Literary + Media deserves much more than a simple thank-you, but I suppose it will have to do: Director of filmed entertainment, Richie Kern, and editorial assistant Jessica Felleman. The foreign rights team: Kristen Neuhaus and Heidi Gall. The contracts team: Dierdre Smerillo, Melissa Moorhead, and Hayley Burdett. And the agency's finance folks: Sara DeNobrega and Alex Rice. Thank you so very much.

I have to thank my parents, too, and in particular my father. I asked my dad to read the first chapter of *The Rift Uprising* when we were on a plane together coming home from Singapore (talk about a captive audience—ha!). He read *the entire book* en route. He's not the kind of dad who says something is great just to make you feel good. That's why, when he told me that he loved it, I really knew I was onto something special. Since then he has been beyond supportive. So Dad, thank you for your wise counsel and your undiluted enthusiasm. To my sisters—thank you. Somebody in the family has to be the big nerd. I happily take up the mantle and I am grateful you guys get that that's just who I am.

The team at the William Morrow imprint of HarperCollins. Wow. I am so lucky to have you. My incredible editor, David Pomerico, who treats everything that happens in Battle Ground like it's nonfiction, which is beyond awesome.

Liate Stehlik, Shawn Nicholls, Jennifer Brehl, Pamela Jafee, Jessie Edwards, Angela Craft, Doug Jones, Carla Parker, Austin Tripp, Carolyn Bodkin, Katie Ostrowka, Jeanne Reina, Shannon Plunkett, Ivy McFadden, Kathleen Go, and Rebecca Lucash.

Juliet Grames was my first editor. She was my first champion and continues in that role. Thank you, Juliet, for all your advice and wisdom. It's weird that you're actually younger than me (by a lot), because you have always been a mentor.

In that vein I'd like to thank *all* my early readers. Leigh Wright, Jennifer Ambrose, and Elaine Lui. Lainey, you especially have a ton of sage advice on many fronts. Is there anything you don't know? I have other amazing friends who read various and sometimes all the drafts of this book. Lisa Rockower in particular—you've been right there with me since the very beginning. You might have read this book more times than I have! I adore you. My NSLP Sheryl Zentner, Melissa Sher, and Claire Coffee. A special shout-out to all my Portland pals—you know who you are. *Besos.*

My Nashville crew: Kristin Russell, Shelly Fairchild, and Kristin Barlowe. Barlowe, you get a special thanks for being literally the coolest girl I know. Also, you have my undying gratitude for being such a talented photographer and always making me look a hundred times better than I do in real life and for refusing to take a dime for doing so. That's a true friend.

I have to thank my musical family. Stephanie Cox at Kobalt—how lucky am I to have such a good friend and plugger in crime? Thank you for supporting *all* my writing. Also at Kobalt, Jesse Willoughby and Chris Lakey. Michael Bublé, my might-as-well-be brother—in so many ways, none of this would be possible without you. You read this book the day

I sent it to you in its early stages when you were at your busiest. Your friendship and support mean so much to me. To all my musical collaborators, thank you for putting music to my words. There's always music when I write, and that is invaluable.

My producing partners took this project to a whole other level. Michael Sugar and Ashley Zalta and Anonymous Content. Ivan Rietman and Ali Bell at Montecito Pictures. Thank you and fingers crossed.

I also got help from a couple of actual experts who have my complete gratitude for not ever laughing at any of my weird questions: Jack Bennetto for all the physics stuff, and Lieutenant Colonel Matt Fandre from the 101st Airborne.

Finally, I have to thank my family. Matt, my dear sweet husband. Thank you for your patience. Thank you for holding down the fort so I can run away from home every so often and be a crazy writer lady. Thank you for your English degree and your tolerance when I present you with yet another draft. I love you. And to my children, Mikaela, Eva, and Vaughn. I don't know who I'd be or where I'd be without you. Love doesn't even begin to cover it.